Improving Clinical Communication

Ernesto Gil Deza

Improving Clinical Communication

A Clinician's Guide to Building Better Skills and Patient Outcomes

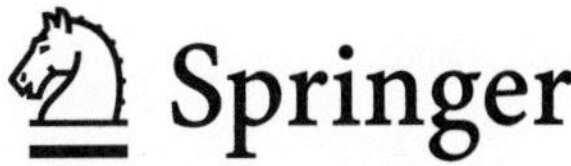 Springer

Ernesto Gil Deza
Facultad de Medicina
Universidad del Salvador
Buenos Aires, Buenos Aires, Argentina

Director of Teaching and Research at the Instituto Henry Moore
Buenos Aires, Argentina

ISBN 978-3-031-62448-3   ISBN 978-3-031-62446-9   (eBook)
https://doi.org/10.1007/978-3-031-62446-9

This Springer imprint is published by the registered company Springer Nature Switzerland AG
The registered company address is: Gewerbestrasse 11, 6330 Cham, Switzerland

If disposing of this product, please recycle the paper.

Preface

Dear reader, the book you have in your hands is aimed at all members of the health team.

It is based on a simple premise: communication with the patient is a fundamental tool that can be learned and perfected throughout one's professional life.

The text has been organized into 12 sequential chapters that address the fundamental topics of communication in the doctor's office.

Its pages reflect the author's profession as a medical oncologist and it does not have the ambition of being a text based on erudition but rather on experience, on the daily challenges that interaction with patients presents in modern medicine.

All errors are attributable only to the author, and I assume full responsibility for them, since the text is a distillation of 30 years of work, with all its triumphs and also its mistakes, which are the ones that teach us the most and are not easily forgotten.

It is my hope that you find it useful and that you enjoy reading it as much as I enjoyed writing it.

Buenos Aires, Buenos Aires, Argentina   Ernesto Gil Deza
February, 2024

Contents

Chapter 1
Introduction

What do you think of communication in everyday human interaction?

What do you think of communication in the medical field?

How much do you value communication with your doctor, nurse, or provider when you are sick?

How much do you value communication as a healthcare professional?

The answers to these questions will be crucial in order for you to decide if the book you hold in your hands is worth your time.

Most communication skills are classified as "soft skills", in contrast to "hard skills," which are the core scientific and technical foundations of knowledge for a particular medical specialty. (Note that throughout the text I will use the term "doctor" as a way of referring to the entire team of professionals involved in the healthcare industry. That is to say, the content of this book is valid for doctors, nurses, psychologists, social workers, and all other healthcare professionals.)

However, if we reflect on the reality of the current state of doctor–patient relationships, we will see that it has changed more in the last 30 years than in the last 30 centuries! This is because many of these "hard skills" have ceased to be the sole domain of the medical professional in various ways:

1. Medical knowledge, both accurate and inaccurate, is readily available on the Internet.
2. Many of the diagnoses are nowadays carried out by pathologists.
3. Determining the stage of various diseases is, in many cases, up to image specialists.
4. What kind of therapy is required is also readily available online.
5. The success of the treatment is attributed mostly to the drugs involved rather than the professional administering them.
6. At the same time, the efficacy of these drugs is determined by complex statistical analysis (the well-known Big Data).

© The Author(s), under exclusive license to Springer Nature Switzerland AG 2024
E. Gil Deza, *Improving Clinical Communication*,
https://doi.org/10.1007/978-3-031-62446-9_1

We can see this outlined in Fig. 1.1. Therefore, the underlying question we need to ask ourselves is: What is the doctor's nowadays? How has it evolved, and what will it become? I propose that doctors in the twenty-first century and beyond will be human, and therefore they should be skillful communicators most of all or else they will be a hindrance.

The truth of the matter is that all skills are "hard." It is not too long after starting our professional careers that we realize that knowing *how to do* something is just as important as knowing *how to say it*.

As with many other things, how you perceive communication itself may have an impact on your ability to improve your communication skills.

Do you believe that communication is a gift, that is to say, something you are born with and cannot be changed?

Or do you believe that communication is a skill, something that can learned and perfected with use?

Or perhaps you believe that communication is a tool, and like all tools it has times and uses it is suited for, but others where it is not?

The use you get out of this book will depend heavily on how you answer these questions.

I believe that communication, by which I mean both the gestures and the words with which we relate to each other, is all three things at once: a gift, a skill, and a tool.

Allow me to explain: it is a gift, for it is undeniable that some people have an easier time communicating than others. We have all known people who are the

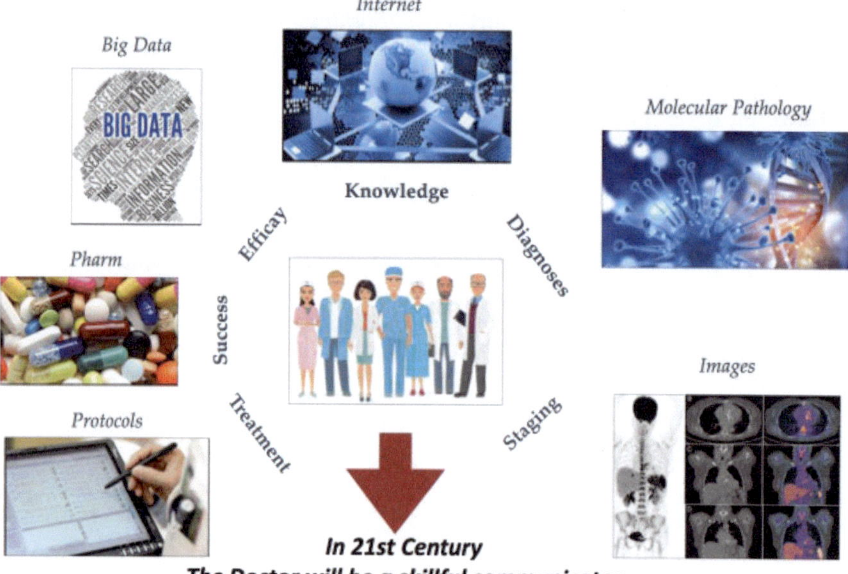

Fig. 1.1 Role of the doctor in the twenty-first century

center of every party, charismatic, and who easily and readily convey their ideas or experiences; while others are shyer, or uncouth, or otherwise have trouble getting their points across.

However, I am convinced that most of us, no matter how gifted, are not using our communication skills to the fullest.

Therefore, in my view, it is also a skill: practice makes perfect, as they say.

Learning to communicate, understanding our limitations, training ourselves daily to develop the skills we lack or to perfect the ones we have, is a central point of our professional development, just as much as our technical and scientific knowledge.

Finally, it is a tool. Or rather, it would be better to say communication is a *variety* of tools. A toolbox, if you will.

There are those who can communicate better with children than with adults; with women than with men; with terminally ill patients than with curable ones; with demanding people than with timid people; with extroverted people than with shy people. What comes naturally to us, or what we learn more easily (that is to say, what *tools* we are most comfortable and familiar with), is one of the things that guided us each to our respective specialty.

Therefore, before you continue reading, I invite you to reflect on the two aspects that we are going to develop throughout the book:

(a) What do you think communication's role in medicine, for each member of the health team, is in the twenty-first century?
(b) Do you consider yourself particularly gifted in communication? Do you think you have developed your natural communication skills as much as you can? And finally what tool (or tools) do you use the most?

Throughout this book, we will delve into many topics: the origin of the human word; the word as medicine; the historical evolution of medical communication; the differences between information and communication; nonverbal communication; empathy and communication; communication strategies according to the evolution of the disease (although we will be using cancer patients as a model, the strategies here are perfectly suitable for other medical specialties); communication with marginalized groups such as the LGBTQ community; the communication experience during the pandemic; communication and prevention of burnout; and the development of a personal communication kit and the teaching of communication skills in undergraduate and graduate studies [1–14].

This book is intended for a great variety of readers: patients (and their families); students in one of the many healthcare fields; and professionals in these fields.

Each chapter has recommendations that will be of use to each of these types of readers.

If I have managed to convince you to join me, I invite you to proceed to the first chapter, where we will discuss the origin of the human word, and how it is likely that the first words were sung.

References

1. Buckman R. Words that make a difference: enhancing the "how" in "how we say it". Support Cancer Ther. 2006;3:127.
2. Parekh AK. Winning their trust. N Engl J Med. 2011;364(24):e51.
3. Hollander JE, Carr BG. Virtually perfect? Telemedicine for Covid-19. N Engl J Med. 2020;382(18):1679–81.
4. Back AL, Arnold RM, Baile WF, Tulsky JA, Fryer-Edwards K. What makes education in communication transformative? J Cancer Educ. 2009;24:160–2.
5. Derse AR. The physician–patient relationship. N Engl J Med. 2022;387(8):669–72.
6. Stone JH. Communication between physicians and patients in the era of E-medicine. N Engl J Med. 2007;356(24):2451–4.
7. Jain SH. Practicing medicine in the age of Facebook. N Engl J Med. 2009;361(7):649–51.
8. Baile WF, Aaron J. Patient-physician communication in oncology: past, present,and future. Curr Opin Oncol. 2005;17:331–5.
9. Flores G. Language barriers to health Care in the United States. N Engl J Med. 2006;355(3):229–31.
10. Zwingmann J, Baile WF, Schmier JW, Bernhard J, Keller M. Effects of patient-centered communication on anxiety, negative affect, and trust in the physician in delivering a cancer diagnosis: a randomized, experimental study. Cancer. 2017;123(16):3167–75.
11. Parker PA, Ross AC, Polansky MN, Palmer JL, Rodriguez MA, Baile WF. Communicating with cancer patients: what areas do physician assistants find most challenging? J Cancer Educ. 2010;25(4):524–9.
12. Srivastava R. Dealing with uncertainty in a time of plenty. N Engl J Med. 2011;365(24):2252–3.
13. Back A, Tulsky JA, Arnold RM. Communication skills in the age of COVID-19. Ann Intern Med. 2020;172(11):759–61.
14. Lensink MA, Jongsma KR, Boers SN, Bredenoord AL. Better governance starts with better words: why responsible human tissue research demands a change of language. BMC Med Ethics. 2022;23(1):90.

Chapter 2
The Therapeutic Origin of the Human Word

2.1 The Word and Mankind

What is the most important human attribute?

We are born extremely vulnerable. We lack any kind of protection, such as an exoskeleton or osteoderm. We lack claws or sharp teeth. We lack strength or agility.

How then do we survive in an adverse environment?
What is our evolutionary advantage?
What is the outstanding feature of our species?
There is no doubt that one of the outstanding characteristics of mankind is its communal lifestyle.

Individually we are very vulnerable, but we can act together in a way that makes us almost undefeatable.

This kind of lifestyle requires communication and for this we were endowed with three formidable conditions: intelligence, memory, and speech.

Intelligence has often been reduced to reason; however, the name itself gives us a clue that this is not so. Intelligence etymologically derives from *interlegere*, which means *to read between the lines* [1]. This implies much more than simply *reasoning*, it also requires *feeling*. This is how a great Spanish philosopher of the last century, Xavier Zubiri, described it in his book *Inteligencia sentiente* [2].

Every time we think, we feel; and every time we feel we also think, because thinking and feeling are one and the same in the human being.

Memory has been one of the most studied subjects of both the previous and current centuries, fundamentally guided by Alzheimer's disease. One of the most interesting findings in this regard was the evidence supporting the existence of two systems: thought and memory, both of which Daniel Kahneman reflects in his book *Thinking, Fast and Slow* [3]. In it, he masterfully summarizes the experiments he has carried out during his extensive and prolific scientific career.

© The Author(s), under exclusive license to Springer Nature
Switzerland AG 2024
E. Gil Deza, *Improving Clinical Communication*,
https://doi.org/10.1007/978-3-031-62446-9_2

In this text, Prof. Kahneman demonstrates that system 1, or *fast*, is designed for our survival: it analyzes reality in a way that is both biased and heuristic, which allows us to make decisions quickly, but perhaps not accurately.

The second system is slower, consumes more energy, and allows us to analyze the peculiarities of each case and therefore make better decisions.

From this perspective, a very interesting find is that memory prioritize three kinds of experiences: the very first experience of any kind, the most intense moments (positive or negative) of any given experience, and finally, the way in which an experience *ends*. Our memory then summarizes these experiences and classifies them as either positive or negative, depending mainly on the intensity of the experience and its end.

Last but certainly not least comes the way we share our knowledge and experiences.

Learning, and therefore teaching, are essential activities for survival. We are all aware that the more you know, the better you teach, and the more you teach, the better you know. Clearly, for the transmission of knowledge, the word is an unmatched evolutionary advantage.

Human beings develop because we cultivate these three characteristics: our ability to comprehend the world (i.e., to intellectively understand it), to memorize experiences (i.e., to remember it), and transmit these to our community (cultivate, educate, teach, communicate).

Among many, the one who expressed this idea most clearly is Aristotle, probably the most important philosopher in history. In his book, *Politics*, he says the following about man:

> And why man is a political animal in a greater measure than any bee or any gregarious animal is clear. For nature, as we declare, does nothing without purpose; and man alone of the animals possesses speech. The mere voice, it is true, can indicate pain and pleasure, and therefore is possessed by the other animals as well, for their nature has been developed so far as to have sensations of what is painful and pleasant and to indicate those sensations to one another, but speech is designed to indicate the advantageous and the harmful, and therefore also the right and the wrong; for it is the special property of man in distinction from the other animals that he alone has perception of good and bad and right and wrong and the other moral qualities, and it is partnership in these things that makes a household and a city-state. [4]

This distinction between voice (sound) and speech (logos, reason) is crucial to be able to research what the first word might have been.

Let us note that Aristotle maintains that the *voice*, the ability to emit sound, is a characteristic shared with other animals and expresses pain and pleasure: the human scream, the growl, the bray or the neigh, are fundamentally not so different. It is not that sound that makes us different from other living beings.

On the other hand, *speech* is proper to man.

When was the first word of humanity spoken?

What was its speaker like?

What distinguished this word from other sounds?

For what purpose was it spoken?

All of these questions bring us to our next topic

2.2 In Search of the Original Word

In order to imagine the first word, we must first discuss the concept of evolution.

This is a relatively easy task in the current age, largely due to the scientific, social, and political influence of Charles Darwin's book *On the Origin of Species*, published in 1859.

In fact, the word *evolution* has had a notable impact on both science and society. Today we know about the evolution of the universe (from the Big Bang to the present). The evolution of matter (from hydrogen) to all the elements of Mendeleev's periodic table (the completion of which was itself a century spanning project). The evolution of ideas, words, politics, and economics and much more.

But this was not the case until the beginning of the nineteenth century. In those times, the accepted standard was fixism, creationism, and the "status quo." The world had been created as it was known at the time, relatively recently, and was extremely stable and predictable.

In the beginning of the nineteenth century, several inconsistencies between geological timeframes and the timeframe presented in the Bible began to crop up.

The age of both the earth and stones seemed significantly older than the age attributed to the origin of creation according to the literal interpretation of the book of Genesis, which is the first book of the Bible.

The most daring of the time considered that the earth's creation had been carried out at most few thousand years ago, but geological ages were *much* older.

In addition, a great variety of fossils were discovered. Many of them belonged to beings that did not exist anymore, but others were very similar to known species.

This then led to the idea that there was a relationship between the environment and the characteristics of the living things we observed. According to Jean-Baptiste Pierre Antoine de Monet, chevalier de Lamarck (more commonly known today simply as Lamarck), animals adapted to the environment by directly inheriting physical characters acquired by their parents. Later on Charles Darwin added to this his idea of *survival of the fittest*, better known today as *natural selection:* in any given population, some individuals who possess advantageous characteristics will reproduce more, passing down those characteristics and, in the long run, change the makeup of any given species. However, both Lamarck and Darwin were wrong in one crucial fact: acquired characteristics are *not* inherited.

A few years later, an Augustinian monk named Georg Mendel who worked in the garden of a convent in the city of Brünn, near Austria, postulated that what was inherited was not the acquired characters themselves but rather the *information* that gave rise to the appearance of those characters. Without naming them, he described in broad strokes what we know today as *genes* and in doing so set the foundation for the entire branch of biology known as *genetics*.

Because history is fond of hiccups, Mendel sent a letter with his discovery to the most important botanist of his time, Carl Näegeli, who did not put much, if any, stock in it. So this 1865 discovery remained hidden until the beginning of the twentieth century. Thus, Darwin died without knowing that the answer that validated his theory had been found, Mendel died without knowing that he had made one of the most important discoveries in the history of biology, and Näegeli died without any remorse at having dismissed such an important discovery.

Mendel's work, once it was rediscovered in the twentieth century, reinvigorated Darwin's theory, generating what is called Neo-Darwinism.

Today natural selection is accepted as the most solid theory to explain the evolution of species, although we know now that it is far more complex than Darwin thought. Nevertheless, there is no doubt that genes, and their transmission, take center stage.

As Jorge Wagensberg maintains: "The old dilemma of what came first, the chicken or the egg, has been solved for a long time: it was the egg, although of course, it wasn't a chicken's egg" (Aphorism 116) [5]. The main point expressed in this statement is that genetic changes precede the expression of new characters.

The enormous diversity of life is a direct consequence of evolution. All life on earth comes from small bacterium that arose in the depths of the warm seas 3800 million years ago. Their remains are represented by the stromatolite fossils found in Greenland, dated to around 3700 million years ago [6], which is very close to the currently best models of genetic evolution, which traces the origin of life on earth to around 4000 million years [7].

Therefore, when we observe nature with the eyes of biologists, we cannot but admire the beauty, diversity, variety, and creativity of marine and terrestrial life, microscopic and macroscopic, plant or animal, its shapes, colors, sounds.

Now let us ponder that this all boils down to inheriting genes. Let us imagine from the evolutionary perspective what it means to be capable of speech. Human beings are not only capable of transmitting genes, but as Daniel Dennett, a philosopher who studies consciousness, says, we are also capable of transmitting "memes," words, concepts, and culture.

From this perspective, the word represents a remarkable evolutionary advantage. This is what Yuval Noah Harari, professor of history at the Hebrew University of Jerusalem, proposes in his book *Sapiens: A Brief History of Humankind.*

What allowed us to evolve were not only genes but also communal life and the establishment of culture, which led to the domestication of animals (such as the reindeer—the first animal domesticated by man—the wolf, the donkey, the camel, and many others) and vegetables such as wheat, corn, or soybeans. Traditions, values, and education have a larger impact on our survival than genetics itself.

And all of these things require speech.

Today we are so immersed in the world of communications and words that it seems incredible that there was a time when we did not have speech.

We are capable of transmitting so many "bytes" of information that we forget that we were once nonspeakers.

That is why our first approach to the origin of the human word will be through fossils.

2.2.1   *The Evolution of the Vocal Apparatus*

The evolution of the vocal apparatus is something truly wonderful.

First of all we must consider that the ability to emit sounds (exhalations, trills, snorts, grunts, neighs, shouts, etc.) came about much later than the ability to *perceive* sounds (in the form of vibrations).

Perhaps this should already tell us that we should listen more and talk less. The more we respect biology, without falling into a naturalistic fallacy, the more we will take advantage of our innate abilities.

Let us start, then, with the ability to hear.

As we have discussed previously, life arose in the sea. Marine life is full of vibrations because the liquid medium is extremely suitable for transmitting them. Furthermore, the deeper we go, the darker it gets and the less one can rely on other senses to survive.

Therefore, we can find many living beings that have organs that specialize in detecting changes in pressure, chemical composition, or temperatures of the environment that surrounds them.

Bacterial chemoreceptors are probably among the first kind of sensory organs to appear in the evolution of life.

Certain chemicals are able to attract or repel flagellated bacteria by stimulating movement of the flagellum. This process is called chemotaxis.

It has been discovered that there has been very little variation in these chemoreceptors between the first living beings of the domain called "Archea"and the bacteria we know today. In fact, while current Gram-positive bacteria have different flagella structures to those of ancient specimens, the receptor is practically the same [8].

From these first receptors evolved all the others that we see in living beings.

Marine flora and fauna have a wide variety of receptors that are capable of sensing what is happening around them.

If we take a look at fish, for example, we can see they have great sensitivity to detect pressure changes that can tell them (among other things) if a predator is approaching, and some can even detect very subtle changes in electrical or thermal signals.

In amphibians and insects that spend time outside of water, we can see the development of specific sensory organs that allow them to perceive the aerial environment that surrounds them with great clarity and sharpness. Birds, reptiles, and mammals that descend from amphibians show further specialization in sensory organs.

How, then, did the ear as we know it today appear?

The study of the auditory apparatus present in different species is fascinating because it shows a great variety of designs perfectly adapted for their primary function. This research has also been remarkably improved with the addition of genetic studies [9].

For example, Johnston's organ is an ear located externally on the antennae of fruit flies [10] that is specifically tuned to the sound frequency caused by the vibration originating from the male fly's wings in order to facilitate mating.

Crocodiles use their hearing, much more than their sight, to sense when prey has approached to drink as they lie at the bottom of muddy streams and lakes [11].

The spatial awareness that comes from possessing bilateral auditory organs is a very useful evolutionary trait for both hunter and prey [12].

The evolution of the auditory system in mammals has been extensively studied. [13–19]But it can be summarized in the evolution of three elements: the eardrum, the ossicles, and the cochlea. If I were to boil it down to its essentials, it consists of a spectacular feat of engineering that manages to internalize a large antenna (ossicles and cochlea) and protect an exquisite microphone exposed to the elements (the eardrum).

Let me explain by reviewing the physiology of hearing.

The ear is an organ specialized in detecting sounds, that is, pressure changes of an air wave, which moves a membrane (the eardrum), which through the ossicles in the middle ear (Hammer—Anvil and Stirrup) transform this movement of air into a liquid wave in the inner ear (in the chlochea or cochlea of the temporal bone). There it moves specialized cells in Corti's organ (hair cells) that vibrate according to the wavelength or frequency of the sound and transform the liquid wave into an electrical impulse that is transmitted through the acoustic nerve (eighth pair) to the cerebral cortex and we perceive sound.

We can imagine that these cells, located in the cochlea, are like a piano rolled up on itself, from right to left, in such a way that the high-pitched sounds at the base of the snail and the low ones are at the apex or tip of the snail, which is known as tonotopic organization.

And if we want to see how it works I recommend the audiovisual *Auditory Translation Animation* by Brandon Pletsch, Medical College of Georgia, winner of the inaugural 2003 Science and Engineering First Prize display Challenge and which   can   be   accessed   at   https://www.youtube.com/watch?v=PeTriGTENoc&ab_channel=BrandonPletsch.

The smallest wavelengths, that is, sounds with the highest number of cycles per second, of higher frequency, press the keys that are closest to the stirrup, while the longer wavelengths, with the lowest number of cycles per second (and therefore the lowest frequency), press the keys that are furthest from the stirrup.

The frequency of a wave is measured in Hertz (in honor of Heinrich Rudolph Herz). One Hertz (Hz) represents one cycle per second.

The human ear is capable of perceiving sounds ranging from 20 Hz to 20,000 Hz; sounds with a frequency less than 20 Hz are called *infrasounds* and those with a frequency greater than 20,000 Hz are called *ultrasounds*.

Despite the wide amplitude range, the human ear is most sensitive to sounds between 2000 Hz and 5000 Hz, which is the range of the human voice.

Not only do we have greater capacity to pick up certain frequencies, but we also have preferences for certain voice intensities depending on the circumstances. [20]It has been shown that we are better able to understand auditory cues from people we are close with, such as being able to determine whether laughing or crying is genuine. [21, 22] Similarly, it has been shown that males prefer female sounding voices [23].

So before we dive into the ability to speak, we must honor the enormous evolutionary effort that endowed us with the ability to detect environmental cues, the wonders of auditory development, and the sense's astounding discernment ability by developing our own mindful listening.

Now let us move on to the ability to make sounds.

How did the animal world become an orchestra?

Insects are capable of making a great variety of noises: with their wings, with their legs, with their jaws, but none have the ability to make sounds by flowing air through a tube called the *trachea*.

In vertebrates (excluding fish), we can see two large groups: birds have an organ that vibrates called the *syrinx* [24] located in the lower part of the trachea where it joins the bronchi. In all the others, from the crocodiles to turtles, geckos, frogs, and so forth and even in humans, the organ is located at the other end of the trachea and is called the *larynx* [25–29].

We could therefore think of this biological orchestra as having two large sections: on the one hand, we have the percussion instruments represented by insects, while, on the other hand, we have the woodwind section represented by many vertebrates.

In order for vertebrates to produce sound, we must have three separate but related structures: a bellows (lungs) that can expel pressurized air through a tube with a vibrating membrane (trachea and larynx) and a resonator apparatus that amplifies sound. The creativity with which nature has solved this problem is amazing and admirable.

In the case of humans, the anatomical structures to produce sounds can be seen in Fig. 2.1.

When we talk about anatomical descriptions, Aristotle is the father of comparative anatomy, and although it is unknown if he ever carried out any human dissections, his descriptions of animal dissections are numerous. He laid the foundations of an anatomical description that was based on finding the *why* of any given structure, which was itself to be found in the function of the said structure [30].

This was later taken up by Galen, whose anatomical descriptions were used for a long time in Western medicine, all the way from the first century to the sixteenth.

The problem with many of Galen's descriptions was that they were based on animal, not human, anatomy. Galen mainly used wild apes and pigs for his descriptions since these were the specimens provided to him by the emperors he served.

In the sixteenth century, Andreas Vesalius, who had studied at the University of Padua, wrote the first systematized anatomy text *De Humani Corporis Fabrica*, which was a very advanced text for the time. Not only did he describe with great accuracy the steps that had to be followed when dissecting a corpse, but his explanations were also accompanied by very detailed illustrations.

This was the first time that dissections could not only be repeated following the instructions outlined in the text, the organs found could be compared to their

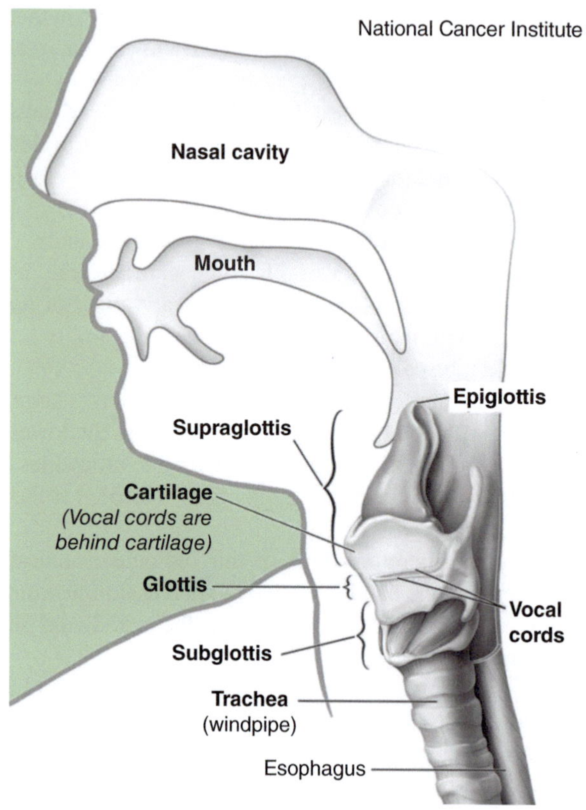

Fig. 2.1 Anatomical structures for vocalization. (Extracted from https://picryl.com/media/larynx-and-nearby-structures-b9ff8f. Under Creative Common LisencesLicenses)

illustrations. In a way, we could say that it was the first multimedia anatomy text. Those interested in delving deeper into this subject are encouraged to read *Doctors: The illustrated History of Medical Pioneers* [31] by Sherwin B. Nuland.

The names of anatomical structures, most of which are derived from Greek or Latin origins, refer to elements of military or everyday life.

The laryngeal structures in particular have an exceptionally rich etymology [32].

Just as a small sample I will show here a few terms, extracted from what is in my opinion one of the best texts on this topic: Henry Alan Skinner's *The origins of Medical Terms* [33]:

"Epiglottis: Greek π, *upon*, plus γλωττα, the Attic form of *tongue*."

"Glottis: Greek γλωττα, which is the Attic form of γλῶσσα, the *tongue*. Also the name for the reed of a wind instrument."

Chord or cord (both spellings are correct): "From Greek. ορδη, a string of gut used for musical instruments. Latin Chorda, also corda. Spanish 'cuerda.'"

"Trachea: Greek. χεια, rough, feminine formo of τραχυς, *rough*. The ancients thought that the arteries contained air, hence the term artery which means *air vessel*. The trachea or windpipe was also an air tube and the Greeks called it the *rough artery*."

"Lungs: Anglo-saxon—lunge, which Skeat says is allied to lungre, meaning quickly or lightly and he thus sees a connection which suggests that the lungs were named for their lightness, their ability to float in water, etc."

"Diaphragma: Greek διαφραγμα, a partition. From δια, through or across, plus φραγμαα wall or a fence."

As you can see, these names describe a structure's form, function, or both.

Having all the elements to emit sounds, to have a voice, is necessary but not enough to have speech.

For *that* you have to control the air flow very carefully. And to do that, you need to be able to control your breath.

2.2.2   The Evolution of Breath Control

Why do humans have so much control over our own breathing?

Hominids, unlike our first cousins (chimpanzees, gorillas, and orangutans, which, together with humans, make up the great apes), are born prematurely.

The causes of this premature birth are still unknown, but it is thought that the main culprit is the size of our brain relative to our body. The brain's development reaches such a volume that the human pelvises would be too narrow for safer births if we were born at a later stage.

This condition of "prematurity" is accompanied by a face with less development of the maxillary bones, which is why humans have a flatter face. This makes our tongue, which does not change in size, relatively large for our oral cavity, which is why both the hyoid bone and the larynx descend [34].

The consequence of all these changes is that we gain control over the opening and closing of the upper part of the larynx (epiglottis), which functions as a small lid that closes to allow food to pass into the digestive tract and opens to allow air to enter and exit our lungs [35].

As we learn to control the frequency with which we open and close the epiglottis, so too are we better able to control the flow of air through the larynx and, finally, the vibration of our vocal chords.

Our tongue is also able to modulate the sounds we produce both by changing shape and coming into contact with teeth in specific ways. Finally, we can further refine sound thanks to the *orbicularis labia,* which is a facial muscle highly developed in humans due to breastfeeding [36–40].

Along with developing these features, humans have also developed several resonating structures: the nasal cavity, palate, and paranasal sinuses (frontal, ethmoid, sphenoid, and maxillary).

All these features together are what allow us to produce human sounds. Each human's voice is unique and develops throughout their life.

If we study the phonetic structures of other primates, we will find that there are some that are endowed with all the elements to produce words [41, 42]; however, they cannot do it. Why?

Because in addition to having the cartilaginous, muscular, and nervous structures to be able to emit a controlled sound, they need to develop brain structures that allow them to do so.

Knowing the complexity of the vocal apparatus explains why it is so difficult to know when man began to speak, but it allows us to get closer.

Allow me to explain: fossil remains are, with a very few exceptions, composed only of bones and similar structures. Soft tissues, such as nervous, muscular, and cartilaginous structures, do not survive the fossilization process. As a consequence of this, we are limited to studying mostly the bones and what features we might find on them: the foramina (holes) through which nerves or blood vessels emerge; the ridges, valleys, or deformities where the muscles attach; and any other impressions that may have been left by soft structures.

It is an arduous task that requires not only a keen deductive intellect but also more than a bit of artistic interpretation.

For all these structures (larynx, lungs, tongue, muscles, etc.) to function in a coordinated manner, they need to be profusely innervated.

And it is here that we begin to approach an answer to our original question: When did humans develop nerves of sufficient size to be able to control the muscles related to the emission of sound?

The nerves related to the structures of breathing and, by extension, speech exit the central nervous system through the foramina at the base of the skull, while the spinal cord is located in the canal formed by the vertebrae, the neural foramen.

The ribs and intercostal muscles are innervated by nerves that leave the spinal cord when two vertebrae articulate. The size of both the neural foramen and the smaller foramina present at each junction provide us with an idea of the "neuromuscular domain" (that is to say, how many nerves and muscles are involved) of respiration.

At this point, we are getting even closer to our answer.

The comparison of hominid skulls, as well as neural and junction foramina, allows us to infer at what time humans would have possessed the required nerves to operate the vocal apparatus.

This time was approximately 80,000 years ago [27, 39, 43].

However, even with the muscles and nerves necessary to operate the apparatus, something must coordinate those movements if it is to produce anything. And that something is the brain.

2.2.3 The Evolution of the Brain

Our nervous system not only allows us to perceive the world around us; gives meaning and coherence to what we observe; detects threats and opportunities; anticipates events that may occur but it also regulates our temperature, humidity, hormonal, and chemical balance, and it even allows us to dream while we sleep.

But how does it achieve all of this?

Through specialization and interconnection.

The nervous system evolved from the small chemoreceptors found in unicellular beings, leading first to specialized cells capable of transmitting impulses, which would, much later, become the nervous system we know today, divided into the central nervous system (composed of the spinal cord, medulla, pons, cerebellum, and brain) and the peripheral nervous system (composed of the sensory and motor nerves, as well as the sympathetic and parasympathetic nervous system, which regulates the functions of the viscera without conscious thought).

The brain is the most complex, interesting, and intricate organ known to us.

Consider, for example, that in an average human it weighs just over a kilogram and yet the number of connections it has is greater than the number of particles in the entire universe [44].

The evolution of the brain was from the bottom up, from the inside out, and from the back to front.

Unlike many other organs in our bodies that atrophied during our evolutionary journey (such as a vestigial tail on the coccyx, the vermicular appendage in the cecum of our ascending colon, among others), our brain instead continued accumulating control functions, developing newer structures on top of older ones as it grew in complexity. The most recent of these structures is the cerebral cortex, which is a small, thin dark-colored layer on the outside of the brain. Of particular interest was the development of the frontal cortex, which is responsible for what we call higher brain functions: planning, self-control, and voluntary decisions.

According to the triune brain model proposed by Paul MacLean in the 1960s, the modern brain can be subdivided into three parts: the *reptilian brain* (formed by the medulla and the cerebellum) responsible for our survival, which developed hundreds of millions of years ago; on top of it we find the *old mammalian brain or limbic system,* where negative (distance) and positive (approach) emotions reside, which developed tens of millions of years ago; and finally, on top of the limbic system we find the neocortex, which developed two or three million years ago and is, of the three parts, the only distinctly human one (see Fig. 2.2).

This model was superseded at the beginning of the twenty-first century [45]and is seen as a pedagogical simplification of how the brain functions. It is, however, a very clear schematic of the evolution of the nervous system in humans.

The brain is itself "specialized," that is, within it there are certain groups of neurons that are in charge of carrying out specific tasks or regulating specific bodily functions.

Bilaterality could be considered the broadest degree of specialization.

The fact that we have a "left" brain (rational, objective, mathematical, detailed, scientific) and a "right" brain (emotional, subjective, musical, gestalt, artistic) is something we can also see in birds and reptiles.

Having brain bilaterality is a huge evolutionary advantage, both for prey and predators.

For prey, with lateralized eyes, bilaterality allows them to pay attention to what they are eating with one eye and to perceive the surroundings with the other eye, so that they may flee at the first sign of danger.

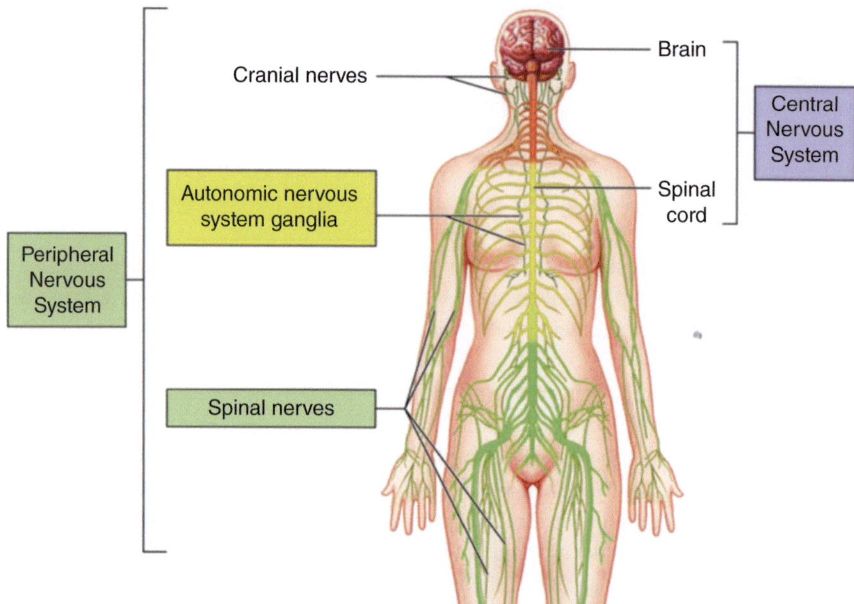

Fig. 2.2 Organization of the human brain. (https://pressbooks.ccconline.org/bio106/chapter/nervous-system-levels-of-organization/)

For predators, with frontal eyes, bilaterality allows them to accurately calculate the distance to their target and thus save energy by arriving exactly where their prey is.

In addition to this bilateral organization, each of the hemispheres holds discrete neuron islands (nuclei) that perform a specific function (vision, smell, taste, hearing, tactile perception), including one area described by Peter Paul Broca (1824–1880) [33],who was a great French surgeon and anthropologist.

Broca described an area of the brain, located in the third left frontal convolution, which is related to speech.

Broca could be considered a very peculiar man. Firstly, he was born with all his teeth (this neonatal dentition is a situation that is seen in less than 1 in 3000 births, and the ancient Egyptians considered it an important omen). Secondly, he was a child prodigy, having enrolled in medical school at the age of 17 and graduating at the age of 20. In addition to being a great surgeon, he was a great anthropologist and mathematician.

In Broca's time, infectious diseases were calamities that were very difficult to control, the concepts of asepsis and antisepsis were just developing, and overcrowding in cities favored the proliferation of these ailments in both rich and poor (though as is often the case, the poor had it much worse).

Oral hygiene was particularly poor, and this led not only to the loss of teeth but also frequently to dental abscesses, which in many cases became chronic and could give rise to abscesses in other parts of the body, including the brain.

Depending on which part of the brain was affected by an abscess, hemorrhage, or a tumor, patients could suffer any or all of the following: loss of consciousness, seizures, loss of strength, sensitivity alterations, or difficulty in carrying out a task.

This is how the inability to speak was first described: an alteration called *aphasia*, masterfully described by Dr. Broca.

Broca's first case was a patient whom he followed for 10 years and who progressively developed a *softening* of the second and third frontal convolution. Broca published this case, and his observations on it, in August 1861.

A few months later, he published a second case, reported in the *Bulletin de la Societé Antomique* in November 1861.

This case was more important than the first for two reasons: (a) it confirmed the findings of the first case since the patient was an 84-year-old man who suffered a loss of consciousness around Easter 1860 and was left with acute aphasia. (b) It was a more recent, smaller, and localized lesion, exactly in the place predicted by his first observation of a patient with *aphemia*, as Broca first called the condition. He later changed the term to *aphasia*, which is a neologism formed by two Greek terms meaning "no word."

In his story from November 1861, which I invite you to read, Broca describes with exquisite sensitivity the nonverbal communication capacity of an 84-year-old man, who has worked all his life making roads, and whose oral ability is limited to five words: yes (oui), no (non), three (trois), still (toujours), and Lelo (because his last name was Lelong). However, combining this limited vocabulary with body language, he was able to explain what his job was, how old he was, his sex, and how many children he had. Upon dying as a result of a fractured femur worsened by his advanced age, Broca carried out an autopsy and found the brain injury he suspected.

Let us stop for a moment to contemplate the enormity of what we have just read.

Here is a 37-year-old doctor, who has been practicing surgery for 17 years, who has had a patient with a chronic condition that has led him to postulate the existence of a language-specific area of the brain. He publishes his findings and theories for all of French society to read in the French summer. Not 3 months later he meets a patient, an 84-year-old farmer with a fractured femur, affected by an aphasia that began during Easter the previous year. When that patient dies, he finds a brain injury in precisely the same area he had postulated the existence of not even 3 months earlier.

In 1861, French medicine was probably the most developed in the world, although it was beginning to have severe competition from German medicine, especially due to the recent appearance of a new rising star: Rudolph Virchow. It was not yet at the same level though.

In the beginning of the nineteenth century, a great school of medicine arose in France due to the influence of Jean Nicolas Corvisart (1775–1821). This school was known for systematizing clinical semiology (the study of the signs and symptoms of patients). In addition to the observation and palpation that came from the Greeks, it incorporated the percussion described by Leopold Auenbrugger (1722–1809), a Viennese doctor, and later in 1816, the auscultation described by René Théophile Hyacinthe Laennec (1781–1826).

With all these techniques in hand, patients at the French school were scrupulously examined through anamnesis, inspection, palpation, percussion, and auscultation. Any findings were carefully recorded in a clinical history and, if the patient died (which unfortunately was very common in hospitals at the time), the same doctor who examined the patient would perform the autopsy.

We can see then where Broca developed his way of doing research.

Keep in mind that this examination seeks to detect the clinical evidence of the lesions that we would observe in the autopsy. The virtue of the clinician was to be able to connect the data provided by the history of the patient's illness (symptoms) with the doctor's findings (signs) and infer the types of lesions and their locations in order to explain both phenomena.

We owe this idea of the locations of diseases in certain organs to an Italian, Giovanni Baptista Morgagni (1682–1771), who, shortly before he died, published one of the most influential books in the history of medicine: *De sedibus et causes morborum per anatomy indagatis*, where he detailed the findings of around 700 clinical histories and their corresponding autopsies.

Thus, Broca came to demonstrate the existence of an affected area in aphasic patients.

In the mid-nineteenth century, the study of the internal environment described by Claude Bernard (1813–1878) was added to the above by means of laboratory analysis of blood, urine, or other fluids.

At the beginning of the twentieth century, images based on the works of Wilhelm Konrad Roentgen (1845–1923) were incorporated into the medical arsenal, which have had an extraordinary development in the modern age.

Today we are in a position to detect clinical or subclinical (asymptomatic) lesions, and we can also study the function of organs by studying the vascularization or the consumption of certain substances, such as sugar or specific drugs.

This has allowed us to study in even greater depth the brain changes that occur when we observe or listen, but also when we remember, think, or express certain ideas or words.

This is what neuroscience studies tell us.

2.2.4 *Neuroscience and Speech*

The study of the central nervous system is probably one of the most exciting fields of the twenty-first century as the advances in genomics, proteomics, neuroimaging, and neuroethics have all been overwhelming.

For this reason, we must be extremely cautious with the reductionist vision of science. Detecting a biochemical or electrical change is not the same as detecting an idea or a concept. The ideas of historicity, of identity, and even the idea of the mind have been challenged by some of the results of magnetic resonance imaging studies.

Lydia Feito Grande, professor of bioethics at the Universidad Complutense de Madrid, says in her text *Neuroética: cómo hace juicios morales nuestro cerebro* [46]:

Neuroscience—of which we certainly cannot speak in the singular because it encompasses very different approaches—falls within the so-called cognitive sciences .

The six disciplines within cognitive sciences are philosophy, anthropology, psychology, linguistics, artificial intelligence, and neuroscience.

Each of them contributes something that is unique to the study of human knowledge.

It is important to note that the human brain always responds as a whole to stimuli, and therefore in all functional studies, the signal noise must be attenuated in order to detect meaningful fluctuations. Let us remember that in 2012 the Ig Nobel Prize in Neuroscience (https://blogs.scientificamerican.com/scicurious-brain/ignobel-prize-in-neuroscience-the-dead-salmon-study/) was awarded for the functional magnetic resonance imaging study of a dead salmon performed by Bennett et al. [47]

These results at first seem hilarious but quickly make you reflect on the certainty of the fundamentals with which we defend certain positions.

Regardless of the care, precautions, and rigorous standards that we expect from these different studies, it is undeniable that electroencephalography (EEG), magnetoencephalography (MEG), computed axial tomography (CAT scan), positron emission tomography (PET), magnetic resonance imaging (MRI), and functional magnetic resonance imaging (fMRI) have provided a new and challenging landscape in the study of the brain.

One of the most fascinating discoveries, in relation to emotions and speech, has been the discovery of mirror neurons [48–50].

Mirror neurons have the peculiarity of being activated when one performs a specific act or sees someone else perform a certain gesture or act. They were first described by di Pellegrino et al. in the early 1990s. They located them in the F5 region of the ventral promoter area of the brain of a macaque monkey (Nemestine macaque).

What these researchers found is that the same area of the brain was activated when the monkey intentionally performed an act with its hand (catching or holding an object) and also when they saw the researcher do it with their own hand.

This "imitation" in our brain that reacts to actions performed by someone else has several implications: firstly, it helps with learning since seeing another do something helps us understand how to do it ourselves; and secondly, it helps with understanding on an emotional level since when we associate feelings and emotions with specifics actions, we are then able to infer the mood or intentions of our fellow human beings. These findings were integrated into the so-called theory of mind, a field developed from the work of anthropologist Gregory Beatson (1904–1980) in his book *Mind and Nature: A Necessary Unity.* [51]Today the two major areas of study of the Theory of Mind (ToM) are the Affective ToM, which studies the ability to infer the emotional states of others, and the Cognitive ToM, which studies the ability to infer the beliefs and intentions of others. [52]

Speech learning has two main components: affective and cognitive.

Today we know that children can pick out their mother's voice from a group of voices only a few hours after birth and that the identified maternal voice produces different neural responses than the other voices. This relationship between the sound and musicality of the maternal voice is established in the prenatal stage, when the child is still in the womb [53–58].

The relationship between voice, face, and music is much deeper than we think. In fact, we are not yet sure if humans should be called *talking* or *singing* apes since language and music share so many structures in common [59–64].

This deep relationship between voice and musicality explains why every speaker has a *little song* that helps us to identify their place of origin, their sociocultural level, and also, in some circumstances, allows others to tell when they are being dishonest, but sometimes this very same *song* also facilitates deception [65].

The truth is that the another's voice has a great impact on our behavior: we may find it attractive or repulsive, truthful or deceptive, trustworthy or not. This is not only in relation to our own personal experience but also our species as a whole [20, 21, 23, 66–72].

It is very reasonable to think that a crucial element for our evolution and our survival in the context of complex social relationships has a genetic basis. The anatomical structures we have described before (laryngeal, muscular, and neurological) developed from specific genetic information; therefore, the search for the origin of human language and its relationship with other animals has also been carried out in the fascinating world of genomics (the study of DNA), transcriptomics (the study of RNA), and proteomics (the study of proteins) [57, 63, 73–81].

So far we have seen the origin of language from the sensory structures related to sound (cochlea); structures related to the emission of sound (lungs, trachea, and larynx); and the structures that allow us to control our respiratory rhythm and finally the musical modulation of language.

Additionally, we have analyzed the way we learn (maternal voice identification, mirror neurons, theory of mind) and the use of language to trust or distrust a speaker, to select a partner and to establish social relationships.

All this has been achieved through millions of years of evolution, at least three million years culminating between 100,000 and 80,000 years ago when a human spoke for the first time on the planet.

Therefore, with all these previous tools in place, we can now dream.

2.3 The Poetic Origin of the First Word

Poetry is intimately tied with creation, with generation (Poyesis), and in my view, it is the next step toward scientific advancement.

Scientific knowledge, defined as that which is methodologically obtained and systematically organized, is universal and, without a doubt, has managed to change the face of the earth and, by extension, the face of medicine.

But it has two attributes that are both a strength and detriment: in the first place, it must have a very solid foundation (this is the reason why the best scientific knowledge is based on experimental evidence); secondly, it can only answer questions it is actually asked; those questions that cannot be answered by scientific evidence are questions that are not asked at all.

Therefore, the search for the origins of the human word is a scientific task, but imagining the first human word is a poetic task. We can never know if what we imagine or believe is true. That is why I share my own idea.

For me the first human word was **feminine**.

If we imagine our ancestors in the African savannah, or in the Eurasian caves, 80,000 years ago, the distribution of tasks was very clear: men were essentially hunters, with brains oriented to the sequential resolution of problems, concerned with an economy of movement and who communicated with short, low-intensity sounds, gestures, and warning shouts. That is to say, they were relatively simple beings, with a clear focus and mostly silent existence, punctuated by a strong release of adrenaline at the proximity of the prey, followed by rapid muscular discharges and jubilant cheers if the hunt was successful. It was sporadic and often unsuccessful high-intensity work (requiring a great expenditure of energy in a short time).

Women, on the other hand, formed a work network. They were gatherers, caretakers, and hunters of small prey and educators. They would create hierarchies and alliances in order to carry out constant and fruitful work that was of low to moderate intensity (which requires lower energy expenditure over a longer period of time).

In which of these groups would the first word most likely have originated? In which group was it most likely to be heard? And if it was heard, in which group was it most likely to be learned? Therefore, I reaffirm my preference: **the first human speaker was a woman**.

The second choice we must consider is if this word was uttered by a child or an adult. From my perspective, a child experiences many things, but an adult learns. I like to think that the first word was spoken by an adult, heard by a child, and the adult learned the effects it had on the child. **My preference is that the first word was maternal**.

The third choice we must consider is whether the first word was sung or not. I think so, speech and music are perceived better than unconnected syllables. **My preference is that the first word was sung.**

The fourth choice we must consider is for what purpose was the word sung? To inform? I do not think so as alerts are usually expressed with shouts. To point something out? I do not think so as nonverbal language is usually more accurate. To reassure and comfort? Yes I think so. **My preference is that the first word was conjuring, meaning therapeutic**. Spells are the oldest evidence of medical treatment, based on a magical understanding of the world and their purpose is to calm the mind (placebo effect) in the face of nature's wrath, giving us peace and quiet.

If we look at these attributes: feminine, maternal, and conjuring, we can imagine in the mists of time, a mother nursing a crying child, and suddenly the first human voice, guttural and sung, breaks the silence, spontaneously comes out of her larynx. The first lullaby, its tone and cadence unknown, but it soothed the child, the crying subsided, surprise led the child to listen carefully and allowed him to nourish himself, the mother groomed the little one with her hand and he fell asleep peacefully, without the inclement weather or the threats that surrounded him disturbing his sleep.

That was, for me, the first human word.

This turned into an evolutionary advantage, with healthier and stronger children.

It was transmitted to the community that first listened and then imitated. The nights became sung, the crackling of the fire and the singing of the women gave peace to the community.

The learned word began to be exercised more and more frequently. Humans became speakers.

It became a language, initially dominated by women and imitated and learned by men.

Much later it became writing and there history changed ... but that is another story.

What seems crucial to me, in this imagined story, is to recover the therapeutic value of the human word. This conjuring intention translates into a placebo effect in the infant, and this effect in turn has an impact on sleep and health.

Even today the word reassures children when they are upset. Stories help them understand reality and fall asleep. Deep voices give us confidence, shrill voices make us nervous. Soft cadences make us drowsy and high-sounding cadences excite us.

All these effects will be studied in the next chapter.

2.4 Teaching Exercises

1. Individual

    (a) Do you think it is reasonable to think that the cochlea predates the ability to speak?
    (b) If you answered yes, why did you?

        • Because it is a structure present millions of years before it is possible to speak?
        • Because being able to pinpoint a sound's location is more important than producing it?
        • Because both silent predators and silent prey tend to be more successful?
        • Because the cochlea is bilateral and the larynx is not?
        • Because even within human evolution speech is relatively recent?

    (c) Do you think speech is an evolutionary advantage?
    (d) What do you think was the first human word?
    (e) If you had to choose an alternative version of the feminine, maternal, and conjuring word, which one would you choose?
    (f) What are the reasons that led you to choose other features?

(g) Do you exercise your voice?

(h) Do you do impressions or sing? Would you like to do it?

(i) Do you do warm up exercises before speaking?

(j) Are you aware of the effect that your voice has on your listeners?

2. Group

(a) What are the anatomical elements necessary for hearing and phonation?

- Point out the salient features of.

    - The cochlea.
    - The hyoid bone.
    - The larynx.
    - The windpipe.
    - The lungs.
    - The intercostal muscles.
    - The diaphragm.
    - The vagus nerve.
    - Broca's area.

(b) You can speak musically: try imitate accents from your country or other countries.

(c) Select a native speaker of a given dialect and an impersonator. Without looking, have the rest of the group try to guess which is which. Why did they choose the way they did? What tipped them off one way or the other?

(d) Modulate the tone, intensity, frequency of your voice. In which do you feel more comfortable? What is your natural register?

(e) Read a paragraph in a language you are not fluent in out loud.

- What do you find most difficult about it?
- What are the sounds you need to work on the most?
- Do you hear the difference between what you hear, what you think you are saying, and what you are actually saying?
- Why does our recorded voice seem unrecognizable to us?
- Where do we hear our own voice?

(f) Summarize the evolutionary history of life on earth up to the earliest hominids.

(g) Summarize the evolutionary history of the human being, from three million years ago to the present.

(h) What are the outstanding fossil elements that lead us to believe that the first speaking humans appeared between 100,000 and 80,000 years ago?

(i) What do you think the first human languages were like?

(j) Where does the language you currently speak in your community derive from?

References

1. Intelligence|Etymology, origin and meaning of intelligence by etymonline. https://www.etymonline.com/word/intelligence. Accessed 22 Oct 2022.
2. Zubiri X. Sentient intelligence. Publishing Alliance; 1980.
3. Kahneman-Daniel. Thinking-fast-and-slow. New York: Farrar, Strauss and Girouix; 2013.
4. Aristotle. Politics (Gredos Classical Library, ed); 2000.
5. Wagensberg G. If nature is the answer, what was the question? Collection Metathemas. Tusquets Publishers; 2002.
6. Nutman AP, Bennett VC, Friend CRL, van Kranendonk MJ, Chivas AR. Rapid emergence of life shown by discovery of 3,700-million-year-old microbial structures. Nature. 2016;537(7621):535–8. https://doi.org/10.1038/nature19355.
7. Hedges SB. The origin and evolution of model organisms. Nat Rev Genet. 2002;3(11):838–49. https://doi.org/10.1038/nrg929.
8. Faguy DM, Jarrell KF. A twisted tale: the ori in and chemotaxis in prokaryotes. Microbiology. 1999;145:279–81.
9. Michalski N, Petit C. Genes involved in the development and physiology of both the peripheral and central auditory systems. Ann Rev Neurosci. 2019;42:67. https://doi.org/10.1146/annurev-neuro-070918-050428.
10. Eberl DF, Boekhoff-Falk G. Development of Johnston's organ in Drosophila. International Journal of Developmental Biology. 2007;51(6-7):679–87. https://doi.org/10.1387/ijdb.072364de.
11. Bierman HS, Carr CE. Sound localization in the alligator. Hear Res. 2015;329:11–20. https://doi.org/10.1016/j.heares.2015.05.009.
12. Schnupp JWH, Carr CE. On hearing with more than one ear: lessons from evolution. Nat Neurosci. 2009;12(6):692–7. https://doi.org/10.1038/nn.2325.
13. Fritzsch B, Straka H. Evolution of vertebrate mechanosensory hair cells and inner ears: toward identifying stimuli that select mutation driven altered morphologies. J Comp Physiol A Neuroethol Sens Neural Behav Physiol. 2014;200(1):5–18. https://doi.org/10.1007/s00359-013-0865-z.
14. Carey J, Amin N. Evolutionary changes in the cochlea and labyrinth: solving the problem of sound transmission to the balance organs of the inner ear. Anat Rec A Discov Mol Cell Evol Biol. 2006;288(4):482–90. https://doi.org/10.1002/ar.a.20306.
15. Manley GA. Evolutionary pathways to the mammalian cochleae. J Assoc Res Otolaryngol. 2012;13(6):733–43. https://doi.org/10.1007/s10162-012-0349-9.
16. Carr CE, Christensen-Dalsgaard J. Evolutionary trends in directional hearing. Curr Open Neurobiol. 2016;40:111–7. https://doi.org/10.1016/j.conb.2016.07.001.
17. Christensen-Dalsgaard J, Carr CE. Evolution of a sensory novelty: tympanic ears and the associated neural processing. Brain Res Bull. 2008;75(2–4):365–70. https://doi.org/10.1016/j.brainresbull.2007.10.044.
18. Köppl C, Manley GA. A functional perspective on the evolution of the cochlea. Cold Spring Harb Perspect Med. 2019;9(6):a033241. https://doi.org/10.1101/cshperspect.a033241.
19. Albert JT, Kozlov AS. Comparative aspects of hearing in vertebrates and insects with antennal ears. Curr Biol. 2016;26(20):R1050–61. https://doi.org/10.1016/j.cub.2016.09.017.
20. Re DE, O'Connor JJM, Bennett PJ, Feinberg DR. Preferences for very low and very high voice pitch in humans. PLoS One. 2012;7(3):e32719. https://doi.org/10.1371/journal.pone.0032719.
21. Jiang X, Pell MD. On how the brain decodes vocal cues about speaker confidence. Cortex. 2015;66:9–34. https://doi.org/10.1016/j.cortex.2015.02.002.
22. Kosilo M, Costa M, Nuttall HE, et al. The neural basis of authenticity recognition in laughter and crying. Sci Rep. 2021;11(1):23750. https://doi.org/10.1038/s41598-021-03131-z.
23. Jones BC, Feinberg DR, DeBruine LM, Little AC, Vukovic J. Integrating cues of social interest and voice pitch in men's preferences for women's voices. Biol Lett. 2008;4(2):192–4. https://doi.org/10.1098/rsbl.2007.0626.

24. Kingsley EP, Eliason CM, Riede T. et al, Identity and novelty in the avian syrinx. Proc Natl Acad Sci U S A. 115:10209. https://doi.org/10.1073/pnas.1804586115.

25. Russell AP, Bauer AM. Vocalization by extant nonavian reptiles: a synthetic overview of phonation and the vocal apparatus. Anat Rec. 2021;304(7):1478–528. https://doi.org/10.1002/ar.24553.

26. Li Z, Zhou Z, Clarke JA. Convergent evolution of a mobile bony tongue in flighted dinosaurs and pterosaurs. PLoS One. 2018;13(6):e0198078. https://doi.org/10.1371/journal.pone.0198078.

27. Kelemen G. Evolutionary sources of human language. Folia Phoniat. 1964;16:59–66.

28. Zhang YS, Takahashi DY, Liao DA, Ghazanfar AA, Elemans CPH. Vocal state change through laryngeal development. Nat Commun. 2019;10(1):4592. https://doi.org/10.1038/s41467-019-12588-6.

29. Zhou CF, Bhullar BAS, Neander AI, Martin T, Luo ZX. New Jurassic mammaliaform sheds light on early evolution of mammal-LIKE hyoid bones. Science. 365:6450. http://science.sciencemag.org/.

30. Lydiatt DD, Bucher GS. The influence of the final cause doctrine on anatomists of the sixteenth and seventeenth centuries concerning selected anatomical structures of the head and neck. Laryngoscope. 2012;122(SUPPL. 3):S35. https://doi.org/10.1002/lary.23391.

31. Nuland SB. Doctors: the illustrated history of medical pioneers. New York: Black Dog and Leventhal Publisher Inc.; 2008.

32. Lydiatt DD, Bucher GS. The historical Latin and etymology of selected anatomical terms of the larynx. Clin Anat. 2010;23(2):131–44. https://doi.org/10.1002/ca.20912.

33. Skinner HA. The origin of medical terms. Philadelphia: The Williams & Wilkins Company; 1961.

34. Coquerelle M, Prados-Frutos JC, Rojo R, Mitteroecker P, Bastir M. Short faces, big tongues: developmental origin of the human chin. PLoS One. 2013;8(11):e81287. https://doi.org/10.1371/journal.pone.0081287.

35. Titze IR. Human speech: a restricted use of the mammalian larynx. J Voice. 2017;31(2):135–41. https://doi.org/10.1016/j.jvoice.2016.06.003.

36. Matzinger T, Fitch WT. Voice modulatory cues to structure across languages and species. Philos Trans R Soc B Biol Sci. 2021;376(1840):20200393. https://doi.org/10.1098/rstb.2020.0393.

37. Rouse AA, Patel AD, Kao MH. Vocal learning and flexible rhythm pattern perception are linked: evidence from songbirds. Proc Natl Acad Sci U S A. 118:e2026130118. https://doi.org/10.1073/pnas.2026130118.

38. Vernes SC, Kriengwatana BP, Beeck VC, et al. The multi-dimensional nature of vocal learning. Philos Trans R Soc B Biol Sci. 2021;376(1836):20200236. https://doi.org/10.1098/rstb.2020.0236.

39. Belyk M, Brown R, Beal DS, et al. Human larynx motor cortices coordinate respiration for vocal-motor control. NeuroImage. 2021;239:239. https://doi.org/10.1016/j.neuroimage.2021.118326.

40. Michon M, Zamorano-Abramson J, Aboitiz F. Faces and voices processing in human and primate brains: rhythmic and multimodal mechanisms underlying the evolution and development of speech. Front Psychol. 2022;13:13. https://doi.org/10.3389/fpsyg.2022.829083.

41. Boë LJ, Berthommier F, Legou T, et al. Evidence of a vocalic proto-system in the baboon (Papio papio) suggests pre-hominin speech precursors. PLoS One. 2017;12(1):e0169321. https://doi.org/10.1371/journal.pone.0169321.

42. Fitch WT, de Boer B, Mathur N, Ghazanfar AA. Monkey vocal tracts are speech-ready. Sci Adv. 2016;2:1. https://www.science.org.

43. Rosas A. The origins of language: in search for the specificity of large-brained hominin languages. J Anthropol Sci. 2013;91:273–5. https://doi.org/10.4436/JASS.91018.

44. McGilchrist I. The master and his emissary. In: The divided brain and the making of Western World. New Haven: Yale University Press; 2009.

45. Gardner R. The evolutionary neuroethology of Paul MacLean: convergences and frontiers. New York: Praeger; 2002.
46. Feito Grande L. Neuroética. (Plaza y Valdés Editores, ed.). Plaza y Valdés SL; 2019.
47. Bennett CM, Baird AA, Miller MB, Wolford GL. Neural correlates of interspecies perspective taking in the post-mortem Atlantic Salmon: an argument for proper multiple comparisons correction. JSUR. 2009;1(1):1–5.
48. Bonini L, Rotunno C, Arcuri E, Gallese V. Mirror neurons 30 years later: implications and applications. Trends Cogn Sci. 2022;26(9):767–81. https://doi.org/10.1016/j.tics.2022.06.003.
49. Kilner JM, Lemon RN. What we know currently about mirror neurons. Curr Biol. 2013;23(23):R1057. https://doi.org/10.1016/j.cub.2013.10.051.
50. di Pellegrino G, Fadiga L, Fogassi L, Gallese V, Rizzolatti G. Understanding motor events: a neurophysiological study. Exp Brain Res. 1992;91:176.
51. Bateson G. Mind and nature: a necessary Unity. Cheshir: Dutton; 1979.
52. Samuel S, Durdevic K, Legg EW, Lurz R, Clayton NS. Is language required to represent others' mental states? Evidence from beliefs and other representations. Cogn Sci. 2019;43(1):1. https://doi.org/10.1111/cogs.12710.
53. Mehler J, Bertoncini J, Barriere M, Jassik-Gerschenfeld D. Infant recognition of mother's voice. Perception. 1978;7:491.
54. Purhonen M, Kilpeläinen-Lees R, Valkonen-Korhonen M, Karhu J, Lehtonen J. Four-month-old infants process own mother's voice faster than unfamiliar voices -electrical signs of sensitization in infant brain. Cogn Brain Res. 2005;24(3):627–33. https://doi.org/10.1016/j.cogbrainres.2005.03.012.
55. The mirror brain concepts and language.
56. Uchida-Ota M, Arimitsu T, Tsuzuki D, et al. Maternal speech shapes the cerebral frontotemporal network in neonates: a hemodynamic functional connectivity study. Dev Cogn Neurosci. 2019;39:39. https://doi.org/10.1016/j.dcn.2019.100701.
57. Jablonka E, Ginsburg S, Dor D. The co-evolution of language and emotions. Philos Trans R Soc B Biol Sci. 2012;367(1599):2152–9. https://doi.org/10.1098/rstb.2012.0117.
58. Liu P, Cole PM, Gilmore RO, et al. Young children's neural processing of their mother's voice: an fMRI study. Neuropsychologia. 2019;122:11–9. https://doi.org/10.1016/j.neuropsychologia.2018.12.003.
59. Leongómez JD, Havlíček J, Roberts SC. Musicality in human vocal communication: an evolutionary perspective. Philos Trans R Soc B Biol Sci. 2022;377(1841):20200391. https://doi.org/10.1098/rstb.2020.0391.
60. Scherer KR. Expression of emotion in voice and music. J Voice. 1995;9:235.
61. Sterelny K. Language, gesture, skill: the co-evolutionary foundations of language. Philos Trans R Soc B Biol Sci. 2012;367(1599):2141–51. https://doi.org/10.1098/rstb.2012.0116.
62. Dehaene-Lambertz G, Montavont A, Jobert A, et al. Language or music, mother or Mozart? Structural and environmental influences on infants' language networks. Brain Lang. 2010;114(2):53–65. https://doi.org/10.1016/j.bandl.2009.09.003.
63. Masataka N. Music, evolution and language. Dev Sci. 2007;10(1):35–9. https://doi.org/10.1111/j.1467-7687.2007.00561.x.
64. Abrams DA, Chen T, Odriozola P, et al. Neural circuits underlying mother's voice perception predict social communication abilities in children. Proc Natl Acad Sci USA. 2016;113(22):6295–300. https://doi.org/10.1073/pnas.1602948113.
65. Guyer JJ, Briñol P, Vaughan-Johnston TI, Fabrigar LR, Moreno L, Petty RE. Paralinguistic features communicated through voice can affect appraisals of confidence and evaluative judgments. J Nonverbal Behav. 2021;45(4):479–504. https://doi.org/10.1007/s10919-021-00374-2.
66. Marin MM, Rathgeber I. Darwin's sexual selection hypothesis revisited: musicality increases sexual attraction in both sexes. Front Psychol. 2022;13:13. https://doi.org/10.3389/fpsyg.2022.971988.

67. Pisanski K, Cartei V, McGettigan C, Raine J, Reby D. Voice modulation: a window into the origins of human vocal control? Trends Cogn Sci. 2016;20(4):304–18. https://doi.org/10.1016/j.tics.2016.01.002.

68. O'Connor JJM, Fraccaro PJ, Pisanski K, Tigue CC, Feinberg DR. Men's preferences for Women's femininity in dynamic cross-modal stimuli. PLoS One. 2013;8(7):e69531. https://doi.org/10.1371/journal.pone.0069531.

69. Gray RD, Atkinson QD, Greenhill SJ. Language evolution and human history: what a difference a date makes. Philos Trans R Soc B Biol Sci. 2011;366(1567):1090–100. https://doi.org/10.1098/rstb.2010.0378.

70. Pisanski K, Oleszkiewicz A, Plachetka J, Gmiterek M, Reby D. Voice pitch modulation in human mate choice. Proc Biol Sci. 2018;285(1893):20181634. https://doi.org/10.1098/rspb.2018.1634.

71. Apicella CL, Feinberg DR. Voice pitch alters mate-choice-relevant perception in hunter-gatherers. Proc R Soc B Biol Sci. 2009;276(1659):1077–82. https://doi.org/10.1098/rspb.2008.1542.

72. Biederman I, Shilowich BE, Herald SB, et al. The cognitive neuroscience of person identification. Neuropsychologia. 2018;116:205–14. https://doi.org/10.1016/j.neuropsychologia.2018.01.036.

73. Berwick RC, Friederici AD, Chomsky N, Bolhuis JJ. Evolution, brain, and the nature of language. Trends Cogn Sci. 2013;17(2):89. https://doi.org/10.1016/j.tics.2012.12.002.

74. Fisher SE. Evolution of language: lessons from the genome. Psychon Bull Rev. 2017;24(1):34–40. https://doi.org/10.3758/s13423-016-1112-8.

75. Davila-Ross M, Dezecache G. The complexity and phylogenetic continuity of laughter and smiles in hominids. Front Psychol. 2021;12:12. https://doi.org/10.3389/fpsyg.2021.648497.

76. Schmidt ERE, Polleux F. Genetic mechanisms underlying the evolution of connectivity in the human cortex. Front Neural Circuits. 2022;15:15. https://doi.org/10.3389/fncir.2021.787164.

77. Bennett MS. Five breakthroughs: a first approximation of brain evolution from early Bilaterians to humans. Front Neuroanat. 2021;15:15. https://doi.org/10.3389/fnana.2021.693346.

78. Benítez-Burraco A, Barceló-Coblijn L. Hominin interbreeding and language evolution: fine-tuning the details. J Anthropol Sci. 2013;91:277–90. https://doi.org/10.4436/JASS.91020.

79. Christiansen MH, Kirby S. Language evolution: consensus and controversies. Trends Cogn Sci. 2003;7(7):300–7. https://doi.org/10.1016/S1364-6613(03)00136-0.

80. Benítez-Burraco A, Barceló- CL. Paleogenomics, hominin interbreeding and language evolution. J Anthropol Sci. 2013;91:239–44. https://doi.org/10.4436/JASS.91012.

81. Żywiczyński P, Wacewicz S, Lister C. Pantomimic fossils in modern human communication. Philos Trans R Soc B Biol Sci. 2021;376(1824):20200204. https://doi.org/10.1098/rstb.2020.0204.

Chapter 3
The Placebo Effect of the Medical Word

3.1 The Placebo Effect in the History of Medicine: History of Medical Knowledge (Abbreviated Epistemology)

Nowadays we live in the era of scientific medicine. However, from the therapeutic point of view, the history of *medicine* has been the history of the *placebo* for most of human existence.

In order to delve into this subject, we must study medical epistemology, that is, the foundations of medical knowledge. The definition of diseases, patients, and therapies throughout the history of medicine.

Epistemology is defined as "the doctrine of the foundations and methods of scientific knowledge" (Dictionary of the Royal Spanish Academy, Ed. XXII).

In this chapter, however, we will not limit ourselves only to scientific medical knowledge, but to the study of the foundations and methods of medical knowledge in general.

The reason for broadening our horizons to medical knowledge without scientific foundation is due to the fact that, if we look at medical practice today, we can see an overlap of knowledge from different origins and obtained with different degrees of rigor.

This differentiates medicine from the hard sciences, in which new knowledge displaces old knowledge and, for this very reason, we can trace a linear and progressive development toward complexity, assertiveness, and predictability.

Let us take physics as an example: today physics as a whole is considerably more complex than it was in Newton's time, but it is also more precise and can accurately determine the place where a projectile will hit, the flow of a river, the speed of a particle, the passage of a comet, etc. On the other hand, astrology is no longer accepted as part of serious astronomical studies, the same way phlogiston is no longer accepted as part of thermodynamics.

E. Gil Deza, *Improving Clinical Communication*,
https://doi.org/10.1007/978-3-031-62446-9_3

If we try to do the same in medicine, we will see that instead of being linear, progress has been fractal.

This means that theories do not always replace each other, but often coexist, are revisited, reformulated, and developed asymmetrically. It is as if everything in medicine were alive and in transformation, even old ideas may not completely die, resurfacing in unpredictable ways long after they had been considered outdated.

For this reason, we will study the seven orders of knowledge that coexist in modern medicine, just as I described them in my book *On Cancer and its Demons* [1]:

Magical.
Clinical.
Anatomopathological.
Assisted.
Predictive.
Coercive.
Wishful.

We will develop each of them in order to understand the placebo effect and the role of the doctor in each of them.

This will be crucial to understand communication in the doctor–patient relationship.

In the history of medicine, the first knowledge of which there is evidence is magical knowledge.

3.1.1   *Magical Knowledge in Medicine [2–15]*

We summarize this field of knowledge in Table 3.1.

The prehistoric evidence for cults of the dead or talismans carved in stone, as well as the medicine practiced both by ancient peoples, by some tribes isolated from civilization (wild) and by human groups with their own codes of knowledge in civilized society (urban) was all based on magic.

But what do we mean by magic?

That they have no scientific basis for their claims and that they basically have four main characteristics:

Table 3.1 Characteristics of magic medicine

- Prehistoric evidence
- "Urban" and "wild" tribes
- Imposed diagnosis
- Spell therapy
- Esoteric knowledge
- Hereditary transmission of knowledge

3.1.1.1   Imposed Diagnosis

The diagnosis of a disease or condition is not a consequence of semiology, rather there are a series of conditions that are used to define what happens to a subject: *it is bad luck, they have done something wrong, he has the evil eye, he is intoxicated, he is envious, the disease of the moon, he is a werewolf, it's black magic* ... How do you arrive at these diagnoses? Without any method. A person is assigned a condition by a "healer," "shaman," or similar figure, and this is not discussed or verified further, only accepted.

3.1.1.2   Spell Therapy

The diagnostician possesses the gift (or art) of conjuring the forces of nature and changing the course of a disease from bad to good. Through a public or private ritual, with prayers or sacrifices, sometimes putting the subject in an altered state of consciousness, by using concoctions, incense, enchantment, seduction, or hypnosis; that is how healing, expiation, or restoration is achieved.

3.1.1.3   Esoteric Knowledge

When one investigates how illness or healing is produced, the answers that one receives always end in mystery. Even though many of these phenomena can be attributed to hysteria (sometimes collective) or to the placebo effect, the truth is that neither the sufferer nor the healer knows the causes of their conditions or powers.

3.1.1.4   Hereditary Transmission of Knowledge

The healer or shaman transmits their knowledge or power in a hereditary fashion. They select a person from the community whom they train in spells and the art of healing. This person "inherits" such a condition or gift, sometimes congenitally (when there are families of shamans), sometimes not.

There is a tendency today to disparage magic in developed societies, but we will soon see how prevalent it is even today.

What is *medical intuition* but the halo of magic that surrounds a good diagnostician?

Based on what objective parameter do we select our doctor if not guided by the social "magic" of word of mouth?

Why do we always think that a more expensive drug is more effective?

Why are alternative treatments successful?

Why is the greatest consumption of *antibiotics* used to treat *viral* diseases, such as seasonal flu, even though they are useless for that purpose?

What are the criteria for prescribing vitamins for fatigue or poor academic performance?

Why do serious newspapers keep publishing astral horoscopes?

Does phosphorus really increase our IQ?

All these questions have magical ideas as an answer.

The problem with magical thinking is that it has no error; therefore, it is not perfect. It is knowledge that is not falsifiable (according to Popper) and has no set methodology for being obtained.

This does not mean that beliefs do not influence our health.

The placebo effect (beneficial) and the nocebo effect (harmful) are evidence that what we believe in affects the way we act and our biology, and are two of the many reasons human beings are so complex. The human person is not only biology but also biography (experiences, beliefs, values, choices) but we will delve into that later.

Continuing with the historical order of medical epistemology, the second order of knowledge to appear was that of scientific knowledge.

3.1.2   The Scientific Knowledge of Medicine Is the Second to Appear

For reasons related to its influence in the Western world, we attribute the origin of scientific medicine to Greece [16–25], and especially to the Hippocratic school of the island of Kos, but they were not the only ones: Chinese, Indian, Babylonic, and Egyptian medicine, which were the four great contemporary medical schools of the fifth century BC, also evolved into scientific during this time. Medicine. I have summarized its outstanding characteristics in Table 3.2.

The characteristics that correlate with the birth of scientific ideas in medicine are

3.1.2.1   Empiricism

In other words, the search for truth in observation, that is, the importance of sensory data and the detection of functional or structural alterations in the patient's body. That is why the first evident progress occurs in the treatment of wounds, surgical techniques, immobilization, and bandages; this is where a change is first seen in coping with and solving medical problems.

Table 3.2 Characteristics of scientific medicine

- Empirical
- Rational
- Experimental
- Exposed diagnosis
- Universal knowledge
- Institutionally transmitted

3.1.2.2   Rationality

That is to say, the diagnosis is not the consequence of a hidden revelation, an oracle, or an inspiration, but as a consequence of establishing a causal relationship between the circumstances, the environment, and the appearance of the symptoms or ailments. Once again, physical injuries, their causes, and how to handle them were the first evidence of this human activity.

3.1.2.3   Experimentation

We can trace the first written evidence of human experimentation to the *Book of the Prophet Daniel* (Chap. I), written around 530 BC, which narrates the adventures of the people of Israel under the reign of Nebuchadnezzar (600 BC). In this chapter, in Daniel's dialogue with the eunuch Ashpenaz, they establish "a dietary regimen based on legumes and water, so that the Israelites are not contaminated with impure foods" for the law and after 10 days they "compare their countenance" with other young people to determine if they should continue receiving that diet or not. Despite the fact that this text showed a creative and innovative way to obtain medical knowledge, it took more than 25 centuries for it to be applied as a standard method in medicine. For more modern examples, we can consider the studies on vitamin C in the seventeenth century, as well as the study of the major and minor blood circulations by William Harvey in the fifteenth century. Both of these serve as examples of experimental studies of human physiology. Resorting to experimentation to obtain knowledge is a crucial step in scientific epistemology.

3.1.2.4   Exposed Diagnosis

The medical diagnosis consists of the integration of the symptoms that afflict the patient and the signs that the doctor detects in the patient's examination; this allows one to qualify the patient's ailments. The study of diseases is known as nosology (nosos = disease; logos = study) and includes etiology (*cause* of diseases), pathogenesis (*how* the disease manifests itself), semiology (*signs and symptoms* of diseases), pathology (the clinical, histological, or cytological lesions of the diseases), therapeutics (the treatment of the ailments), and prognosis (possible evolutions of the conditions). All of this make it possible to organize knowledge in a systematized way. One can trace the origin of a disease in the history of medicine, from the first time it was exposed to the present day: the study of fevers, neurological, cardiac, gastrointestinal, renal, pulmonary problems, etc. Each discovered disease has its own story.

3.1.2.5 Universal Knowledge

This systematization of medical knowledge made it universal; the scientific knowledge of a disease is valid throughout the world. For this reason, it is the most valued knowledge and at the same time the most basic. The scientific knowledge of medicine is the one that is demonstrable, methodically obtained, and systematically organized; it is the foundation of any fact in medicine; and it is the one that is obligatory to teach and know.

3.1.2.6 Institutional Transmission

This scientific knowledge based on the exposed diagnosis and experimental therapy can be taught and learned objectively. That is the foundation of medical schools and institutions. The programs of the different schools may vary, their ways of teaching may differ slightly, but the core of what a medical student should learn is quite similar all over the world, and indeed the programs are easily comparable between different institutions both locally and internationally.

These two orders of knowledge, magical and clinical, were maintained throughout 25 centuries in the West until a third order of knowledge appeared in the mid-nineteenth century.

3.1.3 Anatomopathological Knowledge

We already saw when we analyzed the case of Broca how in the French medical school the clinician who carried out the clinical record and treatment was the one who also carried out the autopsy, following the steps that Giovanni Battista Morgagni (1662–1771) had elaborated in his book *De sedibus et causis morborum per anatomy indagatis,* which was a real revolution for its time.

Under this paradigm, the role of the clinician was to detect in a living patient organic lesions using semiology; the same lesions that he himself might later discover in the autopsy of the same patient.

Therefore, the autopsy was seen as an instance of additional learning, perfecting what the clinician had been unable to detect or what they had detected wrongly.

In the German school, on the other hand, the doctor who carried out the autopsies was someone completely different from the general practitioner or surgeon who had carried out the medical history and the medical or surgical treatment.

This doctor was the pathologist, who, in addition to the macroscopic examination of the corpse, used the microscope, invented several centuries ago by Dutch shopkeeper Antonie van Leeuwenhoek (1632–1723), for the study of tissues and cells [26–29].

Table 3.3 Anatomopathological knowledge

• Two diagnostic moments: Clinical + determination.
• The birth of specialized knowledge
• Based on the body–mind (soul–mind) dichotomy

This is how the third order of knowledge was born. I have summarized it in Table 3.3.

We say that it is the third order of knowledge because of the way it was practiced in Germany, whose most famous pathologist was Rudolf Virchow (1821–1902), the biopsy or autopsy was done by a different professional, and therefore two diagnostic moments appear: the one carried out by the clinician and the one carried out by a different doctor (the pathologist), who often does not know the patient, has not made a clinical history and, nevertheless, is determining the clinician's success or error.

Thus, a new field of specialized knowledge was born.

The pathologist is a specialist in injuries, and therefore, for the first time in medicine, there is an expert in diseases who does not see a patient, does not operate on a patient, does not treat a patient, and does not directly cure anyone.

But its impact went further. For the first time in medicine, diseases for which there was a detectable lesion (such as diseases of the *body*) and diseases without obvious lesions (such as diseases of the *mind or soul*) were separated.

This dichotomy did not previously exist.

This German model was considered the highest form of medical science and art and was incorporated, among others, by William Osler (1849–1919), who was commissioned to write Virchow's eulogy in the *New England Journal of Medicine*. But Ostler is also one of the four founders of the Johns Hopkins University School of Medicine, which in 1910 was named the best School of Medicine in Canada and the United States by the Flexner report, carried out by Abraham Flexner (1866–1959), written in 1909 and subsequently published by the Carnegie Foundation for the Advancement of Teaching in 1910.

From that moment on, all the medical schools in the world modeled their teaching methods on those of Johns Hopkins University and anatomopathology was definitively incorporated into medical epistemology.

As we can see, this order of knowledge contributes rigor and systematics to the study of human diseases while at the same time creating a distinction between different types of conditions that a person can suffer and, above all, adding a confirmatory step. When this step reaffirms that the doctor is correct, it can be reassuring, but when it shows that a clinical or surgical diagnosis is wrong, it can be a source of doubt and grounds for legal action.

3.1.4 Assisted Knowledge

Even though we can trace this order of clinical knowledge to the use of the senses to study the excreta (in fact, the word diabetes is more than 2500 years old and its name derives from the fact that the urine was sweet), it was at the end of the nineteenth century, after the work of Claude Bernard (1813–1878) and his description of the body's internal environment, that biochemistry became part of the diagnostic process [30–32].

The study of the functioning of the liver, blood, kidneys, endocrine glands, immune system, and all the organs of our body can be analyzed by searching for quantitative or qualitative variations in the body's many substances.

This was complemented at the beginning of the twentieth century, with the birth of medical images from the discovery of X-rays by Wilhelm Roentgen (1845–1923) [33–38].

The discovery of X-rays made it possible to observe bone structures for the first time. In fact, the first X-ray was of the hand of Roentgen's wife, who fainted when she saw it due to the shock of seeing her own skeleton while being alive (Fig. 3.1).

This was complemented by the discoveries of Marie Curie (1867–1934) and her husband Pierre Curie (1859–1906), with the discovery of radium and the series of radioactive ions that gave rise to the scintigram, followed by the discovery of radar and the development of ultrasound scanners; the improvement of radiography toward linear, axillary, and finally axial computed tomography (CAT scan), which we use today on a daily basis. The appearance of magnetic resonance and the fusion of tomography and scintigraphy in positron emission tomography (PET scan) is extremely useful in oncology.

This order of assisted knowledge (which relies on lab results and images) is summarized in Table 3.4.

With assisted knowledge, scientific knowledge gains another layer: the first layer is that of clinical knowledge, motivated by the patient's illnesses and detected by the doctor's senses; the second layer is that of anatomopathological knowledge, more rigorous and certifying of histopathological lesions; to these two we add the third layer, that of alterations present in lab results (functional) or organ structure (images).

Each of these layers has its own sensitivity and specificity; when the three layers of knowledge are in agreement, the patient and the doctor can be confident in the veracity of the information, but when the results inconsistent (e.g., there are symptoms without alteration of the laboratory or of the images; there are imaging changes without symptoms; there are laboratory changes without symptoms or images), this conflict generates restlessness and mistrust.

What significance do these findings have?

What is the evolution of these alterations?

Will they be correct?

What should we do?

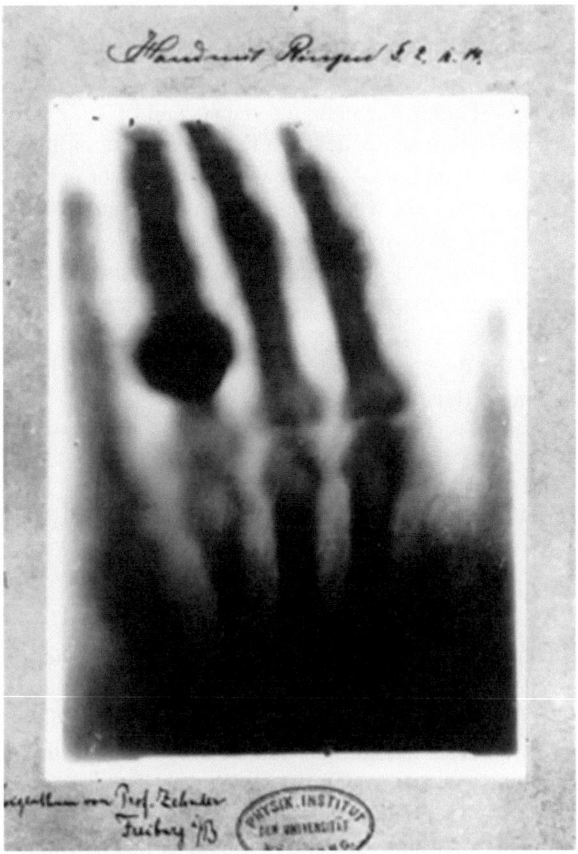

Fig. 3.1 (Hand mit ringer. https://en.wikipedia.org/wiki/X-ray#/media/File:First_medical_X-ray_
by_Wilhelm_R%C3%B6ntgen_of_his_wife_Anna_Bertha_Ludwig's_hand_-_18951222.gif)

Table 3.4 Assisted knowledge

• Three diagnostic moments: Clinical + complementary studies + confirmation
• Each moment provides its own information
• Incidental lesions (those without signs or symptoms) are first seen
• Biochemical alterations without evident lesion (preclinical and prepathological) are first seen
• Population screening studies are implemented (diabetes–tuberculosis–cancer)

All the answers to these questions are controversial, and the evidence on which they are based is less reliable the more the three layers disagree with each other.

The incorporation of lab results and images gave rise to secondary prevention, that is, the research of diseases in the initial stages of development: laboratory alterations in endocrine disorders such as diabetes or hypothyroidism and the implementation of population imaging studies for tuberculosis screening and cancer.

The most important impact of this knowledge consists in the incorporation of subclinical or preclinical diseases. This leads to the paradox of patients who enjoy excellent health and yet are affected by an eventually incurable and fatal disease.

In oncology, the CAT scan, magnetic resonance, and PET-CT have notably modified the profile of disseminated patients in numerous tumors: lung, breast, colon, melanoma, kidney, and lymphomas. These went from a poor performance status to an excellent performance status, which was unheard of as late as the 1980s but today represent more than 70% of disseminated patients.

This has a huge impact on communication, prognosis, patient selection, and interpretation of clinical trials, where highly selected patients have extraordinary results that are not reproduced in office practice.

In the middle of the twentieth century, a fifth order of knowledge was incorporated: predictive knowledge.

3.1.5 Predictive Knowledge

Prediction in medicine is called prognosis; it was the most valued art of the Hippocratics 2500 years ago, and it is still the most difficult art of modern medicine.

Two thousand five hundred years ago, prognosis was key to defining therapy since diseases were divided into those that were curable and those that were not. The doctor had to focus on treating curable diseases, but he had to be very careful to use his science or his art in dealing with incurable ones as this could be interpreted as a sin of hubris, that is, excessive pride and defiance of the gods, a sin for which he could be severely punished.

Until the middle of the twentieth century, prognosis was focused on how a condition would develop (what is known as the natural history of a disease) and objective variables began to be established for the medical prognosis: in oncology, the TNM (tumor, nodes, and metastases) scale and the Karnofsky activity scale are two examples of this effort.

However, halfway through the deciphering of the genetic code carried out by James Watson (1928) and Francis Crick (1916–2004) (winners of the 1962 Nobel Prize in Medicine and Physiology), a fifth order of knowledge appears: predictive knowledge [39–43].

This knowledge is based on the study of the genetic code that each cell has in DNA (genomics), in the study of RNA or the part of DNA that is transcribed to synthesize proteins (transcriptomics), and the study of proteins themselves (proteomics). That is, in the study of the information necessary to form the different components of the cell. If that information is altered, it is possible that cell structure or function is also altered.

To delve deeper into this subject, we will focus on the human being.

Today we know that the information with which a human cell is built functions and repairs itself is encoded in a large molecule called deoxyribonucleic acid (DNA) that is found in the nucleus (nuclear DNA). There is also mitochondrial DNA but for now we can leave it aside.

DNA is made up of complex chemical structures called bases: adenine, cytosine, thymine, and guanine (ACTG). These bases are attached to a sugar (deoxyribose) and the sugars are linked to each other through phosphate bonds; the bases are distributed in two chains and a base of one chain is joined with a complementary base of the other chain in a very specific way: A is joined with T and C is joined with G. Therefore, by knowing the distribution of bases of one chain we can know the composition of the other. These chains spiral into progressively denser structures until they form chromosomes. When the cells have to reproduce, they loosen (forming chromatin), the DNA is copied, and then distributed to the newly formed cells in order to transmit the information they possess.

Therefore, we can find DNA in different states: as loose DNA, as chromatin, or as a chromosome, depending on whether the cell is functioning or dividing.

In each of our cells, there is a single nuclear DNA molecule made up of 3.2 billion base pairs (or 6.4 billion bases), arranged in a certain sequence for each gene or unit of genetic information.

If we wrote those six billion letters on A4 paper, single face, single spaced, in Times New Roman font, size 12, and left a margin of two centimeters on each side, this sequence of letters As, Cs, Gs, and Ts would form a pile about 60 meters high.

In other words, every time you walk and see a 20-story building, think that in the nucleus of each cell in your body, from the sidewalk all the way to the top, the sequence of bases of your DNA, which determines how your body was formed, how your body works and many of the diseases that you will suffer, is written page by page.

This is what is called predictive medicine.

Regarding genomic studies, we must distinguish two aspects: the first aspect encompasses research that seeks information about a certain condition or disease. We can think of this aspect as assisted knowledge, that is, it provides additional information about a disease, but it is not strictly speaking a new *type* of knowledge. The second aspect encompasses research into probabilistic information, such as the risk of suffering from a disease or developing a disease given certain conditions. This constitutes the fifth order of knowledge.

In other words, we are dealing with a healthy person but their genetic code or RNA or some cellular proteins indicate that they are at greater risk (in some cases, *much* greater risk) of developing a certain condition than the general population. This information can also be applied in a slew of situations, as shown in Table 3.5.

Let us recap what this new order of knowledge means: until now we had magical (what we believe in), clinical (what we perceive through our senses), anatomo-pathological (what can be observed through the microscope), and assisted (changes in lab results or images). Excluding the first order of knowledge, all the others concern themselves with, and provide, objective and concrete evidence of functional or structural changes.

Table 3.5 Predictive knowledge

- Genomic: Study of the DNA base sequence
- Transcriptomics: Study of messenger RNA synthesized from a DNA sequence
- Proteomics: Study of the structure or function of proteins synthesized from a DNA sequence and a messenger RNA.

It is used for

- – Genetic studies (individual and population)
- – Forensic medicine
- – Filial determination (such as paternity tests)
- – Selecting embryos for implantation
- – Studying endocrine diseases
- – Studying oncological diseases
- – Studying neurological diseases
- – Assessing cardiovascular risk
- – Studying the methods of aging
- – Selecting a dietary regimen

This new knowledge, on the other hand, is *probabilistic,* and based on the detection of either an alteration of the genetic code itself or the product of that code (RNA, proteins).

The main problem with this type of knowledge is that only its successes can be confirmed. Firstly, because the lack of an expected result due to an alteration may be delayed (that is to say, it has not happened *yet,* but it may still happen), and secondly, the problem of considering that a given alteration will *inevitably* lead to a given result. This last idea is called genetic determinism.

Perhaps an easier way to understand the problem of genetic determinism in medicine is to use an allegory. Below I share the musical allegory I wrote to explain the problem of genetic determinism in oncology.

I transcribe the core of that article below:

In order to get closer to understanding this phenomenon, and above all to be able to communicate it to patients, since many of them lack the necessary biological knowledge to ponder this information, in my practice I frequently use a musical allegory that is the following:

1. **The phenotype** is the executed piece. What we see at the cellular level or at the organism level. It is the final piece, the expression of all variants and variations. Phenocopy (by mimicry or plastic surgery) is plagiarism, which may deceive us, but it is not genuine.

2. **The chromosomes** are the lecterns, the supports of information (remember that it is an allegory). They may be broken, joined in an anomalous way, altered in number. The scores of each instrument may be mixed up or placed in an inappropriate way. This does not necessarily mean that the work will be executed poorly, but it does imply an additional difficulty in the execution.

3. **Genomics** is the score (First DNA according to J. Enríquez). The sequence of symbols that represent the notes and rests. There is almost everything, but there is no sound. Nature copies with some imperfection the letters from parents to children —about 50–100 letters out of a total of 6 billion between one generation and another.

4. **Genomic editors** (CRISPR and the like) are copyists that can quickly modify the original text.

5. **The exomics** are the playable DNA fragments, since not the entire score will be played.

6. **Epigenomics (Second DNA)** are the arrangements that activate or silence certain exomic sequences and allow them to be executed or not. It is responsible for tissue differentiation, a part of it is heritable and another is modifiable through diet and habits. In fact, the difference between queens, drones and workers in a bee hive is given by epigenomic changes due to larval feeding with royal jelly or honey.

7. **Transcriptomics** (RNA) is the study of orchestral instruments. It is not sound yet, but it is the execution of the score necessary to be so.

8. **The post-transcriptional changes** are instrumental variations that allow the same instrument to produce enormous amounts of different sounds. In this way, with a single DNA sequence, different RNAs can be generated that will give rise to different proteins.

9. **Proteomics** is sound. The primary, secondary, tertiary, and quaternary structure of the protein molecule will be the note and intensity of the sound of life.

10. **The kinomics** will mark the speed with which that sound produces effects in the cell.

11. **Metabolomics will** coordinate sounds into the rhythm of the symphony of life and aging.

12. **The microbiome** (DNA of the bacteria that live in and with us (Third DNA) will be the bacterial orchestras that will modulate the sounds of our cells and tissues. The microbiome is easily and rapidly modifiable through diet and antibiotics.

13. **The virome** (viral DNA of the viruses that live in and with us—Fourth DNA) is rapidly modifiable through diet, vaccines, and antivirals.

14. **The biome** (DNA of all living beings that inhabit the planet) are the other rooms that are playing other pieces of music.

15. **The environment** is the theater where all the music of life takes place.

When we understand the complexity of interpreting genetic information, in which there are at least eleven salient points of uncertainty and unpredictability, we can understand the relativity of exhaustive statements.

If we are sure that it has this alteration susceptible to treatment, why does the tumor not respond? Why, if we are sure that it expresses this aggressive variant, does it behave in a more benevolent way in this person?

All of us are capable of listening countless times to the same score masterfully executed by different instrumentalists, orchestras, and conductors or by the same agents, but in different theaters or moments, and each time understanding the beauty of the harmonic variations that are produced. Will we be able to do the same in genetics? [44]

At the end of the twentieth century, a sixth order of knowledge appeared: coercive knowledge.

3.1.6 Coercive Knowledge

This order of knowledge is very old and is related to the promotion of fake medicines or attributing healing properties to ineffective potions (quackery). Why then should we incorporate it as new knowledge? Because of the impact that new information channels have on medicine and among the patients.

We must remember that the pharmaceutical industry was born at the end of the nineteenth century or the beginning of the twentieth century (with the foundation of Bayer). Until then medicine was produced by individual pharmacies and their quality could vary wildly. The pharmaceutical industry initially began to provide certified, good quality active ingredients to these pharmacies; later it began to provide the medicine itself, marked with a specific brand; today it provides not only the drugs, but also information on their use and the necessary tests to justify its use (in some specialties such as oncology, independent efficacy studies have essentially disappeared, since practically all the clinical trials of the last 50 drugs have been sponsored and supervised by the industry that produces them). This is how in less than a hundred years the pharmaceutical industry went from providing technical assistance to doctors to being medicine itself.

This has been extensively studied by Ray Moynihan in his extraordinary text *Selling Sickness* [45–50].

What is the difference, then, between the old style of quackery and the current pharmaceutical industry "selling" sickness?

Are they the same? No.

There are quite a number of differences.

Coercive medicine uses a "scientific" methodology for its claims. It shares its results through "serious magazines." Its findings are proclaimed at "symposiums" of the many medical societies by prominent professionals. Its claims are disseminated through "serious" journalism. Its products are approved by government agencies and are sold legally [51–57].

We can easily see that its influence is notably more extensive, its techniques are much more persuasive, and its effects much more harmful than a traveling quack because it is very difficult for the average doctor to assess these claims with healthy skepticism, which leads to them to prescribe something convinced that it benefits the patient out of trust in these institutions. Unfortunately, we can find countless cases where either the patient does not need the medication, the expected benefits are wildly exaggerated, or in the worst case they suffer great harm, whether physical or financial [58–60].

In Table 3.6, we can see some of the most notable examples of this type of knowledge.

In all these cases, the origin of the whole process comes from a medication that can indeed have a beneficial effect, but later this benefit as well as the risk of not treating the condition are exaggerated to such a degree that normal, everyday situations that could be left untreated without any issue end up being turned into serious health problems.

Table 3.6 Coercive knowledge

• Hair loss treatments (particularly for males)
• Diagnosis and treatment of hypoactive sexual desire disorder (HSDD)
• Hormone replacement therapy for menopause
• Preventive treatment of osteoporosis
• Pharmacological treatment of low hypercholesterolemia
• The oncological risk of irritable colon
• Using medication for nonapproved situations (*off-label*) based on anecdotal evidence

Example 1

Treatment of male [61–63] alopecia (hair loss)

Male alopecia is fundamentally related to testosterone levels and aging.

Finasteride shows a desirable side effect (most drug side effects are problems, but not all): men who take it for benign prostate problems report that their hair has grown back.

After this is discovered, a trial is designed to determine finasteride's efficacy in treating alopecia: the result is that in those with incipient baldness, hair loss is delayed or stopped.

This favorable result is presented as the only proven treatment that prevents hair loss; while at the same time baldness is presented as the main cause of discrimination against the males: women prefer men with hair, studies show that bald men perform worse than those with hair, and even the divorce rate is higher if you have less hair.

This is widely shared and suddenly alopecia is (a) much more frequent, (b) much more severe, and (c) its treatment is more successful.

All of this is publicized by all available means, scientific and educational meetings on finasteride treatment are sponsored, and patient groups are organized to lobby for government agencies to make sure insurance covers this new hair loss prevention drug.

Example 2

Treatment of female HSDD

A drug designed for the treatment of pulmonary hypertension, sildenafil, showed a highly desirable side effect in some trials: male patients who suffered from sexual impotence were able to recover their erectile function.

Thus, Viagra was born and revolutionized male sexuality [64–66].

So we have a drug designed to produce pulmonary artery dilation and thus lower pulmonary hypertension, except it also produces vasodilation of the penile arteries, which results in improved blood flow to the penis and increases erectile capacity and erection duration.

This was not expected by the researchers but was a welcome side effect, and it is a highly effective drug for treating male impotence.

No problem so far.

Coercive knowledge arises when they decide to use Viagra to treat HSDD based on the fact that if the clitoris receives better blood flow, women's sex drive and sexual gratification will improve.

Study groups are organized to corroborate the importance of the clitoral orgasm for female sexual satisfaction. The relationship between frigidity and insufficient clitoral stimulation is remarked upon. The impact of HSDD on depression is highlighted, and female Viagra is proposed to solve this problem.

All the evidence generated is at least questionable if not outright fallacious, as demonstrated by later studies.

The only goal here was to sell Viagra to the other half of humanity.

Example 3

Hormone replacement therapy for menopause

Menopause is a condition in which ovarian function ceases and therefore plasma estrogen levels drop.

It can occur naturally between the ages of 50 and 55, but there are also early menopauses, in which the ovaries stop working at earlier ages.

In other situations, menopause is caused by the removal of the ovaries (surgery), irradiation of the ovaries (radiant), or inhibition of the ovaries (hormonal) for different reasons. For the latter (hormonal) case, the two most frequent reasons are oncological treatment (for prevention in BRCA mutated patients; as an adjuvant treatment; or as definitive diagnosis of breast cancer) and transition therapy (transmen remove their ovaries or suppress them so that testosterone can work better) [67, 68].

The earlier, more abrupt and more complete the menopause is (such as surgery in young patients), the more severe are the symptoms it produces, such as hot flashes, decreased libido, vaginal dryness, pain or discomfort during sexual intercourse, insomnia, irritability, and depression. It can also lead to calcium loss, osteoporosis, and increased hip fractures. Finally, the estrogen/androgen quotient is altered, and this can lead to heart issues.

The discovery of estrogens, as well as the ability to acquire large quantities of them naturally by processing mare urine or by synthesizing them in laboratories, opened the door for estrogen to be considered as a therapy for menopause. It was later combined with progesterone, becoming known as menopausal hormone replacement therapy. Estrogen is used on its own in people without a uterus, but it is combined with progesterone in people with a uterus because the first adverse effect observed is an increase in endometrial cancer if estrogen is used on its own (the risk is between 20 and 30 times higher compared to the untreated population).

This hormone replacement therapy was the most prescribed treatment in the United States in the 1970s and 1980s.

Where do we find coercive medicine? Firstly, by aggravating the effects of menopause. While the symptoms are definitely real, their severity is seen in fewer than one in five women. For these few women, the treatment produces real and significant relief from their conditions and significantly improves their quality of life. Secondly, it was falsely reported that this therapy also protected against osteoporotic fractures, but later clinical trials showed the effect was marginal. Thirdly, it was claimed that this therapy provided protection from cardiac risks: not only was this false, it was later proved that it slightly increased them.

Finally, although it was initially thought that there was only increased risk of endometrial cancer, it was later discovered that women undergoing this therapy for more than 5 years also showed a marked increase in the risk of breast cancer.

The end result is that today this therapy is recommended only for those patients with severe symptoms and low risk of breast cancer, for a short time, with the aim of reducing the symptoms since all the other benefits have not been proven.

There are numerous other examples, but for space reasons and in order not to bore you or overwhelm you with evidence of lies, half-truths, manipulated or exaggerated truths, I invite you to look at drug adverts, where you will see how the large and small print differs greatly.

In general, coercion revolves around exaggerating both the benefits of the drug and the risks of not treating the sickness while minimizing the adverse effects of a treatment.

What this culminates in is that both doctor and patient have a similar thought process: *"I now have a safe and effective new weapon to solve this problem with. Sure, at first the problem seemed minor, but now I see that it's serious. Better safe than sorry."*

This has led to the medicalization of our civilization, in some cases from a very young age.

The problem is that while it is true that it is better to be "safe than sorry" when it comes to serious issues with proven, safe solutions, the saying rings far less true when both the risk and treatment of a condition are provided by the same person selling you the cure.

3.1.7   Wishful Knowledge

This seventh order of knowledge was born in the twenty-first century.

That is not to say that it did not exist before, but rather that for a long time the patient's desire had to conform to the standards of medicine at the time, lest it be considered deranged. This is the foundation of medical paternalism: the professional (and thus, medicine) knows what is best for the patient. If the patient is intelligent and understands it, they should adapt to this new knowledge; and if the patient is ignorant or does not understand it, they have to accept it because they are in no position to choose.

This thought process was applied not just to medicine, but also to laws and morality: doctors, judges, and priests possessed the knowledge of what was just, good. and healthy, citizens and patients had to conduct themselves according to those rules.

This paradigm was widely applied in the case of mental illness (or things considered to be mental illness), and while we consider this experiment is repulsive nowadays, we must not forget that the inventor of the lobotomy was awarded a Nobel Prize, or that treatments closer to torture than to medicine, such as aversion treatments that were used to treat homosexuality, were used even in highly developed countries until relatively recently. In England, for example, homosexuals were actively persecuted by the police until the late 1960s, leading many of them to commit suicide, including, among others, the man who had helped them win the war, the father of computing: Alan Turing.

This type of behavior as well as the discovery of the experiments in the Nazi death camps, the discovery of the Tuskegee study, the Willowbrook study, the experiments at the Jewish Chronic Hospital of New York, the experiments carried out in Soviet gulags and the experiments of Japan's Unit 731 in Manchuria. All of these experiments, which were carried out without respecting human rights, generated a movement focused on the liberation of the patient, a movement seeking to reaffirm the patient's authority over themselves.

This was reflected in the fundamental document of modern bioethics, the Belmont Report, produced by the bioethics commission convened by US President Jimmy Carter.

From then on, the doctor–patient relationship began to change and the autonomy of the patients, that is, the freedom and wishes of the patient, had primacy. Initially to consent to research practices but soon this became the ability to consent to any medical practice and currently in many cases to generate medical practices based on the wishes of the person.

In Table 3.7, we can see examples of this order of knowledge.

What all these examples have in common is that it is the patient's desire that generates a medical act, which does not necessarily have the objective of curing any illness but rather satisfying a person's desire.

This is applicable to the interruption of a pregnancy because it is the woman who chooses to do so; to assisted suicide or euthanasia because it is the patient who requests it; and so on and so forth. The reasons will vary from individual to individual, but it is always the *patient* who asks for a given procedure.

One could say none of these examples are particularly new. What has changed then?

What has changed is the extent and acceptability of these (and other) examples: what once infrequent is today a much more common occurrence, what was once an

Table 3.7 Desirative knowledge

• Voluntary termination of pregnancy.
• Assisted suicide
• Sex reassignment surgery
• Bariatric surgery (obesity treatment)
• Aesthetic orthodontics
• Cosmetic surgeries

intimate and personal decision is today in many cases publicly spoken about, and what was once seen as a whim is now considered a right.

But it is not just in these examples where we can see the weight a patient's wishes carry in current medical practice. Consider the cases in which there are several therapeutic alternatives. Which one should we choose? The one that suits the desires and values of the patient.

This is part of Sackett 's evidence-based medicine tripod: the best scientific evidence, together with the greatest medical experience in respecting the patient's values.

We began by seeing how in medical paternalism the patient's desire was despicable and we saw how, in the span of a couple of decades, it became one of the pillars of the ethics of decision-making in medicine.

3.1.8   How Do These Orders of Knowledge Interact in Practice?

They are permanently present in every medical act.

We start with magic and end with the patient's desire, and it is like that, always and in all cases.

That is why the first step is to recognize them.

The magic often translates into the patient's expectations. None of our patients choose us scientifically, in the best of cases they choose us for our prestige, but we must not forget that prestige is what those who do not know us think of us, while respect is what those who do know us think of us. Therefore, we must be humble when believing that they choose us for our science or our technique. Those patients are few and far between.

Clinical, anatomopathological, and assistive knowledge are all part of our daily art or, as the Greeks would say, our *phronesis*, what we do (or *should do*) well.

Predictive medicine is present in many specialties and will soon be part of all of them, which is why we must incorporate it carefully and rigorously.

Coercive medicine has an impact on the beliefs of patients based on what the media shares (which, according to a very dear colleague: "they make oddities out of everyday things"), but also on our own beliefs as doctors. Which is why today, more than ever, doctors must be experts at interpreting the information they receive by exercising a healthy skepticism.

Wishful medicine is a crucial element of modernity. We may disagree with what our patient wants, but we should always be respectful about it. The doctor's autonomy should not be imposed on the patient, or vice versa. Learning to deliberate together with the patient implies that we must explain our difficulties and doubts regarding certain actions, which is an act of honesty that most patients deeply appreciate.

Therefore, in order to communicate properly, we must always keep these seven channels in mind and make them evident to the patient. Countless difficulties can be smoothed out in this way, particularly because several conflicts in communicating arise due to patient and doctor being on different wavelengths.

A classic example is trying to combat magical knowledge with scientific knowledge.

Science does not go against magic or faith but rather credulity [69–72].

It is very important to make sure the patient understands this.

Magic or faith are part of each person's beliefs. Credulity, on the other hand, is the attitude of someone who assumes something to be of scientific value when it is not.

Magic and faith are an affirmative choice, the person chooses an answer to that for which science has not yet provided one.

Credulity is a resignation, in a way. It is to consciously fail to rigorously examine what we believe to be a scientific answer.

This is why our next step will be to analyze with scientific rigor one of these magical aspects: the placebo effect.

3.2 The Mechanisms of the Placebo and Nocebo Effects: Modern Science in Service of an Old Problem

The scientific literature on placebos today is very extensive. Just to give us an idea: if we search the "Pubmed"publication base for the terms "Placebo effect, " we have as of December 31, 2022, one hundred one thousand eight hundred and ninety-two nine articles. If we limit the search to articles that are research papers or systematic reviews, published in English in the last 10 years and that have free access to the full text, the number is "reduced" to fourteen thousand six hundred and sixty-nine articles.

When the magnitude of the information is so overwhelming, one must select the most important referents and start with them.

If one wants to study the placebo effect, the first obligatory reference is the book by Arthur and Elaine Shapiro published in 1997 *The Powerful Placebo* [73]. It records the research on this topic carried out by Dr. Shapiro from 1953 until 1995 when he passed away. This text is the most rigorous and complete synthesis of what has been published on this topic up to that date. To update the information to the present day, there are two more highly recommended authors: Fabrizio Bendetti with his book *Placebo Effects* published in 2014 [74]and the wonderful placebo research carried out at Stanford by Dr. Alia Crum [75–82].

The first thing we must understand is that both the placebo effect and its counterpart, the nocebo effect, refer to the effects that our beliefs have on our health.

But how do we define the placebo effect?

The placebo effect is the result that beliefs, expectations, and previous experiences have on our health. These are closely related to suggestion and conditioning.

The origin of the word placebo can be found in verse 9 of Psalm 116: *"I will walk in the presence of Yahveh through the land of the living"*; in Hebrew *"I will walk before"* is written *ethalekh,* which was translated into Latin as placebo. The complete verse of the psalm in Latin reads "Placebo Domino in regione vivorum," and it was recited during Mass honoring the departed. It was incorporated into English in the thirteenth century with a more generic meaning: " to please , to give pleasure , be approved , be pleasing , be agreeable , acceptable , to suit , satisfy ." [73]

From 1785, the use of this word as a pharmacological effect is documented according to the *Dictionary of Medical Terms of the Royal Academy of Medicine of Spain.*

What then does the placebo effect consist of? In essence, it refers to the well-being and better health that a patient experiences when they believe that the procedure being performed or the medicine being administered is good for their ailment. This effect is so powerful and universal that it can occur even if the procedure is useless or the drug administered has no active substance [72, 83–99].

It is important to note three things:

(a) The placebo effect is universal and is closely linked to suggestion, both from the doctor and the patient themselves.
(b) It occurs in medicines with or without an active ingredient.
(c) The opposite effect, called the nocebo effect, is just as powerful as the placebo effect [100–106].

You may reasonably wonder just how powerful the effect of belief is?

In subjective matters such as pain, anxiety, insomnia, and depression, a notable beneficial effect has been observed. Of course, analgesics, anxiolytics, hypnotics, and antidepressants are more effective since they have been studied against a placebo and have shown to be better, but in all the trials to date we can find a group of patients (sometimes very large) that show improvement in their in symptoms simply by believing that they are taking an active medication.

The same is true for toxicity or intolerance when the patient believes that they are receiving a less effective, less safe, or lower quality medication [103, 105].

But then what about objective variables?

For example, could the metabolism of carbohydrates be impacted if the patient believes that they are eating food with more or less calories?

The answer seems to be *"yes."* [76]

Is it possible that the extent of an allergic reaction or the speed of its resolution is greater if the patient believes that he is being administered an antiallergic than if he believes he is only being administered saline solution even though he is being given saline solution in both cases?

The answer seems to be "yes." [78]

And what about the response to stress? Or to physical exercise? Or to genetic information? Or to information provided in medicine and food packaging? All of these and more seem to change according to our expectations and moods [79–81, 107–112].

In cancer patients, mental state has proven to be very important in multiple aspects: how well they tolerate chemotherapy, how well the post-treatment rehabilitation goes, even their quality of life [75].

The mechanisms of both the placebo effect and the nocebo effect have not been fully elucidated, but different neuroscientific studies point to a cognitive, emotional, and cultural response (which means there is a social aspect to the effects) [89, 113–117].

Elements that influence our feelings of well-being include the tablet's color, its taste, its shape. All of this is well known by the pharmaceutical industry. But we can also be influenced by way in which a given drug or treatment's effects are communicated to us, the environment in which this information is given, and also who is administering this treatment or drug.

All the knowledge we have accumulated over so many years regarding the placebo effect shows us that it is the most human of therapeutic reactions.

We are not mere biological machines that respond only in a biochemical way. We are much more complex beings, and our body's responses can be influenced by not only the active ingredients of the drugs, but also our beliefs, our expectations, our trust in the professional, and our current state of mind.

Diseases, therefore, have a biographical and cultural component, which is why the twenty-first-century doctor has to be, in addition to an expert in the technique, an expert in humanity.

Which opens the doors to the next topic.

Can the doctor himself be a placebo?

3.3   The Doctor as a Placebo

The doctor–patient relationship continues to be the best way in which medicine is practiced.

A large number of medical utopias have tried to replace it without success.

Medicine will only ever be as good as the relationship of a particular doctor with a particular patient.

The purpose of the doctor–patient relationship is always therapeutic.

It is in this scenario where medicine finally has a face, body, and voice: that of each doctor.

Can you be a placebo or a nocebo? The answer is yes. Undoubtedly yes. And this has been widely demonstrated [118–126].

If the effects that benefit or harm a patient depend, in part, on their beliefs and expectations, there is nothing that generates expectations quite like the first time you see a doctor.

A very common mistake is to believe that the patient who comes to see us for the first time has chosen us. In fact, the patient has truly chosen us only if they choose to return. It is the second consultation that shows that our patient has chosen us. The first is just the opportunity it gives us to be among those eligible.

As Will Rogers (allegedly) said: *You never get a second chance to make a good first impression* (https://www.forbes.com/quotes/9717/).

What is valid in business is also valid in the first doctor–patient encounter.

You are the most important medicine and you are administered through your words.

If this idea ends up being your only takeaway from this book, I will consider my objective fulfilled.

It is because you are the most important medicine that you must take care of yourself: everything, from the way you are dressed, to the care with which you conduct yourself, the attention you pay to your patient, and how you record the information given to you, influences the patient greatly. Patients can perceive their doctor's state in a much deeper and more subtle way than you think.

There are two or three central aspects in which it is impossible to deceive a patient: whether you are genuinely interested in helping them and whether or not you are paying attention to them.

You can do your best to fake a great many things, but the indifference and inattention that patients report when meeting their doctors are generally very credible: "I felt like a number," "The doctor was thinking of something else," "He was talking on his cell phone while looking at my studies," and "He was in a hurry." These are only some of the statements I collected when I was in charge of the quality control at the institution where I work.

These situations show a lack of professionalism, but they begin with a lack of awareness regarding the role the doctor himself has in patient care.

In systems that are not centered on a single doctor–patient relationship, such as those with residents or fellows, each meeting must highlight that it is a supervised system, in which all professionals act under the careful eye of people with greater experience, and furthermore that careful record keeping is taking place.

In this case, interpersonal trust is transferred to the "system" and often to "institutional prestige." Even so, patients often choose a particular doctor as their point of reference in order to feel more protected.

Now, if the doctor is the most important medicine and the way to administer it is through the word, the question arises: How do words become a placebo?

3.4 The Word as Placebo

The Therapy of the Word in Classical Antiquity [127] was a text published by Don Pedro Lain Entralgo in 1958, and we will use it to evaluate the role of the medical word since it continues to be an excellent instrument in the hands of good doctors.

In this text, Lain Entralgo developed three Homeric therapies of the word: catharsis, spell, and placebo.

Catharsis, washing, purification, or liberation is an act in which the spoken and heard word relieves the patient of his sufferings. Many patients feel that they have been released from a burden when they find a doctor who listens to them.

The spell or enchantment is the role that the word has on the faith professed by the patient. It dates from the time in which doctor, shaman, and priest were the same thing. Today in modern medicine this is seen as prescientific, protoscientific, or simply quackery. However, we must be aware that patients are attentive to our words to such an extent that many years later they can repeat them almost exactly, like someone repeating a litany. Imagine how many times a patient will have recreated that dialogue within themselves to be able to repeat it several years later almost perfectly.

Finally, the use of the word as a placebo, as recreation, so that it cooperates with the therapy. They are the anecdotes, stories, and tales that help the patient to be more comfortable.

In the modern medical meeting, the purpose of a conversation goes beyond the mere practical need to acquire medical information. Its true purpose is to get to know each patient in depth as the unique being each is.

For me this has additional practical utility.

I confess to all my patients during the first meeting that it is very difficult for me to put a face to a name until at least the third or fourth meeting. That is why during our first meeting I extract from each patient an outstanding characteristic that makes them unique to me, and later works as a trigger to help me remember the medical history of each patient. Examples such as *prima ballerina, ginger, captain, painter, cheese and salami* are some of the nicknames patients have asked me to call them. As well as helping me remember, I also ask each patient to identify themselves as such when they call me, which also makes *them* feel unique.

But I also use this time to find out what the disease means for the patient, how they discovered it, what they think the cause is, what they think could happen, and how they would like us to act if certain events come to pass.

This allows us to transcend biology and approach biography. To asses the impact that the disease has not only on the body but also on the history of our patient.

In fact, the use of the word in the Hippocratic corpus is more extensive than that described for Homer, as Laí Entralgo himself demonstrates:

(a) The word as prayer (page 151): "[...]in *book IV of the work On Diet 'Thus , after having determined the celestial signs' it is stated in respect to dreams in which torments appear, 'the physician will take precautions, will follow the indicated regimen and will raise prayers to the gods'"*. Many doctors today continue to pray for their patients, each according to his belief, but every one of them asks for his prescriptions to work well. Moreover, many agnostic doctors are unaware that the *Rp* with which they begin their prescriptions is nothing more than the Latin adaptation of the eye of Horus, with which the ancient Egyptian doctors implored the god's protection in their scrolls.

(b) As a question (page 152): *"The communicative speech of the doctor becomes a «question» or «inquiry» (ereuna , eróthesis) in the anamnesis."*

(c) As a vehicle for the prescription (page 153, 154): *"The word of the Hippocratic physician is, in other cases, « prescription », a means to inform the patient of what he must do in the treatment of his disease (ta prospheroména: Epid. , I,*

L. II, 670)." This is the culminating moment in which the word of the doctor becomes a placebo. I do not prescribe anything that I do not believe to be effective. I must be the first one convinced that the medicine can be useful, otherwise it is difficult for the patient to believe it as well. I may be wrong, but I never lie on this point. If I do not believe in it, I do not prescribe it.

(d) Prognostic judgment (page 154): *"It is necessary to tell the prior conditions, to know the present state, to predict the future, the Epidemics teaches (L. I I , 634). In the case of patients who do not feel their malady, 'it is up to the physician to predict what is threatening them', warns the work On the joints (L. IV, 100)."*. At this point, it is up to the physician to take care of the therapeutic and prognostic expectations of their patients [88].

(e) Finally as an instrument of prestige (154) and as a means of illustration (155). The word continues to be the vehicle by which the doctor builds his prestige: the prudence of his statements, the accuracy of his diagnoses, and the humanity with which he communicates an adverse prognosis are among the elements most valued by patients [128].

Therefore, having now seen the reality of the placebo effect, the role the doctor plays in it and the impact of his word, it is now worth asking how we may enhance this effect.

3.5 How to Enhance the Placebo Effect

Knowing about the placebo effect and the power the medical word can have when it comes to healing the sick should lead us to use that power, based on the trust placed upon us by the patient, with greater responsibility [129, 130].

What are, in my view, the three most important elements for the medical–patient encounter to be an effective placebo?

Firstly, we must treat each patient as an absolutely unique person, and in order to do this we must take advantage of the time we have between patients, in order to fully focus on whoever our next patient is. Taking a moment to prepare ourselves will help us receive the new patient in the best way possible.

Secondly, we must treat medical truth as though it was one more drug, one which has indications and contraindications, doses, forms of administration, and desirable and undesirable effects. Drugs are not administered the same way to all patients, and neither should medical truth.

Therefore, the first step is to listen carefully to what the patient wants to know, needs to know, or should know about his illness and his possible fate.

Whatever is said must be said with respect, prudence, and affection.

For this, we have to develop a series of processes, which we will analyze later in this book, in order to (1) know what to say, (2) know why we say it, (3) know what we say it for, and finally (4) know how to say it.

But fundamentally, the interpersonal communication model assumes that the doctor (a) is **prudent**, that is, he thinks before he speaks; (b) is **honest**, that is, he says what he thinks; and (c) is **empathetic**, that is, he feels what he says.

Our experience shows that everything can be said, but you cannot say everything the same way.

This care in using the medical word and the way of communicating ailments to the sick has had great variations throughout the history of medicine, which is why in the next chapter we will develop the history of the word and medical words.

3.6   Teaching Exercises

1. Individual

   (a) Can you identify the seven orders of knowledge outlined in epistemology?
   (b) In which of them can you observe the placebo effect?
   (c) Do you remember your last doctor's visit? Which of your doctor's attitudes gives you peace of mind? Which worried you?
   (d) What are the reasons that lead you to choose "your doctor"?
   (e) Do you exercise the placebo effect in your practice?
   (f) Do you think it is correct to use it?
   (g) Do you think it is wrong to use it?

2. Group

   (a) Discuss each of the epistemological features in medicine.

      - Point out the outstanding characteristics in the current practice of:

         – Magical thinking.
         – Clinical thinking.
         – Anatomopathological thinking.
         – Assisted thinking.
         – Predictive thinking.
         – Coercive thinking.
         – Wishful thinking.

   (b) What does the group think about the placebo effect? It is real? Is it negligible?
   (c) Do you consider the use of placebos in medicine to be immoral?
   (d) In which cases would you consider it reasonable to use a placebo and why?
   (e) Do you think that medical communication can be a placebo or a nocebo?
   (f) Do you think that the doctor, by reporting the undesirable effects of a treatment, could worsen the patient's tolerance of it?
   (g) What does the group think about handling medical truth like a drug?
   (h) What aspect of handling the truth carefully seems most important for a patient?

References

1. Gil DE. On cancer and its demons. Authorship: First Edition; 2019.
2. Anon. The astronomers of the Esagil temple in the Fourth Century BC. In: If a man builds a joyful house: assyriological studies in honor of Erle Verdun Leichty; 2021. https://doi.org/10.1163/9789047408239_006.
3. Stiefel M, Shaner A, Schaefer SD. The Edwin Smith papyrus: the birth of analytical thinking in medicine and otolaryngology. Laryngoscope. 2006;116(2):182. https://doi.org/10.1097/01.mlg.0000191461.08542.a3.
4. Utinans A, Ancane G. Belief in the paranormal and modern health worries. SHS Web Confer. 2014;10:00048. https://doi.org/10.1051/shsconf/20141000048.
5. Wein S. Cancer, unproven therapies, and magic. Oncology. 2000;14(9):1345.
6. Lightner AD, Heckelsmiller C, Hagen EH. Ethnomedical specialists and their supernatural theories of disease. Rev Philos Psychol. 2021;14:611. https://doi.org/10.1007/s13164-021-00589-8.
7. Reynolds EH. Hysteria in ancient civilisations: a neurological review: possible significance for the modern disorder. J Neurol Sci. 2018;388:388. https://doi.org/10.1016/j.jns.2018.02.024.
8. Lambarri Rodriguez A, Flores Palacios F, Berenzon GS. Folk healers, discomfort, and sorcery: a social interpretation. Salud Mental. 2012;35(2):123.
9. Heinz S. Nature as magician: on the Paracelsus heritage of modern medicine. Acta Hist Leopoldina. 2010;55:39.
10. Angutek D. Homeopathic medicine and magic. Med Nowozytna. 2007;14(1-2):29.
11. Luiker H. The persistence of magic and religion in contemporary medicine and psychotherapy. Group Analysis. 2019;52(4):532. https://doi.org/10.1177/0533316418823156.
12. Gilman A. Cunning folklore: the meaning of "superstition" in early modern Europe. Elements. 2010;6(2):1. https://doi.org/10.6017/eurj.v6i2.9036.
13. Spiegel D, Greenman R, Simon V, Cardeña E. Mesmer minus magic: hypnosis and modern medicine. Int J Clin Exp Hypn. 2002;50(4):397. https://doi.org/10.1080/00207140208410113.
14. Carod FJ, Vázquez-Cabrera C. Magical thinking and epilepsy in traditional indigenous medicine. Rev Neurol. 1998;26(154):1064.
15. Picard-Amí LA. Placebo, culture and magic. Rev Med Panama. 1989;14(3):154.
16. Santacroce L, Charitos IA, Topi S, Bottalico L. The alcmaeon's school of croton: philosophy and science. Open access Maced J Med Sci. 2019;7(3):500. https://doi.org/10.3889/oamjms.2019.072.
17. Rhee KB. Empedocles' influence on Hippocratic medicine: the problem of hypothesis and human nature. Kr J Med Hist. 2013;22(3):879. https://doi.org/10.13081/kjmh.2013.22.879.
18. Hippocrates. Greek Medicine—The Hippocratic Oath. U.S. National Library of Medicine.
19. Stefanakis G, Nyktari V, Papaioannou A, Askitopoulou H. Hippocratic concepts of acute and urgent respiratory diseases still relevant to contemporary medical thinking and practice: a scoping review. BMC Pulm Med. 2020;20(1):165. https://doi.org/10.1186/s12890-020-01193-9.
20. Reiser SJ. What modern-physicians can learn from hippocrates. Cancer. 2003;98(8):1555. https://doi.org/10.1002/cncr.11565.
21. Mirrione C. Aristotle's mixture in its medical and philosophical background: the Hippocratic of victory and the Aristotelian of generation and corruption. Peitho. 2021;12(1):69–84. https://doi.org/10.14746/10.14746/PEA.2021.1.8.
22. Čiurlionis J. Heraclitus and Hippocrates: the paradigm of the elements. Problems. 2021;100:50–61. https://doi.org/10.15388/PROBLEMS.100.4.
23. Calves JA. Science, philosophy and tekhne . The Presocratic influence on the biological philosophy of the Hippocrates. lull. 2020;43(87):11. https://doi.org/10.47101/llull.2020.43.87.01alsina.
24. Group LD. Humility and respect: Core values in medical education. Mid Educ. 2014;48(1):53. https://doi.org/10.1111/medu.12269.
25. Cruz-Coke MR. Hippocratic philosophy. Rev Med Chil. 1999;127(5):611.

26. Buja LM. The cell theory and cellular pathology: discovery, refinements and applications fundamental to advances in biology and medicine. Exp Mol Pathol. 2021;121:121. https://doi.org/10.1016/j.yexmp.2021.104660.
27. Ventura HO. Rudolph Virchow and cellular pathology. Clin Cardiol. 2000;23(7):550. https://doi.org/10.1002/clc.4960230717.
28. Lin JI. Rudolph Virchow as viewed by Gross and Osler. Pathologist. 1985;39(11):1480.
29. Hajdu SI. A note from history: Rudolph Virchow, pathologist, armed revolutionist, politician, and anthropologist. Ann Clin Lab Sci. 2005;35(2):203.
30. Gross CG. Claude Bernard and the constancy of the internal environment. Neuroscientist. 1998;4(5):380. https://doi.org/10.1177/107385849800400520.
31. Caponi G. A key text by claude bernard: "on progress in the physiological sciences". Metatheoria. 2021;11(2):25. https://doi.org/10.48160/18532330me11.275.
32. Normandin S. Claude Bernard and an introduction to the study of experimental medicine: 'physical vitalism', dialectic, and epistemology. J Hist Med Allied Sci. 2007;62(4):495. https://doi.org/10.1093/jhmas/jrm015.
33. Sprawls P. X-ray medical imaging—a centennial perspective. Phys Med. 1997;13:193.
34. Hsieh J, Flohr T. Computed tomography recent history and future perspectives. J Med Imaging. 2021;8(05):052109. https://doi.org/10.1117/1.jmi.8.5.052109.
35. Siemens Medical Solutions. Computed tomography its history and technology innovations for people. CT Basics. 2013.
36. Viard A, Eustache F, Segobin S. History of magnetic resonance imaging: a trip down memory lane. Neuroscience. 2021;474:474. https://doi.org/10.1016/j.neuroscience.2021.06.038.
37. Ramsey NF. Early history of magnetic resonance. Phys Perspect. 1999;1(2):123. https://doi.org/10.1007/s000160050012.
38. Fowler JS. 18F-FDG radiosynthesis: a landmark in the history of PET. J Nucl Med. 2020;61(12):105S. https://doi.org/10.2967/jnumed.120.250191.
39. Fertig EJ, Jaffee EM, Macklin P, Stearns V, Wang C. Forecasting cancer: from precision to predictive medicine. Honey. 2021;2(9):1004. https://doi.org/10.1016/j.medj.2021.08.007.
40. Baranov VS. Genomics and predictive medicine. Sibirsky J Kliniceskoj Exp Med. 2021;36(4):14. https://doi.org/10.29001/2073-8552-2021-36-4-14-28.
41. Longo UG, Carnevale A, Massaroni C, et al. Personalized, predictive, participatory, precision, and preventive (P5) medicine in rotator cuff tears. J Pers Med. 2021;11(4):255. https://doi.org/10.3390/jpm11040255.
42. Valet GK, Tárnok A. Cytomics in predictive medicine. Cytometry B Clin Cytom. 2003;53(1):1. https://doi.org/10.1002/cyto.b.10035.
43. Elemento O. The future of precision medicine: towards a more predictive personalized medicine. Emerg Top Life Sci. 2020;4(2):175. https://doi.org/10.1042/ETLS20190197.
44. Gil Deza E. https://pensar.org/2022/03/la-alegoria-musical-contra-el-determinismo-genetico/.
45. Moynihan R, Heath I, Henry D. Selling sickness: the pharmaceutical industry and disease mongering. Br Med J. 2002;324(7342):886. https://doi.org/10.1136/bmj.324.7342.886.
46. Angel K. Sex, lies and pharmaceuticals: how drug companies plan to profit from female sexual dysfunction, by Ray Moynihan and Barbara Mintzes. Psychol Sex. 2013;4(2):1. https://doi.org/10.1080/19419899.2013.774169.
47. Moynihan R. Doctors' education: the invisible influence of drug company sponsorship. BMJ. 2008;336(7641):416. https://doi.org/10.1136/bmj.39496.430336.DB.
48. Schwartz LM, Woloshin S, Moynihan R. Who's watching the watchdogs? BMJ. 2008;337:337. https://doi.org/10.1136/bmj.a2535.
49. Moynihan R. The marketing of a disease: female sexual dysfunction. Br Med J. 2005;330(7484):192. https://doi.org/10.1136/bmj.330.7484.192.
50. Robertson J, Moynihan R, Walkom E, Bero L, Henry D. Mandatory disclosure of pharmaceutical industry-funded events for health professionals. PLoS Med. 2009;6(11):e1000128. https://doi.org/10.1371/journal.pmed.1000128.

51. Parker L, Bennett A, Mintzes B, et al. "There are ways … drug companies will get into DTC decisions": how Australian drug and therapeutics committees address pharmaceutical industry influence. Br J Clin Pharmacol. 2021;87(5):2341. https://doi.org/10.1111/bcp.14636.

52. Davari M, Khorasani E, Tigabu BM. Factors influencing prescribing decisions of physicians: a review. Ethiop J Health Sci. 2018;28(6):795. https://doi.org/10.4314/ejhs.v28i6.15.

53. Spielmans GI, Parry PI. From evidence-based medicine to marketing-based medicine: evidence from internal industry documents. J Bioeth Inq. 2010;7(1):13. https://doi.org/10.1007/s11673-010-9208-8.

54. Fox NJ, Ward KJ. Pharma in the bedroom... And the kitchen.... The pharmaceuticalisation of daily life. Sociol Health Illn. 2008;30(6):856. https://doi.org/10.1111/j.1467-9566.2008.01114.x.

55. Verbaanderd C, Rooman I, Meheus L, Huys I. On-label or off-label? Overcoming regulatory and financial barriers to bring repurposed medicines to cancer patients. Front Pharmacol. 2020;10:10. https://doi.org/10.3389/fphar.2019.01664.

56. Anon. Beware those bearing gifts: Physicians' fiduciary duty to avoid pharmaceutical marketing. Kan Law Rev. 2016;57:491. https://doi.org/10.17161/1808.20087.

57. Willis E, Delbaere M. Patient influencers: the next frontier in direct-to-consumer pharmaceutical marketing. J Med Internet Res. 2022;24(3):e29422. https://doi.org/10.2196/29422.

58. Gil Deza E, Nacul MJ, Garcia Gerardi CF, Morgenfeld EL, Rivarola EGJ, Gercovich FG. Freakoncology: is there an optimistic denial in the ipilimumab publications? J Clin Oncol. 2015;33(15_suppl):e20122. https://doi.org/10.1200/jco.2015.33.15_suppl.e20122.

59. Negro A, Rivarola EGJ, Gil Deza E, et al. Off-label prescriptions in cancer: who should pay for them? J Clin Oncol. 2011;29(15_suppl):e16559. https://doi.org/10.1200/jco.2011.29.15_suppl.e16559.

60. Rivarola EG, Gil Deza E, Negro A, et al. Standard therapy deviations in the practice of clinical oncology. J Clin Oncol. 2007;25(18_suppl):6504. https://doi.org/10.1200/jco.2007.25.18_suppl.6504.

61. Andy G, John M, Mirna S, et al. Controversies in the treatment of androgenetic alopecia: the history of finasteride. Dermatol Ther. 2019;32(2):e12647. https://doi.org/10.1111/dth.12647.

62. Ganzer CA, Jacobs AR. Emotional consequences of finasteride: fool's gold. Am J Mens Health. 2018;12(1):90. https://doi.org/10.1177/1557988316631624.

63. Irwig MS. Finasteride and suicide: a postmarketing case series. Dermatology. 2020;236(6):540. https://doi.org/10.1159/000505151.

64. Dinsmore WW, Hodges M, Hargreaves C, Osterloh IH, Smith MD, Rosen ARC. Sildenafil citrate (Viagra) in erectile dysfunction: near normalization in men with broad-spectrum erectile dysfunction compared with age-matched healthy control subjects. Urology. 1999;53(4):800. https://doi.org/10.1016/S0090-4295(98)00586-X.

65. Danchin N. Sildenafil, the cardiac patient and the cardiologist. Arch Mal Coeur Vaiss. 1999;92(10):1339.

66. Loe M. Fixing broken masculinity: Viagra asa technology for the production of gender and sexuality. Sex Cult. 2001;5(3):97. https://doi.org/10.1007/s12119-001-1032-1.

67. Marsden J. British menopause society consensus statement: the risks and benefits of HRT before and after a breast cancer diagnosis. Post Reprod Health. 2019;25(1):33. https://doi.org/10.1177/2053369119825716.

68. Nappi RE, Cassani C, Rossi M, Zanellini F, Spinillo A. Dealing with premature menopause in women at high-risk for hereditary genital and breast cancer. Minerva Ginecol. 2016;68(5):602.

69. Romm J. IX. Reason, credulity, and faith. In: Herodotus. New York: Yale University Press; 2022. https://doi.org/10.12987/9780300146684-011.

70. Biltoft CN. The anatomy of credulity and incredulity: or, a hermeneutics of misinformation. Harvard Kennedy School Misinform Rev. 2020;1:1–11. https://doi.org/10.37016/mr-2020-016.

71. Pittenger F. From an epistemology of faith to everyday understanding. J Humanist Psychol. 2014;54(3):377. https://doi.org/10.1177/0022167813510206.

72. Worcester E, McComb S, Coriat IH. Faith and its therapeutic power. In: Religion and medicine: the moral control of nervous disorders. Moffat: Yard & Company; 2011. https://doi.org/10.1037/13069-016.

73. Shapiro AK, Shapiro E. The powerful placebo. From ancient priest to modern phyisician. Baltimore: The Johns Hopkins University Press; 1997.

74. Benedetti F. Placebo effects. Second. Oxford: Oxford University Press; 2014.

75. Heathcote LC, Zion SR, Crum AJ. Cancer survivorship—considering mindsets. JAMA Oncol. 2020;6(9):1468–9. https://doi.org/10.1001/jamaoncol.2020.2482.

76. Crum AJ, Corbin WR, Brownell KD, Salovey P. Mind over milkshakes: mindsets, not Just nutrients, determine Ghrelin response. Health Psychol. 2011;30(4):424–9. https://doi.org/10.1037/a0023467.

77. Howe LC, Hardebeck EJ, Leibowitz KA, Crum AJ. Providers' demeanor impacts patient perceptions of visit length. J Gen Intern Med. 2019;34(2):182–3. https://doi.org/10.1007/s11606-018-4665-6.

78. Leibowitz KA, Hardebeck EJ, Goyer JP, Crum AJ. Physician assurance reduces patient symptoms in US adults: an experimental study. J Gen Intern Med. 2018;33(12):2051–2. https://doi.org/10.1007/s11606-018-4627-z.

79. Crum AJ, Phillips DJ, Goyer JP, Akinola M, Higgins ET. Transforming water: social influence moderates psychological, physiological, and functional response to a placebo product. PLoS One. 2016;11(11):e0167121. https://doi.org/10.1371/journal.pone.0167121.

80. Turnwald BP, Goyer JP, Boles DZ, Silder A, Delp SL, Crum AJ. Learning one's genetic risk changes physiology independent of actual genetic risk. Nat Hum Behav. 2019;3(1):48–56. https://doi.org/10.1038/s41562-018-0483-4.

81. Howe LC, Leibowitz KA, Perry MA, et al. Changing patient mindsets about non–life-threatening symptoms during oral immunotherapy: a randomized clinical trial. J Aller Clin Immunol. 2019;7(5):1550–9. https://doi.org/10.1016/j.jaip.2019.01.022.

82. Evers AWM, Colloca L, Blease C, et al. What should clinicians tell patients about placebo and nocebo effects? Practical considerations based on expert consensus. Psychother Psychosom. 2020;90(1):49–56. https://doi.org/10.1159/000510738.

83. Kradin RL. The placebo response and the power of unconscious healing. London: Routledge; 2008.

84. Dispenza J. El Placebo Eres Tú: Descubre El Poder de Tu Mente.

85. Guess HA. The science of the placebo: toward an interdisciplinary research agenda. London: BMJ Books; 2002.

86. The placebo effect in clinical practice.

87. Talking cures and placebo effects.

88. van Vliet LM, Francke AL, Meijers MC, et al. The use of expectancy and empathy when communicating with patients with advanced breast cancer; an observational study of clinician–patient consultations. Front Psychiatry. 2019;10:10. https://doi.org/10.3389/fpsyt.2019.00464.

89. Jubb J, Bensing JM. The sweetest pill to swallow: how patient neurobiology can be harnessed to maximise placebo effects. Neurosci Biobehav Rev. 2013;37(10):2709–20. https://doi.org/10.1016/j.neubiorev.2013.09.006.

90. Héron A, Leroux C, Dubayle D. Use of placebo in French hospitals: data from polyvalent medicine units. Med Sci. 2019;35(8–9):674–81. https://doi.org/10.1051/medsci/2019127.

91. Benedetti F, Amanzio M. The placebo response: how words and rituals change the patient's brain. Patient Educ Couns. 2011;84(3):413–9. https://doi.org/10.1016/j.pec.2011.04.034.

92. Carlino E, Pollo A, Benedetti F. The placebo in practice: how to use it in clinical routine. Curr Opin Support Palliat Care. 2012;6(2):220–5. https://doi.org/10.1097/SPC.0b013e32835269c1.

93. Miller FG, Colloca L, Kaptchuk TJ. The placebo effect: illness and interpersonal healing. Perspect Biol Med. 2009;52(4):518–39. https://doi.org/10.1353/pbm.0.0115.

94. Tavel ME. The placebo effect: the good, the bad, and the ugly. Am J Med. 2014;127(6):484–8. https://doi.org/10.1016/j.amjmed.2014.02.002.

95. Geers AL, Briñol P, Vogel EA, Aspiras O, Caplandies FC, Petty RE. The application of persuasion theory to placebo effects. Int Rev Neurobiol. 2018;138:113–36. https://doi.org/10.1016/bs.irn.2018.01.004.

96. Kirsch I. Response Expectancy and the Placebo Effect. Int Rev Neurobiol. 2018;138:81–93. https://doi.org/10.1016/bs.irn.2018.01.003.

97. Finniss DG. Placebo effects: historical and modern evaluation. Int Rev Neurobioloy. 2018;139:1–27. https://doi.org/10.1016/bs.irn.2018.07.010.

98. Hashmi JA. Placebo effect: theory, mechanisms and teleological roots. Int Rev Neurobiol. 2018;139:233–53. https://doi.org/10.1016/bs.irn.2018.07.017.

99. Pardo-Cabello AJ, Manzano-Gamero V, Puche-Cañas E. Placebo: a brief updated review. Naunyn Schmiedeberg's Arch Pharmacol. 2022;395(11):1343–56. https://doi.org/10.1007/s00210-022-02280-w.

100. Elsenbruch S, Labrenz F. Nocebo effects and experimental models in visceral pain. Int Rev Neurobiol. 2018;138:285–306. https://doi.org/10.1016/bs.irn.2018.01.010.

101. Mestre TA. Nocebo and lessebo effects. Int Rev Neurobiol. 2020;153:121–46. https://doi.org/10.1016/bs.irn.2020.04.005.

102. Colloca L, Panaccione R, Murphy TK. The clinical implications of nocebo effects for biosimilar therapy. Front Pharmacol. 2019;10:10. https://doi.org/10.3389/fphar.2019.01372.

103. Hansen E, Zech N. Nocebo effects and negative suggestions in daily clinical practice—forms, impact and approaches to avoid them. Front Pharmacol. 2019;10:10. https://doi.org/10.3389/fphar.2019.00077.

104. Ashraf B, Saaiq M, Khaleeq-Uz-Zaman. Qualitative study of nocebo phenomenon (NP) involved in doctor-patient communication. Int J Health Policy Manag. 2014;3(1):23–7. https://doi.org/10.15171/ijhpm.2014.54.

105. Darnall BD, Colloca L. Optimizing placebo and minimizing nocebo to reduce pain, catastrophizing, and opioid use: a review of the science and an evidence-informed clinical toolkit. Int Rev Neurobiol. 2018;139:129–57. https://doi.org/10.1016/bs.irn.2018.07.022.

106. Häuser W, Hansen E, Enck P. Nocebo phenomena in medicine: importance in the clinical everyday. German Doctor's Bl Int. 2012;109(26):459–65. https://doi.org/10.3238/arztebl.2012.0459.

107. Leibowitz KA, Howe LC, Crum AJ. Changing mindsets about side effects. BMJ Open. 2021;11(2):e040134. https://doi.org/10.1136/bmjopen-2020-040134.

108. Smith EN, Young MD, Crum AJ. Stress, mindsets, and success in navy SEALs special warfare training. Front Psychol. 2020;10:10. https://doi.org/10.3389/fpsyg.2019.02962.

109. Turnwald BP, Crum AJ. Smart food policy for healthy food labeling: leading with taste, not healthiness, to shift consumption and enjoyment of healthy foods. Prev Med (Baltim). 2019;119:7–13. https://doi.org/10.1016/j.ypmed.2018.11.021.

110. Crum AJ, Salovey P, Achor S. Rethinking stress: the role of mindsets in determining the stress response. J Pers Soc Psychol. 2013;104(4):716–33. https://doi.org/10.1037/a0031201.

111. Zion SR, Crum AJ. Mindsets matter: a new framework for harnessing the placebo effect in modern medicine. Int Rev Neurobiol. 2018;138:137–60. https://doi.org/10.1016/bs.irn.2018.02.002.

112. Crum AJ, Langer EJ. Mind-set matters: exercise and the placebo effect. Psychol Sci. 2007;18(2):165–71. https://doi.org/10.1111/j.1467-9280.2007.01867.x.

113. Wendt L, Albring A, Schedlowski M. Learned placebo responses in neuroendocrine and immune functions. Handb Exp Pharmacol. 2014;225:159–81. https://doi.org/10.1007/978-3-662-44519-8_10.

114. Enck P, Horing B, Broelz E, Weimer K. Knowledge gaps in placebo research: with special reference to neurobiology. Int Rev Neurobiol. 2018;139:85–106. https://doi.org/10.1016/bs.irn.2018.07.018.

115. Koban L, Jepma M, Geuter S, Wager TD. What's in a word? How instructions, suggestions, and social information change pain and emotion. Neurosci Biobehav Rev. 2017;81:29–42. https://doi.org/10.1016/j.neubiorev.2017.02.014.

116. Quinn VF, Colagiuri B. Using learning strategies to inhibit the nocebo effect. Int Rev Neurobiol. 2018;138:307–27. https://doi.org/10.1016/bs.irn.2018.01.011.

117. Wampold BE. The therapeutic value of the relationship for placebo effects and other healing practices. Int Rev Neurobiol. 2018;139:191–210. https://doi.org/10.1016/bs.irn.2018.07.019.

118. Wojtukiewicz MZ, Politynska B, Skalij P, Tokajuk P, Wojtukiewicz AM, Honn K, v. It is not just the drugs that matter: the nocebo effect. Cancer Metastasis Rev. 2019;38(1–2):315–26. https://doi.org/10.1007/s10555-019-09800-w.

119. Quidde J, Pan Y, Salm M, et al. Preventing adverse events of chemotherapy by educating patients about the nocebo effect (RENNO study)—study protocol of a randomized controlled trial with gastrointestinal cancer patients. BMC Cancer. 2018;18(1):916. https://doi.org/10.1186/s12885-018-4814-7.

120. Foster JC, Le-Rademacher JG, Feliciano JL, et al. Comparative "nocebo effects" in older patients enrolled in cancer therapeutic trials: observations from a 446-patient cohort. Cancer. 2017;123(21):4193–8. https://doi.org/10.1002/cncr.30867.

121. Webster RK, Weinman J, Rubin GJ. Explaining all without causing unnecessary harm: is there scope for positively framing medical risk information? Patient Educ Couns. 2019;102(3):602–3. https://doi.org/10.1016/j.pec.2018.09.014.

122. Nestoriuc Y, von Blanckenburg P, Schuricht F, et al. Is it best to expect the worst? Influence of patients' side-effect expectations on endocrine treatment outcome in a 2-year prospective clinical cohort study. Ann Oncol. 2016;27(10):1909–15. https://doi.org/10.1093/annonc/mdw266.

123. von Blanckenburg P, Schuricht F, Albert US, Rief W, Nestoriuc Y. Optimizing expectations to prevent side effects and enhance quality of life in breast cancer patients undergoing endocrine therapy: study protocol of a randomized controlled trial. BMC Cancer. 2013;13:13. https://doi.org/10.1186/1471-2407-13-426.

124. Chacón MR, Enrico DH, Burton J, Waisberg FD, Videla VM. Incidence of placebo adverse events in randomized clinical trials of targeted and immunotherapy cancer drugs in the adjuvant setting: a systematic review and meta-analysis. JAMA Netw Open. 2018;1(8):e185617. https://doi.org/10.1001/jamanetworkopen.2018.5617.

125. Sanderson C, Hardy J, Spruyt O, Currow DC. Placebo and nocebo effects in randomized controlled trials: the implications for research and practice. J Pain Symptom Manag. 2013;46(5):722–30. https://doi.org/10.1016/j.jpainsymman.2012.12.005.

126. de La Cruz M, Hui D, Parsons HA, Bruera E. Placebo and nocebo effects in randomized double-blind clinical trials of agents for the therapy for fatigue in patients with advanced cancer. Cancer. 2010;116(3):766–74. https://doi.org/10.1002/cncr.24751.

127. Entralgo PL. Healing by the word in classical antiquity. Western Magazine, SA; 1958.

128. Morgenfeld EL, Martin Reinas G, Gercovich D, Gil Deza E, Rivarola EGJ, Gercovich FG. Difficult conversations with terminal patients: palliative care and death at home. J Clin Oncol. 2012;30(15_suppl):9038. https://doi.org/10.1200/jco.2012.30.15_suppl.9038.

129. Feito GL. The ethics of caring. Bioethics Debate. 2002;8(28):1.

130. Feito GL. Los cuidados en la ética del siglo XXI. Ill Clin. 2005;15(3):167. https://doi.org/10.1016/S1130-8621(05)71104-9.

Chapter 4
Medical Words Throughout History

4.1 Introduction

In this chapter, we will analyze the medical word from six perspectives:

(a) The **role of the medical word**, especially the communication of the truth, in the history of the doctor–patient relationship, in order to study the historical dynamic of changes in power and roles that have been evidenced over time.

(b) **Why has the medical word been devalued in the twenty-first century?** If at some point the medical word was indisputable, and the biggest question was related to whether or not the truth should be communicated, but no one doubted the honesty or veracity of the doctor, why is the medical word no longer credible or at least as credible as before?

(c) The **etymology of medical terms**: Studying medicine is not only studying a discipline, that is, a set of specific knowledge, it is also studying an art, that is, a way of carrying out an activity, but above all it is learning a new language, made up of about 20,000 words that we do not use in daily life, many of them polysemous or ambiguous and most of them unknown to the patient. When we think that Greek and Latin are languages with few speakers, we forget about medicine since a very significant number of the terms we use have this origin. Knowing its origin allows us to use that language with greater precision and to be able to explain it to our patient.

(d) The **role of the modern doctor as a translator and humanizer** of the set of information about the health of each patient that is delivered daily.

(e) **The patient's narrative generating new knowledge**: Traditionally, the patient has been considered an expert in his illness and the data provided in the anamnesis as a source of information about the way in which the disease has developed, but recently, narrative medicine also takes the patient as an expert in their life and as a central agent in making correct decisions regarding therapeutic

E. Gil Deza, *Improving Clinical Communication*,
https://doi.org/10.1007/978-3-031-62446-9_4

alternatives for the treatment of their conditions. In fact, this has transformed traditional bioethics into narrative ethics in the most modern currents.

(f) **The patient as evaluator of medical quality**: The quality of services very frequently relies on the patient's perception as a source of information; and what most influences the way they rate their satisfaction with the doctor and the health system is how well they have been treated and communicated with.

We will develop each of these six topics below.

4.2 The Role of the Medical Word Throughout the History of the Doctor–Patient Relationship

We must understand that the doctor–patient relationship has changed more in the last 25 years than in the previous 25 centuries.

The one who has changed the most over time has been the patient.

As a consequence, the doctor changed as well.

By virtue of the fact that both changed, the doctor–patient relationship itself changed.

We are going to take the last 26 centuries in the West to cover from Hippocrates to the twenty-first century.

Let us start with the patient. That is to say, society.

Imagine a common city of the Roman Empire or any of the Greek or Mediterranean cities in the four centuries before the Christian era.

Most people there were born and, some 30 years later, died in the same condition. If you were born poor, then you died poor; and if you were born rich, it was very likely that you would die rich.

Education was a luxury for very few, generally the priestly class and the powerful.

Most free men had three alternatives: the militia, the priesthood, or a craft. Those who were not free were slaves or prisoners, and in many cases the latter condition was a prelude to the former.

Child labor was not only accepted but necessary. When the women were not giving birth, they were doing housework. Adolescence practically did not exist, people passed seamlessly from childhood to adulthood. Often after a social ritual.

If we read Plato's *Republic*, which in some way describes his vision of the utopia of the ideal city, we will see that the most outstanding virtue for citizens, patients, students, or parishioners, that is, for politics, medicine, teaching, and theology is **obedience**.

The discussion revolves around establishing who is in charge, but not how this person should rule.

This is what is known as **paternalism**.

We will accept this name because I cannot think of a better one since the alternative is "obediencism,"but I do not particularly like the term.

What paternalism consists of is that it assumes that goodness, truth, or beauty, which are sublime attributes of **being**, are actually known to few people.

The teachers, the judges, the philosophers, the wise, the powerful, they know these truths with greater clarity and depth and therefore they should lead. The others must trust and be led.

This way of exercising freedom prevailed in the West until well into the seventeenth century of the Christian era.

If we take the Greek (democratic polytheism) and the Jewish (theocratic monarchy) as antinomian political models, we will see that autonomy is not individual in either of them.

In the Greek world, it was exercised by the polis, the **cities** were autonomous, the individuals who commanded themselves were considered *idiotes*, idiots, those who gave themselves their own law.

In the Jewish world, the authority was the Torah, the law, autonomy was interpretive, and was reserved to the priests and teachers (rabbi), ordinary people had to follow their mandates.

If this was the role of authority in society, we will now analyze the second component. What was the role of the doctor? How should they behave?

In a similar way.

The doctor governed their conduct by a heteronomous deontological code that they swore to comply with and acted in dealing with the patient in the same way that the civil or religious authority did with citizens or parishioners.

The doctor "knew" what was happening to the patient both in his body and in his mind, they knew what the course of the disease was going to be, and whether it could be modified or not.

The patient had to abide by the indications and trust in the art of the doctor who treated him.

It was unnecessary to inform the patient further than this because if he was in his right mind, he would consent to what the doctor indicated, and therefore there was an abundance of information. If the patient was not in his right mind, it was not necessary to inform him either because whether or not the patient consented was immaterial.

This model of a wise doctor and obedient patient remained in force until very late in the twentieth century in the West, that is, for 25 centuries.

In fact, if we read Thomas More's *Utopia*, we can see that even in the care of dying patients, obedience to authority was considered key to the legitimacy of an act. Let us see the following passage (pages 110–111):

I have already told you with what care they look after their sick, so that nothing is left undone that can contribute either to their case or health; and for those who are taken with fixed and incurable diseases, they use all possible ways to cherish them and to make their lives as comfortable as possible. They visit them often and take great pains to make their time pass off easily; but when any is taken with a torturing and lingering pain, so that there is no hope either of recovery or ease, the priests and magistrates come and exhort them, that, since they are now unable to go on with the business of life, are become a burden to themselves and to all about them, and they have really out-lived themselves, they should no longer nourish such a rooted distemper, but choose rather to die since they cannot live but in much misery; being assured that if they thus deliver themselves from torture, or are willing that others should do it, they shall be happy after death: since, by their acting thus, they lose none of the pleasures, but only the troubles of life, they think they behave not only reasonably but in a manner consistent with religion and piety; because they follow the advice given them by their priests, who are the expounders of the will of God. Such as are wrought on by these persuasions either starve themselves of their own ac-cord, or take opium, and by that means die without pain. But no man is forced on this way of ending his life; and if they cannot be persuaded to it, this does not induce them to fail in their attendance and care of them: but as they believe that a voluntary death, when it is chosen upon such an authority, is very honourable, so if any man takes away his own life without the approbation of the priests and the senate, they give him none of the honours of a decent funeral, but throw his body into a ditch.

When we read this passage, we cannot forget that we are facing the second most important work of political philosophy in the West, after Plato's *Republic*. The essential question of both works is: What is the best possible society for the human being? How should it be governed? What are the roles of its inhabitants?

In that ideal and perfect Island that More imagined, obedience is also the guiding virtue. In fact, when we read the aforementioned passage, we observe that what legitimizes the patient's action at the end of his life is not the exercise of his will but the approval of the priests.

Even though in the political field the rights of citizens had been exercised for several centuries, at least in a large part of the civilized world, it was not until the mid-1950s that this asymmetrical relationship between doctor and patient began to crack.

The Nuremberg Trials (which we will see in the next section) revealed two things: (a) The Hippocratic Oath was a formality for doctors in authoritarian regimes since they obeyed political power more than the Oath and (b) Nazi doctors had committed atrocious crimes, in the name of science, against Jewish people because they considered them sub-human.

This gave rise to the Nuremberg Code, which was the first Never Again in medicine and established a relationship between researcher and research subject that should be more horizontal.

Thus arose informed consent, which had been enforced in England since the nineteenth century and in Prussia since the beginning of the twentieth century, as a document that should be universal in clinical research, as highlighted in number 1 of the Nuremberg Code:

1. The voluntary consent of the human subject is absolutely essential. This means that the person involved should have legal capacity to give consent; should be so situated as to be able to exercise free power of choice, without the intervention of any element of force, fraud, deceit, duress, overreaching, or other ulterior form of constraint or coercion; and should have sufficient knowledge and comprehension of the elements of the subject matter involved as to enable him to make an understanding and enlightened decision. This latter element requires that before the acceptance of an affirmative decision by the experimental subject there should be made known to him the nature, duration, and purpose of the experiment; the method and means by which it is to be conducted; all inconveniences and hazards reasonably to be expected; and the effects upon his health or person which may possibly come from his participation in the experiment. The duty and responsibility for ascertaining

the quality of the consent rests upon each individual who initiates, directs, or engages in the experiment. It is a personal duty and responsibility which may not be delegated to another with impunity.

And one point, which is in my opinion extraordinary, is article 10 of the Nuremberg Code: the investigator's need for moral suitability must be able to terminate the trial if he detects that the patient may be harmed:

> 10. During the course of the experiment the scientist in charge must be prepared to terminate the experiment at any stage, if he has probable cause to believe, in the exercise of the good faith, superior skill and careful judgment required of him that a continuation of the experiment is likely to result in injury, disability, or death to the experimental subject.

Therefore, this historical document places at the beginning and at the end of the document two safeguards for the dignity, life and health of the patient: their autonomous consent to participate in an experiment and the moral suitability of the researcher who must put the well-being of the patient above the needs of science.

However, one of the criticisms of this document was that it applied only to one of the doctor's roles: the researcher. It did not apply to attending physicians, and in fact it was considered that including such a role was unnecessary.

The doctor–patient relationship outside of research continued to be asymmetric and vertical.

The doctor was unquestioningly obeyed.

In other areas, the citizen was freeing himself: the fight against slavery became a fight for equal rights, the voice of those excluded for reasons of race, religion, sex, or any other condition began to rise up and be heard.

Civil rights, consumer rights, organizations for universal suffrage, and women's liberation mark a rising awareness on the part of citizens of their dignity and freedom. In medicine, the increasingly scandalous evidence of immoral clinical investigations permeated toward a liberation of the patient.

In the mid-1970s, in the West, the patient assumed his autonomy and the doctor–patient relationship became more horizontal.

The informed and participatory patient replaced the obedient patient and paternalism gradually disappeared from medicine to be replaced by an autonomy-based, open and auditable doctor–patient relationship. Office walls were made transparent and medical writing accessible to public scrutiny.

These changes were progressive and, as described by Childress and Siegler [1], there are at least five metaphors that can explain the different modes of doctor–patient relationship throughout the twentieth century (we have altered the original order of Childress and Siegler):

1. Paternal, parental, or paternalism: In which the autonomy of the patient is minimal or nonexistent. The professional is the one who possesses the maximum knowledge and the maximum responsibility. A subtle difference marked by Szasz and Hollender [2] is that it can be seen as the relationship between a parent and a child, to whom practically nothing is explained, or as that of a parent and an adolescent, to whom something is explained and expected to consent, but whose dissent is considered a sign of immaturity or inability.

2. Partnership: He sees the doctor–patient relationship as one of adult colleagues pursuing the same goal. There is a kind of camaraderie between the doctor and the patient.
3. Friendship: This model of the doctor–patient relationship was deeply analyzed by the doctor and historian of medicine Lain Entralgo since he adds to the condition of colleagues an obligation of beneficence, benevolence, and confidentiality on the part of the doctor:

> Insofar as man is a part of nature, and health an aspect of this nature and therefore a natural and objective good, the medical relation develops into comradeship, or association for the purpose of securing this good by technical means. Insofar as man is an individual and his illness a state affecting his personality, the medical relation ought to be more than mere comradeship—in fact it should be a friendship. All dogma apart, a good doctor has always been a friend to his patient, to all his patients. (P. Lain Entratgo, *Doctor and Patient*, trans, from the Spanish by Frances Partridge; New York: McGraw-Hill Book Co., World University Library, 1969), p. 242)

4. Rational contractor: The doctor and patient establish a fluid relationship in which both parties make different contracts according to mutual needs. In this type of relationship, mutual trust is not assured.
5. Technicians: In this relationship, the doctor is seen as a knowledgeable craftsman, not unlike a plumber or an architect. The wishes of the patient and his autonomy are a priority, and the professional duty of the doctor is essentially to satisfy the needs of the patient using the technical resources at his disposal. In other words, the doctor and the patient have a punctual, superficial, and often ephemeral relationship. In this model, the autonomy of the doctor is diminished, to the point that some consider it an abdication on the part of the doctor.

These five relationship models summarize or synthesize the changes produced during the last century.

This shift from the paternal figure to the modern doctor was accompanied by other very significant changes, especially in the present century:

(a) The incorporation of women into medicine, which has been increasing throughout the twentieth and twenty-first centuries. Let us not forget that Johns Hopkins University was the first to admit women to the medical career. This was due not so much to the progressivism of its founders as to their pragmatism since this stipulation came from four women who raised the funds necessary for opening the institution. They were always a minority until the last quarter of the last century when they began to progressively increase in number and today in practically all faculties women predominate. There is still a lack of equity in leadership positions since men predominate as service heads, but balance is gradually being achieved.
(b) Fragmentation of medicine into subspecialties. Today the condition of doctor, without qualifying adjectives, is a transitory stage that the newly graduated students go through. Almost immediately they have to choose between clinic, surgery, pediatrics, obstetrics, gynecology, and within each specialty a subspecialty: clinical oncologist, cardiologist, endocrinologist, etc.; and within each

subspecialty an outstanding practice: clinical oncologist specializing in breast, digestive, sarcomas, etc. So much so that it is commonly said that a general practitioner is one who knows almost nothing about almost everything and a specialist doctor is one who knows almost everything about almost nothing.

The problem is that the fragmentation of the subspecialty means that each doctor deals with a part of the patient and almost no one with the patient as a whole.

(c) The displacement of medical knowledge to the Internet and the globalization of its access. Let us think for a moment that until the late 1990s, most of the updated information circulated through magazines, publishing them was a complex affair, and the magazines arrived several weeks late. Today publication is instantaneous and access to the information is almost immediate. Before it was more difficult to access information than to doubt its veracity, today it is easier to access this information, and a very significant number of the things that are published are biased, making it so it takes more time to analyze the work than to obtain it.

(d) Medical diagnosis has gone from being clinical to being subclinical since images show us the structure and function of internal organs like never before in the history of medicine.

(e) Molecular pathology has displaced the sagacity of pathological anatomy, whose role today is practically limited to asserting the malignancy and invasion of a tumor, but everything else is analyzed molecularly.

(f) The selection of treatments is based on the information provided by the images and molecular pathology, leaving the treating physician to adapt the protocols published on the web to some particular conditions of the patient.

(g) The efficacy of therapy is no longer based on the diagnostic capacity of the clinician or the surgical skill of the surgeon, but on the potency of the medication.

(h) The potency of a drug is based on the analysis of population efficacy through the use of artificial intelligence and big data through studies sponsored and published by the manufacturers.

(i) The biological records carried out by the patients in the personal devices at home (temperature, blood pressure, heart rate, respiratory rate, and movements during sleep) means that the patient can have highly sophisticated information at their fingertips and in their own home, as shown by the article recently published by Itzmailova and Ellis [3].

All this makes the practice of modern medicine heterogeneous to say the least.

In the same community, even more so in the same institution, there are doctor–patient relationships that sometimes resemble classic paternalism, many patients consent to the proposed treatments based on trust and not on the understanding of what they are going to be subject to; others practice a medicine in which the professional functions as a dispassionate and distant adviser, leaving decision-making entirely in the hands of the patient and his family; others practice a medicine in which the emotional commitment makes the doctor seem like a close friend or family member.

However, this heterogeneity does not prevent all doctors from being convinced that the current doctor–patient relationship is open (there is always more than one doctor, sometimes explicitly and other times more subtly, usually Dr. Internet), auditable (everything prescribed by a doctor is reviewed, sometimes by peers, or if not, then by Dr. Internet), and less satisfactory than our teachers reported (owing to higher professional burnout and more professional turnover).

An explanation for this phenomenon can be seen in the offer of professionals and therapeutic alternatives, which the psychologist Barry Schwartz called *The Paradox of Choice: Why More Is Less*. In that text, Schwartz explains the psychological reasons why being unable to choose makes us dissatisfied, which we all understand; less intuitive is the fact that when we have three or at most five alternatives and we choose one, we are very satisfied; but from then on when the alternatives increase to six, seven, or ten, we start to be less satisfied with our choice and we always think that we left the one that was optimal on the shelf and we took a good one, but not the best.

If you have a lot of doctors to choose from, if you have a lot of drugs to use, and you have a lot of protocols to apply, the same thing is likely to happen.

In addition to a problem related to the dissatisfaction of the choice, the second problem in the doctor–patient relationship is the devaluation of the word, which we will analyze below.

4.3   Why Has the Medical Word Lost Value in the Twenty-First Century?

As we have seen in the previous section, in the West in the last 2500 years, the medical figure has been "humanized"; it has gone from being a God (Horus) or a demigod (Asclepius) to being an intermediary (Priest—Shaman) and from there to being a more or less wise father (paternalistic medicine) to end up being an almost unnecessary counselor or employee (autonomous medicine) (artificial intelligence).

As you, dear reader, will understand, this has been due to change on both sides: on the one hand, the loss of prestige of the medical figure and, on the other, the liberation of the patient.

Let us look at the first step. How does a doctor go from being a god to being almost unnecessary?

Here the history of knowledge plays a fundamental role.

For a long time, knowledge of humanity was almost inaccessible to the majority of the population.

With the creation of the printing press and especially due to the French Revolution, knowledge becomes more and more accessible. It is very interesting to know that this democratization of knowledge was resisted by the authorities. Fernando Savater's philosophical dictionary, under the heading "Poisons," cites Colbert, creator of the "literary police" in France in the seventeenth century, who maintains:

"the literary police rests on a conviction that directs its methods: illicit books are dangerous drugs that poison the social body." [4]

That is to say, at that time you could freely put into your body what you got in apothecaries or taverns, but you could not read what you wanted.

The reason for this is that free thinking has always been a problem for power.

This is true for political power, which prohibited the free circulation of books; it is true for religious power that, in the case of Catholicism, was opposed to its faithful reading the Bible, until late in the twentieth century (Vatican Council II in 1960), and it is also true for medical power, which considered that it was better for the patient to ignore his illness and the reasons for treatments, at least until the 1970s when this changed.

In many of the banned texts that circulated, medicine was mocked by the French (Moliere), Spanish (Cervantes), and English (Shakespeare) theaters, and not because they did not hold their personal doctors in high esteem, but because medical practice has always had a questionable side.

If this were not the case, it would have been unnecessary to put in the Hippocratic oath that we were going to respect the secrecy of what we heard or saw, and that we were not going to have sex with the inhabitants of the houses we visited (a stipulation repeated, by the way, in Indian and Chinese oaths, which implies the problem is quite universal), which shows we were never as pretty a picture as we like to paint.

It seems that the practice gossip and exchanging favors, if not outright abuse, go back a long time in our profession.

But if the evidence of our inappropriate behavior in the homes of patients and in our offices were not enough to lower us from the pedestal, undoubtedly the evidence of the encroachment on the human rights of patients in clinical investigations, which ended with doctors convicted in courts at Nuremberg, was what ended what little prestige paternalistic medicine had left. I feel it is wrong to call it paternalistic in this case, abusive would be a more apt descriptor given the circumstances.

This is the thesis that I developed in my book *Truth* Versus *Verdict* [5]; the management of medical truth changed as a result of society becoming aware of the scandalous behavior of doctors in clinical research.

What is that behavior? The one who shows that interest in the answer was more important than respect for the way to obtain it. People are not means, they are ends, but on numerous occasions they have been used to obtain a "scientific" answer to a medical problem.

Below I will cite some of the best-known examples, but those who are interested in more information can look up the Alliance For Human Research Protection's website:

1. **Alcmaeon**

    Excellent clinician of Athens in the fifth century BC. We could say that he was a clinician from the hierarchy of Hippocrates and a contemporary of him. While Hippocrates emphasized first not causing harm, Alcmaeon experimented with death row prisoners. He demonstrated, for example, that the optic nerve was essential for sight. How did he do it? Simple: he pulled one eye out and asked the prisoner: Do you see? Then he cut the nerve and asked again: now you see? He also proved that sperm is not formed in the spinal cord as some contemporaries mistakenly thought, and I will leave it to you to imagine how.

2. **Cleopatra**

The seventh, the Promethean, the sovereign of Egypt who flirted with Julius Caesar and fell in love with Marco Antonio to the point of making him the head and the empire, of colossal beauty and boundless ambition, is also often cited as the first to practice an inhumane science (https://www.realclearscience.com/blog/2021/09/07/was_cleopatra_the_first_mad_scientist_790061.html).

This is reported by Plutarch, who experimented with poisons to see which one was the most powerful, administering it to prisoners. In fact, Cleopatra herself drank Nephentes (a concoction based on sour beer and opium) before being bitten by the asp to end her life.

But one of the most scandalous experiments began with a legitimate question for the time: Are male children and female children formed at the same time in the maternal womb?

This must have been expressed by the queen to one of her viziers, those skinny guys dressed in white tunics who appeared in Hollywood blockbusters, and one of them quickly came out to settle the matter.

They selected slaves that had been pregnant at the same time and therefore had a similar gestation period, killed them, and observed the intrauterine development of their children. Question answered: they develop at the same time.

Cost: a few slaves less, almost nothing, right?

3. **Frederick II of Sicily (1194–1250)**

Called Stupor Mundis (Amazement of the world), was King of Sicily and Jerusalem   and   Holy   Roman   Emperor   (https://en.wikipedia.org/wiki/Frederick_II,_Holy_Roman_Emperor).

He was also one of the most cultured and, to put it mildly, eccentric kings of his time: he spoke nine languages and wrote in seven. He was interested in pursuing the original language, which he thought was Hebrew, and so he conducted an experiment (quoted by the chronicler Franciscan Salimbene of Adam).

What did this experiment consist of?

He isolated a newborn from all verbal contact, so that no one would speak in his presence, with the idea that the primitive language of humanity would arise spontaneously. The experiment failed not only because his hypothesis was wrong, but also because the imposed silence was not observed by the child's nurses.

The second experiment attributed to him is one that arose from a gastroenterological question: Is food digested better after exercise or rest?

How did you solve it?

He invited two gentlemen (though some sources say they were prisoners) to dinner and gave them both the same food. After dinner, he sent one to hunt and the other to rest. Four hours later, he ordered them both killed and their stomachs studied. He rightly concluded that rest facilitates digestion.

From then on, it is said every time Frederick invited someone to dinner, many asked, "Does the emperor have any questions?" (although I was unable to verify the veracity of this particular claim).

4. **Edward Jenner (1749–1823)**

Humanity owes an eternal debt to Dr. Jenner, who discovered the vaccine thanks to which smallpox was eradicated from the face of the earth, and essentially fathered all the research related to vaccines, including those against the recent Covid-19 pandemic, which has saved so many lives and prevented so many hospitalizations and suffering.

However, the vaccine story also has a B-side.

We must not forget that the hypothesis on the efficacy of the vaccine (Cow Pox), that is to say, from cowpox, to protect (immunize) against human smallpox (Small Pox) essentially had a historical or anecdotal basis (it is said that Jenner had a fondness for young milkmaids, whose smooth skin was more attractive than English ladies, most with smallpox scars).

How did he test that hypothesis?

He took a child, John Philipps, who had not been infected with smallpox, and injected him with a concoction made from pus extracted from the cow's lesions (hence the name vaccine). After waiting for 3 weeks, pus was taken from the pustule of a smallpox patient and injected into John. To everyone's astonishment, the child was not infected. This latter procedure was repeated countless times throughout John's life to prove that he was immune.

Let us look at the experiment again, but this time with twenty-first-century eyes.

One can argue this is not good from a scientific standpoint, but it is very useful to do it from a moral standpoint because it also allows us to be hopeful. In many places, enough progress has been made to this day that we find the idea of a researcher endangering the life of a child based on anecdotal evidence to be scandalous.

What is less known is that, reinforcing the saying *Nobody is a prophet in their land*, Jenner was not believed in England, where people refused to get vaccinated. In Spain, however, Spanish doctor Francisco Javier Balmis Berenguer was convinced of the benefits of the vaccine and managed to convince the royal family to not only to vaccinate the subjects of the peninsula, but also to bring the benefits of the vaccine to America and Asia.

To bring protection to overseas territories, the Royal Philanthropic Vaccine Expedition or Balmis Expedition was prepared (https://historia.nationalgeographic.com.es/a/expedicion-balmis-ninos-que-llevaron-vacuna-viruela-a-america_15225).

However, there was a problem. How could the vaccine virus strain be kept alive so that it reached America? Well, it could only be done by passing it from person to person.

How they did it?

Twenty-two orphans from La Coruña were used as live recipients of the virus, they were inoculated in pairs once a week (pairs were used in case one of them died from complications or accidents), according to the Madrid Gazette of the time.

So, the vaccine is wonderful, but we should respectfully remember that its success, at least for America, is built on 23 poor children, Phillips, and 22 forgotten orphans.

5. **Adolf Serturner (1805)**

He is credited with the discovery of morphine (although others maintain that in 1803 Charles Derosne had isolated this component from opium), probably the most extraordinary drug of all those discovered by man. The amount of pain it has alleviated and the unnecessary suffering it has avoided should be enough to call its discoverer a hero.

But just like with Jenner, we need to take a closer look at what his discovery was like. He exposed a solution of opium to an alkaline solution, and the result was the precipitation of some yellowish and sour crystals (from there we get their name: alkaloids). Not knowing what they could cause, he invited some friends to dinner and for dessert offered these new crystals. Its effect was almost immediate; they fell asleep in a deep torpor. The chronicle tells that when they woke up they fled in terror. Seeing the effect it produced, Sertürner called his crystals morphine, in honor of Morpheus, the god of sleep.

To make things clear: Did he know what it was? No. Did he know about their adverse effects? No. Did he know the dosage? No. Could it have killed them? Absolutely.

This experiment questions not only non-consensual research but also Sertürner's concept of friendship.

6. **Horace Wells (1815–1848) and William Morton (1819–1868)**

To these two giants in the history of medicine, we owe nothing less than anesthesia. (https://en.wikipedia.org/wiki/Horace_Wells and https://en.wikipedia.org/wiki/William_T._G._Morton).

Today we are used to seeing immaculate operating rooms thanks to the efforts of Joseph Lister (1827–1912) and his tireless fight for antisepsis, and especially the German school of asepsis, with everything sterilized.

But also if we walk the corridors of an operating theater, we will find that the silence is only broken, in some cases by music, in others by the symphony of metallic noises or the movement of elements.

If a surgeon from 1845 visited us, what is the first thing that would catch their attention, besides the clothing and gloves with which surgeons operate nowadays?

The lack of screaming.

Throughout the history of medicine until 1846, surgery was always accompanied by blood and screams.

During that time, surgeons trained to do their work quickly, in such a way that the patient suffered for the least amount of time. One of the lower limb amputation surgeries was done in 30 s: the technique was called "Turkish style," and the leg was cut with an instrument similar to a very sharp cutlass, in the same way that legs were cut in battlefields.

Why did it take so long for anesthesia to reach the operating rooms?

Because pain was seen as "natural." It was natural for it to hurt and not get better. We will see how this same concept of "natural pain" was applied to cancer and how oncology took until the 1980s to proclaim palliative care and pain relief as therapeutic objectives.

But back to anesthesia.

It was thanks to a sudden state of lucidity in the midst of a chemical drunkenness that Horace Wells discovered the anesthetic power of nitrous oxide and changed the course of medicine and dentistry.

The story goes that nitrous oxide (colloquially known as laughing gas) was a frequent diversion at university parties that took place in different hotels in cities around the world. Morton was a regular participant in these festivities and used to play with nitrous oxide. In one such party, as a result of precarious balance, he fell and lost a tooth. Being a dentist, he observed with surprise that such an accident occurred without feeling the slightest pain. What is more, he kept laughing throughout the whole affair.

The next day, now more lucid, he realized the enormous potential benefit of his discovery and began to apply it to his patients, which increased his clientele and his fame.

William Morton studied at Harvard (although he dropped out before graduating) and listened to the lectures of chemist Charles T. Jackson, who analyzed the anesthetic properties of ether.

Morton began using ether as an anesthetic and demonstrated that it relieved dental extirpations. On October 16, 1846, at the operating theater of the Massachusetts General Hospital, the surgeon painlessly removed a tumor from a patient's neck.

For the first time, the wonder of operating without pain was not a dream.

Unfortunately for the discoverers of anesthesia, a painful struggle began between them in order to patent the invention and win an extraordinary prize from the North American government, which ended up costing them their health and eventually, their lives.

They changed the history of medicine, but their ambitions killed them.

In addition to pain relief in dentistry and surgery, anesthesia came to obstetrics at the hands of Queen Victoria.

Here too we have another example of *natural* pain, only with theological underpinnings: "You will give birth with pain" commands the Bible. It is no surprise then that when the obstetrician proposed that Her Majesty use anesthesia for one of her deliveries, it generated an intellectual and religious contention.

The argument was settled when scholars pointed out that in the story of the creation of women, God first put Adam to sleep before taking out his rib, making God the first anesthesiologist in history.

Anesthesia during childbirth, from then on, became known as "The Queen's Anesthesia."

The important thing about this discovery is to reflect again on the concept of "natural" for a condition: dental, surgical, obstetric, or oncological, and how this prevents or makes it difficult to investigate the means to alleviate it.

This also questions medical prejudices when considering a problem to solve it.

7. **James Marion Sims (1813–1883)**

   Undoubtedly one of the best obstetricians of his time: on his tombstone, it reads "Obstetrician of empresses and slaves."

   This is because he was summoned to assist the Empress of France in one of her deliveries while also assisting slaves obstetrically.

   But with the slaves, he also practiced many of the surgeries that he later carried out among his patients in the community of free men.

   He operated on one slave 36 times, without anesthesia.

   Therefore, while it is true that he assisted both empresses and slaves, it was not in the same manner.

   His statue, erected in Bryant Park, New York, in 1894, was removed in 2018 (https://en.wikipedia.org/wiki/J._Marion_Sims).

   I personally believe that these acts are counterproductive as any history we forget we are doomed to repeat.

   It is better to have a permanent reminder of our mistakes and repudiate what we did in the past than to eliminate that memory because it makes us uncomfortable or ashamed.

8. **-Arthur Wentworth**, a pediatrician in Boston, performed the first lumbar puncture in the history of medicine in 1895. [6] No one doubts the usefulness of the procedure and the number of lives it has saved. What one should find extremely controversial is that in 1896 he performed spinal taps on 29 babies and young children at the Children's Hospital in Boston to determine whether the procedure was harmful.

9. **Giuseppe Sanarelli** in 1897 injected five people without their consent with the causative agent of yellow fever, killing three of them. William Osler publicly rebuked him severely.

10. **Walter Reed** in 1900 injected 22 Hispanic workers in Cuba with the causative agent of yellow fever. It is the first time in the history of recorded medicine that $100 in gold was paid for participating in the research and an additional $100 if they contracted the disease. In this case, the patients signed a contract to be able to participate.

11. **Richard Strong**, Professor of Medicine at Harvard, experimented with cholera on 24 Filipino prisoners, killing 13. The deaths of these prisoners were attributed to an error in the administration of a serum for the bubonic plague. He rewarded the survivors with cigars. This work was cited by the defense of the Nazi doctors as evidence of the way in which research was carried out by doctors of the countries that were judging them.

12. **Luther Emmet Holt** was accused in 1909 of having performed over 1000 tuberculin tests on seriously ill and dying children at New York Babies'Hospital.

13. **Hideyo Noguchi** in 1911 injected 146 children with a syphilis preparation at the Rockefeller Institute for Medical Research to develop a diagnostic skin test.

14. **St Vincent House** in Philadelphia in 1913 tested infants with tuberculin, leaving 15 of them blind.

15. **Mass sterilizations**: Tens of thousands of women were sterilized in the United States and Europe for eugenic reasons to prevent them from fathering offspring with psychiatric problems or alcoholism. The most resonant case was that of Carrie Buck, which was carried out for exclusively ideological reasons and defended even by very respected people like the Harvard-educated eugenicist Oliver Wendell Holmes, who infamously declared, *Three generations of imbeciles are enough.*

16. **Experiments with imprisoned people**: Numerous investigations were carried out on convicts in prisons in the United States, especially on people of Black race and without education. One of the most cited researchers is Dr. Leo Stanley, a surgeon from San Quintin, who carried out studies between 1913 and 1951, one of them being testicle transplants between inmates to study violence and masculinity.

17. **Cornelius Rhoades was an excellent pathologist at Harvard**. In 1931 under the auspices of the Rockefeller Institute for Medical Research, he carried out research in Puerto Rico, which consisted in injecting cancer cells into 13 hospitalized patients. An official commission studied the complaint and hid the facts to protect both Dr. Rhoades and the Rockefeller Institute. Dr. Rhoades was transferred to establish a chemical weapons development center, later participating in the design of radiation experiments on prisoners, patients, and soldiers. A prestigious award from the American Association for Cancer Research carried his name from 1979 to 2002, when it was changed due to the racism expressed by Rhoades in his correspondence.

18. **Experimental vaccination of neonates in Lubeck in 1930**. In total, 240 children aged less than 10 days old were vaccinated with the Calmette vaccine. Virtually all contracted tuberculosis because the vaccines were contaminated and 72 children died. As a result of this experiment, Dr. Julius Moses, a severe critic of unethical human experimentation, wrote the draft of the *Guidelines for Human Experimentation* that were approved in Germany in 1931 and were in force under the Nazi regime. In 1941, Dr. Moses was deported to the ghetto of Theresienstadt, where he later died.

19. **Nazi Investigations**: The discovery of the extermination camps and the genocide carried out on six million Jews, hundreds of thousands of gypsies, and thousands of opponents of the Nazi regime revealed that among the indescribable atrocities to which they were subjected, there were also medical research projects. These projects included things such as suffocation in low-oxygen chambers (the skydiver); ice water immersion; extreme dehydration; phosphorus bomb injuries; typhus and other infections; intravenous gasoline injection, among other aberrations. Twenty-three doctors were tried and sentenced for these experiments at the Nuremberg Doctors' Trial. That is where the Nuremberg Code came from.

20. **Japanese Unit 731**: Occurring simultaneously with the Nazi atrocities, Unit 731 led by Dr. Shiro Ishii in Manchuria did similar things to the Chinese population. Among the inhumane experiments carried out were numerous cases of bacterial or viral contamination, through vectors or contamination of food or water; vivisection of pregnant people; and operations without anesthesia. These crimes were concealed by the American forces, with the results the Unit 731 experiments became military secrets and Dr. Ishii negotiating immunity in exchange for handing over the information. In his last years, he opened a clinic where he treated his patients free of charge, converted to Christianity, and died peacefully in 1969 from throat cancer, according to his daughter Harumi, without anyone ever seeking any reparations from him.

21. **Tuskegee Study** (1932–1972): This was research carried out in the United States conducted under the auspices of health authorities and coordinated by Dr. Clark Taliaferro. The aim of the study was to observe the natural development of syphilis in Black people. Four hundred Black patients with syphilis were followed in a deceptive way, without receiving any treatment for their ailment. This was despite the fact that penicillin, discovered in 1928, had been established as the standard treatment since 1942 and that there was evidence that the evolution of [7]patients under observation, compared to 200 controls, showed that they fared clearly worse. This study remained under the radar of the public until 1972, when the *New York Times* exposed it. This caused a great scandal and led the US President Jimmy Carter (probably one of the most ethical rulers in the world) to form the Ethics Commission that later published the Belmont Report and generated changes in many fields, including medical ethics and bioethics. In May 1997, President Bill Clinton apologized to the eight survivors and the families those who had died during the study: *What was done cannot be undone, but we can end the silence.*

22. **Physiology of iron and calcium in Boston**: We have all studied in physiology how and where in our intestine these two essential atoms for our life are absorbed: one to form hemoglobin that allows red blood cells to carry oxygen to our tissues and the other to regulate our nerve impulses and form bones. What is less known is that this study was carried out between MIT and Harvard University: they gave specific children milk that contained radioactive isotopes of calcium and iron. What condition did these children have? Down syndrome. That is to say, disabled children were exposed to nontherapeutic research in order to obtain medical knowledge. And this happened in the United States *after* the Nuremberg Code.

23. **Jewish Chronic Disease Hospital Study**: This was a clinical trial carried out on patients who were unaware of the experiment in which they were participating: injecting tumor cells. Similar to the one carried out in Puerto Rico by Rhoades in 1931, only in this case it was carried out in New York, and the study was coordinated by Dr. Chester M. Southam of the Memorial Sloan Kettering Cancer Center. The reason cited by the researchers as to why the patients were not informed was so it would not cause them undue fear. Three doctors refused

to participate in the experiment: Avar Kagan, David Leichter, and Perry Fresko; all three resigned when they found out that it had been carried out on 22 patients [8], which later led to a lawsuit against the researchers and hospital authorities by the state of New York.

24. **Willowbrook Study**: Willowbrook was an institution for mentally challenged children. The studies carried out in Willowbrook by Dr. Saul Krugman between 1955 and 1970 focused on the study of hepatitis B. To be admitted to the institution that housed more than 6000 children, parents or guardians had to authorize the institution to carry out experiments on them. This coerced consent allowed the oral transmission of hepatitis B to be studied by feeding children feces with live B viruses; B virus was also injected in order to study the natural development of the disease. Dr. Krugman received numerous awards for his experiments, and in the year 1972 when these abominations came to light, Dr. Krugman was elected president of the American Pediatric Society.

25. **Human Gene Editing in China**.

    As we were informed by *The Guardian* in 2018 (https://www.theguardian. com/science/2018/nov/26/worlds-first-gene-edited-babies-created-in-china-claims-scientist), Dr. He Jiankui of the Southern University of Science and Technology in Shenzhen was the first to genetically edit a human being. He altered the embryos of seven couples that were to be implanted and at least one of them developed properly. It employed a technique called CRISPR, developed by 2020 Nobel Prize winners in chemistry Jennifer Doudna and Emmanuelle Charpentier. Essentially, they described the mechanism by which bacteria defend themselves against viruses through the use of enzymes capable of cutting and joining DNA in a very precise way. This mechanism is used to edit the genome and insert the selected fragment exactly where one wants it. It is easy to see how this technology could be applied to the treatment of a disease, especially those in which a single gene in a somatic cell is affected: such is the case of sickle cell anemia, very common in areas affected by malaria. This technique is cheap, effective, and fast, making it a very powerful tool. The problem arises when, as Dr. He Jiankui did, it is used to incorporate a gene that gives the person immunity against HIV, which is not a treatment of a disease but rather an improvement of the person's condition. This improvement could be applied not only for resistance to a virus, but also for improving school or sports performance, which raises notable ethical challenges, especially when this editing affects germ cells, not just somatic ones. This means many of these changes could be inherited since we would be making a genetic edition that is transmissible to our offspring and we would begin to tip the evolutionary balance not by chance but deliberately. Today we are in a position to modify the human genome in a way we never imagined before; this requires much greater responsibility on the part of researchers and much greater control on the part of society. Dr. He Jianku was sentenced to jail for 3 years by the Chinese government, and he was released in 2023.

I have selected here 25 research examples that allow us to reflect on the communication and care of the person. I have elected to put aside research on radiation, surgery, torture, or mind control because the evidence of what we showed already seemed overwhelming.

What do these inhuman research projects have in common and why do they impact the credibility of the medical word?

What they show is that doctors, or at least some of them, do not always act in accordance with what they have sworn to do and that in many situations they have acted against other human beings as if they were something else.

Kings against subjects. Lords against vassals. Men against women. Adults against children. Whites against Blacks. Aryans against Jews. Japanese against Chinese. Free versus prisoners. Military against civilians. Intelligent versus deficient. Young against old. Born versus unborn.

Every time that the doctor has used some additional condition to that of simply being human in order to justify not treating a patient as a person, they have failed in their duty of care, they have experimented on those people, almost always facilitating their murder or exploitation.

Much of the loss of prestige that we have suffered in the last century is fully deserved due to the inhumane behavior of some colleagues and the complicit silence of numerous medical societies, which, far from punishing those who behaved incorrectly, have rewarded and placed them in seats of honor.

Taking care of our conduct gives credibility to our word. Our first conduct is to care for the sick person regardless of any other condition than simply being human.

Now we will focus on another aspect of the words that doctors use, the history of words through time: the etymology of medical terms.

4.3.1 Etymology of Medical Terms

Learning medicine is first and foremost about incorporating a language that has its roots in Western medicine in Greece, where many of the terms we use today come from; later many Latin terms were incorporated from the power and extension of the Roman Empire. In the last 25 centuries, it has incorporated terms from almost every country and language in the world.

Knowing this language helps us to not only make sense of the terms we use, but also to do justice to those who have preceded us and, on many occasions, it helps explain our findings and treatment options during a consultation.

I am going to select a few terms for each letter of the alphabet, simply to encourage anyone who is interested to go to their local library and consult specific texts on medical etymology, such as the extraordinary book written by Professor Henry Alan Skinner, *The Origin of Medical Terms,* from which we draw most of the etymologies.

We will develop below a minimum etymological recount of common terms:

4.3.2   A

- **A**: The letter a is a prefix of Greek origin that denotes negation: anemia (without blood)—a-cephalus (headless)-a-systole (without systole or heartbeat).
- **Abdomen**: Latin term meaning "containing."
- **Abduct**: Latin term meaning "to get away from" its use for the abductor muscles that move the leg away from the midline or for the sixth cranial nerve. Discovered by Eustachius and called abducens because when contracting the external rectus muscle, it moves the pupil away from the midline.
- **Acetabulum**: Latin term that refers to a small glass of vinegar; it is used to indicate a joint that is rounded and shallow.
- **Abort**: Latin term derived from aborior, to disappear like the sunset. In French, the word *avorter* was used to refer to the termination of a pregnancy and so it passed into English in 1580. Shakespeare uses it in Richard III, Act I, Sc2, "If ever he have child, abortive be it".
- **Achilles heel**: Refers to the Greek hero Achilles, who participated in the Trojan War and whose exploits were sung by Homer in the *Iliad*. The only weak point where he could be mortally wounded him was his ankle, where his mother held him when he was submerged in the waters of the River Styx to make him invulnerable.
- **Achondroplasia**: Term of Greek origin formed by three terms: a (without), chondro (cartilage), and plasia (formation). Disease in which there is no formation of growth plates and leads to dwarfism.
- **Achromatic**: Greek term that combines a (without) with chromatic (color). Devoid of color.
- **Acid**: Latin *acidus,* to be sour or sharp.
- **Acne**: For Hippocrates, it meant everything that emerged on the skin.
- **Acrodynia**: Greek word formed by two terms Acro (extremity) and dynia (pain). Pain in the extremities, very common with certain chemotherapy drugs such as oxaliplatin.
- **Actinic**: Greek term meaning "ray." It refers to the effects of radiation therapy.
- **Acupuncture**: Derived from the Latin *acu,* needle. Treatment technique introduced in China by Huang Ti, in approximately 3000 BC.
- **Aetiology**: Greek word formed by two terms: *Aetio* derived from *Airía*, a cause, and *logos,* reason or study. That is, the discipline that studies the origin or cause of diseases.
- **Alcohol**: Term derived from the Arabic "al-kohl," a fine, subtle, impalpable powder, probably originally referring to the antimony powder that ladies used to beautify their eyes. The transition from impalpable to spirit, just like the spirit of the wine, was easy.
- **Alexia**: From the Greek, a-(without) *lexicon* (word). Inability to read.
- **Amaurosis**: Term of Greek origin meaning darkness. Hippocrates used it for all progressive blindness.
- **Amnesia**: Greek a (without), *mnesis* (memory). Loss of memory.

- **Anesthesia**: Greek, *An* (privative or lacking), *Esthesis* (sensations) originally used to describe a sensory disturbance in some patients by Bailey in 1721. Today it is used mainly for sleep induction, pain control, and relaxation in surgeries.
- **Anaphylaxis**: Greek *An* (without) *Phylaxis* (protection); from this word is derived *phylactery* (guard or protection). Term devised to express lack of protection of the organism in certain circumstances. We owe the modern meaning of the term to Charles Richet in 1902. It is commonly used to refer to an allergic phenomenon that endangers life.
- **Antibiotic**: From the Greek *Anti* (against) *Bios* (life). Contrary to life. It refers to natural products generated mostly by bacteria or fungi that prevent the survival of other microbes. Later the term *chemotherapeutic* was used for anti-infective agents produced **artificially** in the laboratory. Currently, the term *antibiotic* is restricted to the use of drugs against infectious agents, while the term chemotherapy refers to the use of drugs against malignant tumors.
- **Arachnoid**: Greek *Arachnos* (spider) and *Eidos* (similar). It refers to an anatomical structure of the nervous system that looks like a spider web.
- **Asthma**: From the Greek, it means a blow or gasp. Hippocrates already used this term and Celsus in the first century of our era described it as severe respiratory distress, with noisy and wheezing breaths.
- **Atelectasis**: Word of Greek origin formed by two terms: *atelos* (incomplete or imperfect) and *ectasis* (expansion). That is, imperfect or incomplete expansion. Originally it referred to the lung of the newborn (*atelectasis pulmonum*) who has not breathed and had legal value since the child was considered to have been stillborn if the lung did not expand. The test was performed by placing the lung in water, if it floated, it had expanded, otherwise it was considered *atelectasis* and did not float. Today it is applied to the lack of expansion that is observed in the pulmonary segments located after a bronchial obstruction of infectious or tumor origin.
- **Auscultation**: From the Latin *auscultare*: to listen, to hear with attention. Direct or immediate auscultation (supporting the doctor 's ear on the patient's chest) to perceive the sounds of breathing is an ancient practice carried out by Hippocrates. Mediate or indirect auscultation through a device (the stethoscope) was an invention of the French clinician Hippolite Laennec in 1817.

4.3.3   B

- **Bacillus**: Latin term derived from *baculus*, a rod, similar to the one used by shepherds. It is used to identify different types of infectious agents.
- **Balsam**: Derived from the Latin *Balsamum*: fragrant gum. Some attribute its name to *Baal-Shemen*, a royal oil.
- **Basilic**: Name of the internal vein of the elbow crease, is the consequence of a bad translation from Arabic by Avicenna. The original term *Al-Basilik* (median vein) was translated as *basilica*, meaning majestic (it was the name that was

given to the great cathedrals), when in reality it is a smaller vein than the external vein, called *cephalic*.

– **Belladonna**: Term of Italian origin meaning beautiful lady. It refers to the extract of leaves and roots of the *Atropa belladonna* plant. The name refers to the popular belief that ladies used this extract to beautify themselves, dilating their pupils and brightening their eyes. The active principle of this formulation is atropine, which is what produces pupil dilation (*mydriasis*).
– **Beri-Beri**: Term of Sinhalese origin, meaning severely weakened [the repetition of *Beri* (weakness) tries to denote severity]. This condition is caused by vitamin B1 deficiency, nowadays the most frequent cause is alcoholism.
– **Bio**: Prefix of Greek origin meaning life. *Bio*-Chemistry, *Bio*logy.
– **Blepharitis**: Word of Greek origin formed by two terms: *Blefaron* (eyelid) and the suffix *itis* (inflammation). It refers to inflammation of the eyelid, often of bacterial origin.
– **Blood**: Term of Anglo-Saxon origin: *blod*. It is a term common to all Germanic languages (*blut* in German, for example).
– **Bolus**: Term of Latin origin meaning dough or lump, probably originally Hebrew: *balah*, to agglutinate.
– **Borborygmus**: Greek term used by Hippocrates himself, which refers to dull sounds of intestinal origin.
– **Botulism**: Derived from the Latin *botulus,* meaning sausage. It refers to a disease initially described in Germany in people who ate sausages, caused by the toxin of *Bacillus butulinus*.
– **Breast**: Derived from Anglo-Saxon: *breost*. In Germany, *brust*. The term refers to something that sprouts (a bursting; bursting forth or budding) referring to the female mammary gland that appears in adolescence and especially during lactation.
– **Bronchus**: Term of Greek origin meaning wind tube. It refers to the division that occurs in the trachea and carries air to each lung.
– **Bruise**: Term derived from Old French: *bruiser* (to break), a bruise with *ecchymosis* and then discoloration.
– **Bulla**: Latin term meaning bubble. It is used for lesions that form in the lung due to air entrapment or for bullous skin lesions.

4.3.4   C

– **Cachexia**: Derived from two Greek terms: *Kakós* = bad, and the word εξισ = *a hágito*. Probably an old term, already used by Galen to mean malnourished.
– **Cadaver**: Latin term to refer to the dead body. Probably derived from *cadere* = to fall.
– **Caecum**: From the Latin *caecus* = blind. The blind end of the large intestine.
– **Calculus**: A pebble. Diminutive of *clax*, a little limestone. It was used by Celso to refer to a small kidney stone, it is also used for gall stones. The term *calculus*

for mathematics, derives its name from the fact that small stones or beads (as in the Abacus) were used to make the accounts.

- **Calvaria**: Latin term for the vault of the cranium. Probably derived from *calvu* = bald because in older men this part of the head is often hairless.
- **Cancer**: Latin term meaning crab. It was first used by Hippocrates, probably in reference to breast cancer, in which the skin involvement extended from the areola to the base of the breast like the legs of a crab.
- **Canine**: Latin term meaning belonging to a dog. The reference to canine teeth in humans is very old, probably made by Aristotle and refers to the prominence of these teeth in the dog.
- **Carbuncle**: Latin term *carbunculus*, meaning a little live coal. It is a translation of the Greek term for this skin lesion: *anthrax*. It is an inflammation of the skin caused by a highly contagious bacillus.
- **Caries**: In Latin, it means dry rot, probably derived from Chaldean: *Carah*, meaning dead bone. Dental caries applies to the destruction of a tooth.
- **Carina**: Latin term that refers to the keel of a boat. In anatomy, it is related to the union of the right and left main *bronchi* to the *trachea*, as if a keel divided the incoming air into halves, one for each lung.
- **Carpus**: Latin term meaning wrist, which is used for the palm of the hand, but originally it meant the end of the arm, hence carpe diem.
- **Catharsis**: Greek term meaning cleansing or purification. Cathartic drugs were those that produced vomiting or diarrhea to purge the intestines.
- **Catheter**: Greek term used for something that is left or placed inside the body. The first rubber catheter in the history of medicine was invented by Auguste Nélaton in 1860.
- **Cauda**: Latin term to refer to the tail end, can derive both from *cadere* = to fall *coda* = to end.
- **Causalgia**: Word formed by two Greek terms: $\kappa\alpha\nu\sigma\iota\varsigma$ = heat, burn, and *algos* = pain; it refers to a severe pain in which the patient feels that a part of his body is being burned. It is a neuropathic pain that can be perceived after herpetic neuritis or after a limb amputation, as phantom limb pain. The same root $\kappa\alpha\nu\sigma\iota\varsigma$ = heat can be found in **Caustic** = that burns; o **Cautery**: which originally consisted of a hot iron that was used to close wounds.
- **Cell**: Term of Latin origin, *cella* = small room or compartment. Although the term itself is very old, its modern application to refer to biological structure began in 1665 when Robert Hooke studied a section of a cork under a microscope.
- **Cerebellum**: Latin term that is a diminutive of *cerebrum* = brain, that is to say, it means: little brain.
- **Chiasma**: Term of Greek origin $\kappa\iota\alpha\sigma\mu\alpha$ = mark of the letter X, in anatomy the term Chiasma, the reference to the optic Chiasma where the nerve bundles of the optic nerves intersect and allow binocular vision, was made by Rufus of Ephesus.
- **Cholera**: Greek term formed by two words: $\kappa o\lambda\eta$': meaning bile and $\rho\varepsilon\lambda\nu$ = flow. In other words, profuse diarrhea in which a yellowish matter that looks like bile flows unstoppably. It is a bacterial disease that causes great mortality in developing countries.

– **Claudication**: From the Latin *claudicare*, to clean or be licked.
– **Clavicula**: From the Latin *claviculum*, diminutive of *clavis,* a key. It is used to identify the bone that goes from the shoulder to the sternum, which closes the thorax as if it were a key in armor. The term **Conclave**, which is used for the Papal election, refers to the fact that the cardinals will remain in a locked room until the election is finished.
– **Clinic**: From the Greek $\kappa\lambda\iota\nu\eta$ = bed. It refers to the activity of the doctor "at the bed's side." The terms *recumbent or inclined* have the same root.
– **Colostomy**: Word formed by two Greek terms: $\kappa\omega\lambda o\nu$ = colon and $\omega\tau o\mu\alpha$ = mouth. It refers to an artificial opening of the colon to the abdominal wall. It is used temporarily or permanently to resolve an intestinal obstruction.
– **Curriculum**: Latin term meaning a race, from *currere,* to run. *Curriculum vitae* (CV) describes a person's professional life career.

4.3.5   D

– **Débridement**: Term of French origin meaning *de,* plus *bride*, bridle. It was used to describe the cutting away of tissue. It is used above all in the opening of abscesses so that the pus from the multiple cavities flows through internal scars.
– **Decubitus**: Term of Latin origin meaning lay down.
– **Deglutition**: From the Latin, swallowed, the act of swallowing, from *de* (down) plus *glutere*, to swallow.
– **Delirium**: From the Latin formed by the words *De* (from) and the word *lira,* a furrow. It refers to getting out of the groove, like water overflowing from a ditch. In medicine, it is speech that overflows from the normal course.
– **Dengue**: Also called "break-bone fever," is an African term of Swahili origin *dinga,* for sudden cramps or seizure. It is a viral agent transmitted by mosquitoes that mainly affects tropical regions.
– **Depilate**:From the Latin *Depilare*, to remove hair.
– **Detrusor**: From the Latin *detrudo*, to thrust away or down. It refers to the bladder muscle that contracts to make urine flow.
– **Dexter**: From the Latin right. Derived from Sanskrit, the worshiping priests of the sun, when they looked at the rising sun, pointed to the south with their right hand: south in Sanskrit is *dekkan,* and they associated it with the word *dhu,* that is to say, the shining manor, while the left hand, *sinister*, pointed to the cold and dark north.
– **Diabetes**: From the Greek $\delta\iota\alpha\beta\eta\tau\eta\varsigma$ = a siphon, referring to the high urinary flow (*polyuria*) that people affected by this metabolic disorder have.
– **Diaphragma**: From the Greek $\delta\iota\alpha\phi\rho\alpha\gamma\mu\alpha$ = a wall across, refers to the muscle perpendicular to the spine that separates the abdominal thoracic cavity in two, forms the base of the thorax and the roof of the abdomen.

- **Diastole**: Greek term meaning a prolongation or pause and refers to the relaxation period of the ventricular muscle in which it fills with blood, and then expels it through ventricular contraction or *systole*.
- **Diathesis**: Greek term meaning to arrange in order to draw up a plan or an outline of a drawing or painting. Aristotle used this term to refer to a person's body disposition, especially when affected by a disease. The temperament or natural disposition of a person was initially analyzed by Erasistratus, who was said to be a grandson of Aristotle and among many of his discoveries were those of heart valves.
- **Didelphys**: Word formed by two Greek terms $\delta\iota\varsigma$ = twice or double and the word $\delta\epsilon\lambda\phi\upsilon\varsigma$ = uterus. Term that designates the person who has two uteruses. The complete division of the uterus and double vagina in humans is very rare, but not the incomplete division giving rise to a *bicornuate* uterus (with two horns) instead of the normal pear shape.
- **Diet**: Term of Greek origin $\delta\iota\alpha\iota\tau\alpha$. It was used as a lifestyle, a way of living, with respect to food, clothing, and work. Later he restricted himself to a ration of food.
- **Diphtheria**: Term derived from the Greek $\delta\iota\phi\theta\epsilon\rho\alpha$, a leather vellum. It refers to the exudation that covers the pharynx like a veil or a membrane in the bacterial disease that receives this name.
- **Disc**: Greek term $\delta\iota\sigma\kappa o\varsigma$, which was a flat and round piece of metal or stone that was used in competitions, especially in Sparta. The term persisted for all structures that are similar in shape, especially for intervertebral discs.
- **Dislocation**: Latin term meaning out of place, derived from *dislocare* (*dis* = apart and *locus* = place). It has been used since the time of Hippocrates for the displacement of a bone from a joint.
- **Distillation**: Term of Latin origin, *distillatus*, which derives from *destillare*, meaning "to fall in drops." It is described by the Egyptians, in Thebes, and the Arabs used a container called an alembic for distillation. Lately, the coil and a cooling method that increase the efficiency of distillation were added to the still.
- **Doctor**: From the Latin *doctus*, a teacher, derived from *docere*, to teach. The content of this education received the term of *doctrine*.
- **Dose**: Greek term $\delta o\sigma\iota\varsigma$ meaning what is given. It was used by Homer in reference to a gift. Galen used it in its current sense: the amount of a remedy to be given.
- **Duodenum**: Latin term meaning twelve. It is the first part of the small intestine, measuring twelve finger widths and surrounding the head of the pancreas.

4.3.6 E

- **Ecchymosis**: Term of Greek origin $\epsilon\kappa X\upsilon\mu\omega\sigma\iota\varsigma$, meaning extravasation, leakage of blood from the vessels into the interstitium of the tissue, Hippocrates already used it in this sense 2500 years ago.

- **Eclampsia**: Word of Greek origin meaning bright light. It is a clinical condition of toxemia of pregnancy and the patient may have flashes of light seen before the eyes.
- **Ectropion**: Greek word meaning to turn around. In this condition, the eyelid turns upside down and exposes the conjunctiva that covers the inner part.
- **Eczema**: Greek term that designates any hot (inflammatory) eruption that occurs on the skin.
- **Elbow**: Term of Anglo-Saxon origin: *elboga*, the prefix el refers to the L-shape of this articulation and the term *vogue* refers to an arc.
- **Elephantiasis**: Greek term meaning elephant-like. The ancient Greeks applied this concept to leprosy due to the thickness of the skin, but the Arabs applied it to chronic edema of both lower limbs where the accumulated fluid gives them the shape of voluminous columns and the skin acquires a greater thickness.
- **Elixir**: *iksir* is a term of Arab origin, which refers to the medium through which a transformation is carried out. It is applied in pharmacy to the medium in which a substance can be diluted.
- **Embolus**: Word of Greek origin $\varepsilon\mu\beta o\lambda o\varsigma$, to place or throw a stopper through a tube. It is used in medicine to designate a thrombus (blood clot) that has dislodged and travels through the blood.
- **Emesis**: Greek word $\varepsilon\mu\varepsilon\rho\iota\varsigma$, meaning to vomit. It was already used by Hippocrates to designate vomiting and substances that cause vomiting.
- **Endemic**: Word of Greek origin formed by two terms $\varepsilon\nu$ = in and $\delta\eta\mu o\varsigma$, meaning town, that is to say, "in the town," originating in the town, native. Said of the conditions that are constantly present in a certain region or population. The term has been used since the time of Hippocrates, where they described the conditions of the air, water, land, and eating habits of the inhabitants of different regions.
- **Epidemic**: Term of Greek origin $\varepsilon\pi\iota\delta\eta\mu o\varsigma$, formed by two words $\varepsilon\pi\iota$, meaning on, and $\delta\eta\mu o\varsigma$, meaning people. It is applied as popular, prevalent, or current. They are those conditions that occurred seasonally or infrequently and affected the majority of the people (while the endemic ones were constant and could affect few, the epidemics are inconstant and affect many), the great epidemics are called pandemics [the term Pan ($\pi\alpha\nu$ = means everyone as in *Pan*orama = total vision or *Pan*creas = all meat)]. Today its use is restricted to those conditions that affect most of the countries in the world, such as the recent Covid-19 pandemic.
- **Epididymis**: Greek term $\varepsilon\pi\iota\delta\upsilon\delta\iota\mu\iota\varsigma$, meaning over the testicles (the term $\Delta\upsilon\delta\iota\mu o\iota$ means twins and is an ancient term that was used for both the testicles and the ovaries).
- **Epilepsy**: Greek term $\varepsilon\pi\iota\lambda\varepsilon\psi\iota\alpha$, meaning seizure. It was defined that way by Aristotle and has been used since the time of Hippocrates. It was also called a sacred disease as it was interpreted as the result of an abrupt punishment from the gods, in which the person fell and began to move involuntarily, like a puppet being moved by strings. It was also called Hercules disease due to the enormous strength that a person in the middle of an epileptic seizure has in their limbs and jaw.

- **Erotic**: Greek term related to passionate love, sexual desire, unlike *Agape,* which was the Greek term reserved for charitable love.
- **Eunuch**: Greek term *ευνουΧος*, which literally means bed-keeper. This is because they were males who had had their testicles removed and took care of the women's bedroom in the harems. Its Latin equivalent is *castrate* and during the eighteenth and nineteenth centuries in numerous European churches it was used in pre-adolescent youth (*Castrati*) in the choir so that they would preserve the brilliance of their voices and not alter their registers due to the effect of testosterone.

4.3.7 F

- **Falciform**: Term of Latin origin formed by two words: *Falcis* = a scythe and *Form* = shape. The best-known falciform ligament is the one that supports the liver and the anterior wall of the abdomen.
- **Farina**: Term of Latin origin meaning meal, derived from far meaning grain of any kind.
- **Fascia**: Means band or bandage.
- **Fauces**: Latin term to define narrow passages that connect two rooms or enclosures.
- **Febris**: Latin term for fever.
- **Finger**: Term of Teutonic origin, it means digit and probably derives from an ancient way of saying five.
- **Flatus**: Term of Latin origin meaning blowing, from flare a blow.
- **Folium**: Latin term meaning leaf.
- **Foramen**: Latin term meaning hole, drift from outside, to bare a hole.
- **Forensic** : Latin term related to forum, public, or judicial court. Applies to legal medicine.
- **Fremitus**: Latin term derived from *Fremere*, to murmur, to roar. It is a vibration perceived by the hand, both when the patient speaks in the respiratory examination and when there is fibrinous pericarditis detected in the cardiac examination.
- **Fusiform**: Latin term meaning spindle shape, applies to both muscle tissue cells and the shape of certain muscles.

4.3.8 G

- **Galactos**: Term of Greek origin to refer to milk, *γαλαΚτος* = milk. It is used in all terms related to the content of milk (sugar = *galactose*) or the mammary gland or its canaliculi.
- **Gamete**: Greek term with which both the husband and the wife were called since it derives from *γαμειν*, marriage. It is the term used to designate the sperm (male

gamete) and the egg (female gamete), specialized cells equipped with half the chromosomes (23 instead of 46) and destined for fertilization.
- **Ganglion**: Greek term $\gamma\alpha\gamma\gamma\lambda\iota o\upsilon$, used by Hippocrates to define a tumor under the skin. It is caused by the accumulation of synovial fluid in a small herniation of the capsule of a joint, frequently the back of the wrist.
- **Gastric**: Derivative of the Latin *Gastricus*, derived in turn from the Greek $\gamma\alpha\sigma\tau\eta\rho$, stomach or bell. It is named numerous times in the *Iliad* and the *Odyssey* by Homer.
- **Gene**: Term derived from the Greek $\gamma\varepsilon\upsilon\upsilon\alpha\omega$ = I produce. It is used to define a piece of DNA that encodes a hereditary character.
- **Genu**: Term derived from the Latin meaning knee. Probably derived from Sanskrit *anu*.
- **Geriatrics**: Word formed by two Greek terms: $\gamma\varepsilon\rho\omega\upsilon$ = old man and the term $\iota\alpha\tau\rho\varepsilon\iota\alpha$ = medical treatment. It is the study and treatment of diseases of the elderly. Even though the concern about this topic goes back to the first years of the last century, today it is even more important since the elderly increasingly represent a greater proportion of the patients assisted by the health system.
- **Glaucoma**: Term of Greek origin meaning shiny or silvery and was used by both Hippocrates and Aristotle in reference to cataracts. It was only in the nineteenth century that we discovered it was a condition related to increased pressure in the anterior chamber of the eye.
- **Glioma**: Tumor originating in glia, described by Rudolf Virchow in 1869.
- **Glottis**: Greek term that designates the attic of the tongue. Galen used this term to refer to the entire larynx, but in the eighteenth century Morgagni limited the term *Glottis* to the upper part of the larynx where the vocal cords are located.
- **Gluten**: Term of Greek origin, for glue or paste, and refers to the insoluble protein in wheat or other grains. It is the cause of dietary intolerance in celiac patients.
- **Gonorrhoea**: Greek term that literally means flow of semen. It was already described by Aristotle, and Galen later described the flow caused by the bacterial infection of this sexually transmitted disease erroneously as semen flow. It is already described in the *Ebers Papyrus*, the Bible describes it as a disease of the urethra generated after living with an infected woman, and Herodotus described it as a disease of women.
- **Gout**: From the Latin *gutta*, a drop. Also called *podagra*, it was considered to be an inflammation of the joints, especially of the big toe, caused by a distillate that dripped into the joint. It was described by Hippocrates, Galen, and Celsus. It mainly affected wealthy people who ate a diet rich in meat since it is produced by an excess of uric acid.
- **Grippe**: French term to designate influenza. It means convulsive attack due to the abrupt and severe fever that made the patient tremble.
- **Gynaecology**: Word of Greek origin that unites two terms: $\gamma\iota\upsilon\alpha\iota\kappa o\varsigma$ = woman and $\lambda o\gamma o\varsigma$ = treated or study. It is the branch of medicine that is dedicated to the study and treatment of diseases that affect women.

4.3.9   H

- **Haema**: Word of Greek origin αιμα, meaning blood. It is combined in numerous words, mostly of French origin, as a prefix denoting related to blood.
- **Halitosis**: Word of Latin origin, *halitus*, meaning breath or vapor. It is used to denote bad breath.
- **Hallux**: Latin term meaning big toe.
- **Head**: Anglo-Saxon term probably originating from the German: *Haupt*. It is the upper part of a body that is connected to the rest of the body by a neck.
- **Heart**: Term of Anglo-Saxon origin, probably derived from the German *Herz*, and this in turn from the Sanskrit *hrid*. It refers, like the term Hearth, to the origin of heat. For the first anatomists the heart were the ventricles, while the atria (atria) were considered ventricular appendages.
- **Hepa**: Greek term εεπαρ meaning liver. Already used in the *Iliad* and the *Odyssey* by Homer. It is used as a prefix of numerous words that denote a relationship with the liver (hepatitis, hepatoma). Heparin is an anticoagulant compound originally isolated from the liver.
- **Hernia**: Latin term meaning rupture or protrusion.
- **Herpes**: Term of Greek origin, used to describe skin conditions that extend by contiguity (ερπειυ = to creep), and was used by Hippocrates. Galen described three types of herpes, and until the eighteenth century numerous skin conditions were included under this name. Today it is limited to conditions caused by herpesvirus.
- **Hiatus**: Latin term to refer to opening or gap.
- **Hormone**: Term of Greek origin meaning to arouse or set in motion. It was originally used by Hippocrates referring to the vital principle generated in an organism.
- **Hospital**: Term of Latin origin derived from *hospitium*, guest house; although the first hospitals date from Roman times, they reappeared in large numbers during the Middle Ages when they were created by religious orders along the path of the crusades to attend to the pilgrims who were going to or returning from Jerusalem.
- **Hymen**: Greek term meaning membrane. It was not restricted to the use of the vaginal membrane (it was also used for the pericardium and peritoneum); however, *Hymen* and *Hymenaeus* are terms related to marriage. Vesalius limited its use to the vaginal membrane.
- **Hypo**: Greek prefix meaning below or deficient.
- **Hyper**: Greek prefix meaning over or exceeded.

4.3.10   I

– **Ichthyosis**: Term of Greek origin derived from *Ichtios,* meaning fish. It is a scaly skin condition, in which it is covered with scales.
– **Icterus**: Greek term used to refer to a yellow bird. It is another name for jaundice, from the yellow color of the skin and conjunctivae due to the accumulation of bilirubin.
– **Ileum**: Greek term meaning twisted, to refer to the small intestine that gives countless turns in the abdomen, unlike the stomach and duodenum that are relatively fixed and the colon that develops as a frame of the small intestine.
– **Immunity**: Term of Latin origin, derived from *immunitas*, exception. Especially related to the exception to provide a public or military service in Rome. In medicine, it is used as a synonym for protection against infectious diseases.
– **Impetigo**: Term of Latin origin meaning attack or invasion. It is used in relation to acute skin infections.
– **Incision**: Term of Latin origin meaning to cut.
– **Incubation**: Term of Latin origin that means to sit or lie down to wait. It was originally used in Homer's time for practice in the temples of the Aesculapians, where the first stage of healing was to incubate sleep. In the eighteenth century, it was used in the modern sense of the period between contagion and the appearance of an infectious disease.
– **Infarct**: Term of Latin origin derived from *infarcire*: to stuff, to fill up. Originally related to the localized accumulation of a humor. Today we use it to refer to hemorrhage and necrosis secondary to arterial obstruction.
– **Infirmary**: Term of Latin origin meaning weak, formed by two terms *in* = not and *firmus* = strong.
– **In situ**: Two terms of Latin origin that mean *in place*. In pathology, it refers to the alterations of the tissues that do not invade neighboring structures; they remain in their place.
– **Insula**: Latin term for island. Insulin is a hormone extracted from the islet cells (Langerhans cells) of the pancreas, hence its name.
– **Inter**: Latin preposition meaning between.
– **Intra**: Latin preposition meaning inside.
– **Introvert**: Word of Latin origin formed by two terms: *intro* = inside together with *verteré* = to turn. It is used for the mood condition in which the subject is more interested in their own emotions than in their environment.
– **Isotope**: Term of Greek origin formed by two terms: *iso* = equal; *moles* = place. Used for atoms that have the same atomic number (protons) but different atomic weights (neutrons).

4.3.11   J

- **Jaundice**: Term of French origin, derived from *Jaune* = yellow. It refers to the yellow color of the skin and mucous membranes due to the accumulation of bilirubin.
- **Jejunum**: Latin term meaning empty or hungry. *Jejunum* was the first breakfast of the Romans and the first portion of the intestine, immediately after the *duodenum*, was always empty; therefore, both Aristotle and Galen called this portion fasting, which was translated into Latin as *jejunum*.
- **Joint**: Latin term for uniting. Derived from *jungere*, to join.

4.3.12   K

- **Keloid**: Term of Greek origin formed by two words *Keilé* = tumor or hernia and *Eidos* = similar to. It refers to the excessive growth of a skin scar, especially those on the chest, as if it were a tumor.
- **Keratin**: Greek term meaning horn. It is a protein found in *faneras*: oven or nails.

4.3.13   L

- **Labium**: Latin term for lip. Derived from a Greek term that means *to lap up* due to taking or receiving food.
- **Laparotomy**: Greek term formed by two words $\lambda\alpha\pi\alpha\rho\alpha$, meaning soft, and *otomy*, meaning to cut or to open. It is used for incisions made in the abdomen, between the ribs and the hip. Originally performed only on the flank, today most laparotomies are performed along the midline. When the procedure is done only to observe, the term *Laparoscopy* is used, *scopere* = observe. In general, these latter procedures are currently done through small openings with optical instruments.
- **Leech**: Term of Anglo-Saxon origin meaning a healer. It refers to an animal commonly known as "blood sucker" whose therapeutic use dates back to India. In the West, their use has been recorded since the second century.
- **Leprosy**: Term of Greek origin $\lambda\epsilon\pi\rho\alpha$ meaning scaly. Literally means "the scaly disease." Probably the disease that we know today as leprosy has been described in ancient times as *Leontiasis or Elephantiasis*, and many cases of leprosy described in antiquity have been eczema or psoriasis, even with the instructions described for its diagnosis in biblical texts, especially Leviticus.
- **Lethal**: Derived from the Latin *Letum* = death, in turn taken from the Greek *Lethes*, which was the river from which the souls of the dead drank, in their transit to the afterlife, to forget the past.

- **Leukemia or Leucemia**: A term devised by Virchow in which he combines the Latin word *Leuco* = white with *hemia* = blood, to refer to a condition in which abnormal white blood cells are in large numbers in the peripheral blood.
- **Libido**: Term of Latin origin meaning lust or desire. Derived from *libet* = it pleases.
- **Liver**: Term of Anglo-Saxon origin, *Lifer*, whose etymological origin is unknown but probably related to Life.
- **Lumbar**: Latin term to refer to the region related to the loins.
- **Lung**: Term of Anglo-Saxon origin *Lunge*, related to *lungre,* meaning lightly, referring to the ability to float in water.
- **Lupus**: Latin term used to designate wolf. Different authors state that the designation of the disease is due to the fact that it destroys tissues with the voracity of a wolf.
- **Lymph**: Latin term meaning clear water and is a corruption of the Greek *Nymphae*, who were the goddesses of rivers, lakes, and the forest. In medicine, it refers to the clear fluid that comes out of the lymphatic capillaries.

4.3.14   M

- **Macro**: Prefix of Greek origin meaning large or long.
- **Macula**: Latin term meaning small spot or blemish. Probably of Sanskrit origin: *mala* = dirt or Hebrew: *machala* = blemish.
- **Malaria**: Word of Italian origin *mal aria* = bad air. Probably from associating malaria, transmitted by mosquitoes, with the swampy areas where it proliferates abundantly.
- **Malignant**: Word of Latin origin meaning to do anything maliciously (*malus* = bad, *genus* = origin). In pathology, it is applied to tumors that grow uncontrollably and can give rise to metastasis.
- **Mamma**: Term of Latin origin to refer to breast. Derived from the Greek $\mu\alpha\mu\mu\alpha$, with the same meaning and probably derived from the sound of the suckling child "ma-ma "that is common in many languages.
- **Medicine**: Word of Latin origin meaning the art of healing, derived from *Medeor* or doctor, to heal or cure.
- **Medulla**: Latin term for marrow, probably derived from *medius* = middle. The marrow of bones was *in medio ossis*, in the middle of the bone.
- **Meiosis**: Term of Greek origin meaning decrease or loss. Although it was used since the time of Hippocrates to record, for example, the reduction of fever, its modern use dates from 1887 when Weismann postulated that gametes should decrease the genetic content in half before fertilization.
- **Melan**: Greek term meaning black. It is the prefix of numerous terms (*Melan*cholia = depression; *Melan*oma = a skin malignant tumor, *Melaena* = black feces due to intestinal bleeding).

- **Microscope**: Term of Greek origin formed by two words: *micro* = small and *scope* = to see. It consists of the use of lenses to be able to observe the structure of the tissues.
- **Migraine**: Latin term *hemicrania* (half skull), which in medieval Latin became *migraine* and from there became French *migraine*. It is a special type of headache that affects one half of the skull, often beginning with ocular symptoms and ending with vomiting. The post-migraine lull is a moment of ecstasy, which is why some famous migraineurs, such as Goethe, asked their doctors not to treat them.
- **Morphine**: Opium alkaloid, extracted in 1805 by Adolf Sertürner, who invited four friends for dessert after dinner and induced them to a deep sleep, for which he named it *Morphium,* in honor of Morpheus, the god of sleep. It is one of the most useful drugs to calm cancer pain.
- **Mosquito**: Term of Spanish origin diminutive of *mosca*; it means little fly.
- **Myopia**: Greek term meaning to close or shut the eye. Those people affected with myopia looking at a distant object narrowing the lids.

4.3.15 N

- **Naevus**: Term of Latin origin meaning a birthmark. Originally limited to congenital moles. Currently, it has been extended to name any mole on the body.
- **Nausea**: Term of Greek origin meaning ship ($\nu\alpha\upsilon\varsigma$) originally reserved for dizziness and vomiting related to navigation; in fact, Hippocrates reserved this term for sea sickness. Currently, it has been extended to the sensations that precede vomiting, the most frequent cause of nausea in oncology is chemotherapy and radiotherapy.
- **Nephr -**: Prefix of Greek origin meaning kidney or related to the kidney ($\nu\varepsilon\theta\rho o\varsigma$) and is used in numerous terms (*Nephro*logy; *Nephr*ectomy; *Nephr*itis).
- **Neutrophil**: Term formed by a word of Latin origin *Neutro* = neither and the Greek term *philos* = fond. This term was created by Paul Ehrlich to refer to blood cells that did not take any dye, did not stain blue like *basophils* or red like *eosinophils*; therefore, they were neither, *neutrophils*.
- **Node**: Term of Latin origin, *nodus* a Knot. From Sanskrit *gandh*, to grasp. In clinic, the word Node refers to lymph node and is one of the crucial elements for tumor staging: TNM (tumor/node/ =metastasis).

4.3.16 O

- **Oculos**: Term of Latin origin meaning eye.
- **Olecranon**: Greek term to signify the point of the elbow. The superior end of the ulna.

- **Olfactory**: Latin term for smelling, derived from *olfactus* (*olere* = to smell and *factus* = to make).
- **Orthopnea**: Term of Greek origin meaning upright (*orthos*) breathing (*penuma*). The term was used by Hippocrates to describe the condition of asthmatic patients who make the maximum effort to breathe. It is also seen in heart failure.
- **Ovary**: Latin term meaning egg receptacle. We must note that the female gonad did not receive this designation in ancient texts, but was called female testis.

4.3.17   P

- **Paediatrics**: Term of Greek origin that unites two words ραις = a child together with ιατρεια = a healing. In other words, a medical discipline that deals with the study and treatment of children's diseases.
- **Pallid**: Latin term meaning pale, from Sanskrit *palita* = gray.
- **Pallium**: Latin term derived from *pellis* = skin, to refer to a cloak to cover yourself from the elements. From this term derives palliative care whose objective is to alleviate the suffering of incurable patients.
- **Panacea**: Greek term to define a medicine capable of curing everything.
- **Parathyroid**: Word of Greek origin meaning next to the thyroid. It refers to four endocrine glands located next to the thyroid that regulate phospho -calcium metabolism.
- **Parotid**: Greek word to designate the gland that is next (*Para*) to the ear (*otis*).
- **Pastille**: From the Latin *pastillus*, a little loaf, diminutive of *pastus* = food.
- **Pathos**: Greek term used by Hippocrates to describe a state of distress and suffering.
- **Pedicle**: Latin term meaning little foot. Derived from *pedis,* foot.
- **Pellagra**: Term of Greek origin meaning skin disease. Today we know that it is due to a vitamin deficiency.
- **Penis**: Latin term meaning tail. The term is derived from *pendere* = to hang down.
- **Peri**: Greek prefix meaning around (it is used in many terms: *Peri*cardium; *Peri*lymph; *Peri*osteum).
- **Pharmacy**: Word of Greek origin φαρμακον = a drug.
- **Physician**: Word of Greek origin meaning according to natural laws, derived from φυσις = nature.
- **Pill**: Latin word meaning little ball.
- **-Placenta**: Latin word meaning cake. It designates the organ in charge of the nutrition of the fetus during its intrauterine development, which has the shape of a cake.
- **Plague**: Greek term meaning a stroke. Originally it applied to any destructive pestilence that abruptly affected a population.
- **Pleura**: Greek term designating the ribs. It was also used in the current sense to designate the membrane that covers both the ribs (parietal pleura) and the lung (visceral pleura).

- **Prefix**: Many Greek and Latin prepositions have been used to form medical terms. The following is a sample of them: *auto-*(self); *bi-*(two); *contra-*(against); *dys-*(bad); *hemi-*(half); *leuc-*(white); *meta-*(among or after); *pro-*(before); *tri-*(three).
- **Pulse**: Latin term meaning to push or beating. The Greeks correctly related the pulse to the movement of the blood and the movement of the heart, but it was not until the seventeenth century that William Harvey correctly related the pulse to the ejection of blood through the left ventricle.
- **Pus**: Latin word originating from the Sanskrit *pu,* meaning corrupt or putrid. It was not until late in the nineteenth century that Joseph Lister, applying the discoveries of Louis Pasteur, considered that pus was a manifestation of a germ-contaminated wound and gave rise to surgical antisepsis.
- **Pyrexia**: Greek term for feverishness, derived from $\pi\upsilon\rho$ = fire.

4.3.18   Q

- **Quinine**: Term derived from the Peruvian natives, *Kina or Quina*, bark.

4.3.19   R

- **Radiology**: Term derived from the Latin *Radius* and the Greek *logos* = study or treatise. It refers to the study of the diagnostic or therapeutic medical applications of radiation.
- **Rectus**: Latin term for straight or upright. Aristotle described the straight passage from the lower bowel to the anus.
- **Rete**: Latin term for net or mesh.
- **Retro**: Latin adverb meaning backward or behind.

4.3.20   S

- **Sacrum**: Term derived from the Latin meaning sacred or holy. The application of this name to the sacrum bone is not entirely clear; some attribute it to the fact that it is the largest bone in the spine, others to the fact that it is one of the last bones to disappear in the corpse, and others to the fact that it protects the genital organs.
- **Salpinx**: Greek term with which they referred to a straight trumpet. In anatomy, it applies to the Fallopian tube, which exit the uterus and receive the oocyte after ovulation.
- **Scala**: Latin term meaning ladder.

– **Scapula**: Latin term for shoulder blades.
– **Scarlatina**: From the Italian *scarlatto* = scarlet, and this in turn derives from the Arabic *saqarlat*. The disease takes its name from the color of the skin rash.
– **Sciatic**: Latin term resulting from the corruption of the Greek term ισΧιαδικος (Ischiaticos), which refers to pain in the loins.
– **Scoliosis**: Greek term meaning curvature. It is applied to the deviations of the vertebral column.
– **Skeleton**: Term that for the Greeks meant dried. They applied it mostly to bodies mummified by exposure to air and did not use it in the modern sense of referring to human bones.
– **Stenosis**: Greek term meaning narrowing.
– **Suffix**: Numerous suffixes of Greek or Latin origin are used in medical terms. The following list some of them: *-algia* (pain); *-cele* (hernia); *-ectomy* (extraction); *—itis* (inflammation); *-oma* (tumor); *-opia* (see); *-tomy* (cutting); *-phobia* (fear).
– **Surgeon**: Word of Greek origin formed by two terms: Χειρ (hand) and εργου (work). He who works with his hands.
– **Suture**: Latin term meaning a seam. In Greek, the equivalent is *raphe*.
– **Syphilis**: Venereal disease, which took the name of a poem written by Girolamo Fracastoro and published in Venice in 1530: *Syphillis sive Morbus Gallicus*.

4.3.21   T

– **Talus**: Term derived from the Latin meaning ankle, the ankle bone.
– **Tampon**: Word derived from French meaning a bung or a plug. They were used since ancient times, even in the time of Hippocrates but they were called *Pessaries*.
– **Tenesmus**: Term of Greek origin meaning straining.
– **Testicle**: Latin term meaning witness: one who testifies. The presence of the testis was evidence of virility, and under Roman law no man was admissible as witness if they lacked testes.
– **Thrombus**: Term of Greek origin meaning to lump or a clot.
– **Thyroid**: Term of Greek origin meaning in the shape of an oblong shield. It refers to what looks like the shield of the trachea. It is a term used by Homer in the *Odyssey* and was applied to a shield used by Minoan soldiers that covered them from neck to knee.
– **Tibia**: Latin term to refer to pipe or flute. It refers to the leg bone, and it is not known if it received or gave its name to the musical instrument of reference.
– **Tourniquet**: Word of French origin meaning to turn. It is applied to generate compression and stop bleeding in the limbs.

4.3.22   U

- **Ulcer**: Term derived from the Latin *ulcus*: a sore.
- **Ulna**: Latin term for elbow.
- **Unciform**: Latin term for a hook-shaped structure.
- **Urticaria**: Latin term to designate a skin lesion that itches or burns.

4.3.23   V

- **Vaccine: Latin term to describe cow pox.**
- **Vagina: Term derived from the Latin meaning a sheath. It was a common term applied by Roman soldiers to the genitals: vagina for the female and gladius for the penis.**
- **Varicella: Latin term to describe chicken pox.**
- **Variola: Latin term to describe smallpox.**
- **Vector: Latin term to describe one that bears, carries, or conveys anything.**
- **Venereal: Latin term that expresses relative to Venus, the goddess of love.**
- **Veterinary: Latin term derived from veterinarius, a cattle doctor. It is a very old term that goes back to the fifth century of our era.**

4.3.24   W

- **Water**: Anglo-Saxon term derived from the Germanic *Wasser*. Until the seventeenth century, it was considered an elemental substance, then it was found to be made up of hydrogen and oxygen.
- **Whiskey**: Word of Gaelic origin *usquebaugh* or *usque beatha*, water of life.

4.3.25   X

- **Xanthoma**: Word derived from the Greek meaning yellow tumor.

4.3.26   Y

- **Yeast**: Word derived from Teutonic (*jesan or gesan*) meaning fermented.

4.3.27   Z

- **Zero**: Word derived from the Arabic *zefiro or cipher* = an empty thing. It is part of the Arabic numerals and was unknown to the Romans.

As we can see in this brief sample, each word has a history and that history is the legacy of an idea, of very different origins, and for more than 25 centuries they have been expanding the colloquial and medical language.

To this we must add the acronyms that have proliferated in medicine since the second half of the twentieth century and that we can find as common medical abbreviations (https://www.asha.org/practice-portal/professional-issues/documentation-in-health-care/common-medical-abbreviations/): like MRI (magnetic resonance imaging), CAT scan (computed axial tomography), ALS (amyotrophic lateral sclerosis), and many more.

As you can see by going through these acronyms, it would be surprisingly easy to write something that would make a lot of sense to the health team but be completely unintelligible to the patient or their family.

Something like this:

"The patient has been admitted to the A&O hospital with a diagnosis of ALS with involvement of the C5, C6, and D8 metameres on the right side. He came to do an MRI, but on the way to the study he had a VF due to an MI, so he is now in the ICU."

Unless you have taken the trouble to memorize the table of abbreviations, it is quite reasonable that you would not understand anything.

If we put together the medical terms, acronyms, and abbreviations that we doctors, nurses, pharmacists, and other members of the health team use, we would find ourselves with a completely new language with more than 55,000 terms learned by students who finish medicine that are unknown to most people [9].

Hence, one of the most important roles of the doctor in communication with the patient is to translate what is happening to the patient and the results of the studies into an understandable language that can be easily understood by the patient and their relatives.

4.4   The Role of the Doctor as Translator and Humanizer of Health Information

What does translate mean?

Translation is a process by which what was originally expressed in one language is expressed in a different language.

Therefore, the translator has the challenge of selecting the terms that will transmit with greater fidelity what was originally expressed.

Many times a translation that is completely straight (a literal translation) is completely unsuitable to transmitting the intent of the original author (as happens, for example, with puns or wordplay unique to each language). Therefore, between accuracy and clarity, the translator often chooses clarity.

Translating from medical language to the nonmedical language of the patient requires the same effort.

The translator's first gesture must be to know what the patient or their relatives are interested in knowing since medical truth is not a truth that leaves us indifferent, it affects our person, our life, and our decisions. Not everyone agrees that the truth should always be told or that any truth is equally tolerable.

Should we tell a truth even if the person could lose their life because of that information? [10]

Should we tell the truth even when the emotional impact may be devastating at the time? [11]

Should we tell the truth even if the patient is a child? [12]

Should we tell the truth even if a change in treatment is foreseeable but will not necessarily be better? [13]

Should we tell the truth even though the cultural context may indicate that it is not the best idea? [14–30]

When we are going to translate medical truth to a patient, we must take all this into account.

There are three things to remember that we will develop throughout this book:

1. Seventy percent of what you communicate is nonverbal. So before you speak, while you speak, and despite what you say or what metaphors you use, you, your body, and your attitude are communicating to the patient in an indubitable way at the same time [31, 32].
2. The medical truth you want to communicate acts like a drug. You should always reflect on whether it is necessary to use it or not, the dose that you are going to administer, the way in which you are going to use it, the and adjuvants with which you are going to accompany it [33].
3. Everything can be said, but not everything can be said the same way. Communication training seeks to teach you techniques that allow you to say what you wish to say in the best way possible [34].

Practice shows us that when it comes to humanizing medical information there are some crucial points:

1. Carefully explain the difference between terms that are synonymous to the patient: probability and possibility; risk and condition; relative and absolute. Even if your patient is an expert in statistics, these differences are often confused in the application of knowledge in our own lives.

   (a) That something is possible does not imply that the probability of it happening is high. It is possible that a patient with breast cancer of 5 mm of a well-differentiated tumor and without axillary or distant involvement will die due to the spread of their disease, but the probability that this will happen in the following 15 years is less than 10%.

If your patient is 85 years old, this information is less relevant than if they are 35 years old. For the former, it is so improbable that it is practically impossible, but for the latter case the probability is low but not impossible.

(b) Being at risk of suffering from a condition does not mean that said condition will inevitably occur, and yet many times we make decisions incorrectly assuming this to be true.

Prophylactic mastectomy is an intervention designed to reduce risk in people with a family history of cancer and BRCA1 or BRCA2 mutation; however, an increasing number of patients undergoing surgery on one breast for breast cancer are requesting that the breast be removed contralateral to reduce the risk (when there is no evidence that removing the contralateral breast helps cure more patients with this condition).

(c) The relative benefit of a treatment can be very high even though the absolute benefit is very low.

This is seen, especially in the so-called adjuvant treatments in cancer, where the risk of dying from cancer can be reduced by 25% in treated patients compared to those who do not receive treatment. But if the risk of cancer is very low, say 4%, this means that only 1% of the population will benefit from this treatment (25% of that 4%). A very common bias in publications is that the benefits are expressed in relative terms while the adverse effects are recorded in absolute terms.

2. Humanize statistics.

The mathematization of biology has made enormous progress. In fact, we could say that the discovery of the circulation of the blood by William Harvey was the first consistent application of the mathematical method to solve a biological enigma. Harvey, the son of a shopkeeper and trained by his father and brothers from a very young age to solve mathematical calculations, calculated how much blood should be produced and where it would accumulate if the heart pumped about 70 ml per beat. This led him to postulate that the blood had to circulate, somehow it had to return to the heart. And thanks to that, he revolutionized medicine.

Without underestimating, therefore, the enormous benefits of mathematics and exact measurements, we must not forget that biology cannot be reduced to mere parameters.

The use of metaphors and, above all, explaining the inevitable uncertainty around medical truths humanizes the story makes it more understandable and probably more true, even if it is less exact [18, 33, 35–39].

This is particularly important when the values are numerically different but clinically insignificant. Is a blood glucose level of 99 mg/dl clinically different from one of 101 mg/dl? However, one is normal and the other abnormal, one is elevated and the other is not. The same thing happens with all the biochemical parameters, electrophysiological or imaging records.

One of the most intelligent dissertations in this topic is Prof. Greene's book *Prescribing by Numbers* [40].

3. Humanize Communication.

The doctor's self-perception of empathy and the patient's evaluation of such are often in disagreement, according to a study with more than 900 patients and 50 doctors carried out by Dr. Carvalho Filho's team [41].

This means that we are optimistic when evaluating our ability to empathize with the patient.

Therefore, we must act with humility.

1. **PREPARE** what you are going to say.
2. **TAKE** your time.
3. **SIT** next to the patient's bed.
4. **ASK** the patient if he wishes to receive the information at this time or prefers to do so at another time or with a family member accompanying him.
5. **LISTEN** to the patient's questions or concerns.
6. **THINK** about what you are going to say and why you are going to say it.
7. **FEEL** what you are going to say and if it is bad news, prepare the patient for what you are going to communicate: "What I am going to say is painful…"; "What I am going to tell you is difficult …", "The study did not go as well as we expected …." There are some ways to prepare the patient; it is not taking a detour, it is giving humanity to bad news.
8. **SAY IT SLOWLY AND RESPECTFULLY**.
9. **WATCH** what happens as you say it [42].
10. DO NOT UNDERESTIMATE THE INTELLIGENCE OF YOUR PATIENT, DO NOT DISTORT THE TRUTH AND DO NOT TREAT THEM LIKE CHILDREN [43–45].

To humanize the information is to allow the patient to incorporate the narrative of the disease into the narrative of his life and exercise his existential autonomy [46].

Understanding the impact of the narrative on the life and health of the patient is to understand that the patient not only contributes biological but above all biographical data to the doctor–patient encounter.

4.4.1 The Patient's Narrative Generating New Knowledge

The humanization of medicine is an imperative of our time.

Throughout the history of medicine, the dehumanization of the doctor lay in his deification. He himself or his contemporaries considered his successes as a manifestation of an extraordinary gift and either minimized or forgot his failures.

Today we are experiencing a reverse movement, there is a feeling that a human doctor is less and less important and sometimes an impediment. The idea that artificial intelligence can replace interpersonal dialogue, that records can avoid clinical examination, and that pharmacogenomics and molecular pathology can select the most effective and tolerable treatment is not a fantasy; it is part of the belief of many patients, providers, and unfortunately doctors [35].

The way to recover the therapeutic role of the medical–patient encounter is the humanization of the doctor, a humanization that begins with recovering the importance of listening in order to personalize diagnoses and therapy [47].

This is true personalized medicine. The one who understands that whoever gets sick is a person. That the disease is an event in a biography and that the biography is a story that deserves to be told and heard.

The person who has made the most efforts to make this medicine a reality is Rita Charon, and this is attested by numerous works and books published on the subject [48–66].

Fundamentally, what does this skill consist of? It consists of recognizing that the disease develops in the context of a life, and that if the doctor is an expert in diseases, the patient is an expert in their own life.

This means we must develop the ability to listen to what the disease means to the patient, what they understand about their condition, what they expect from treatment, and what their wishes and values are. All these things are as important or more than the PET-CT findings, or what the molecular profile of the tumor is.

The clinical history understood in this way is then like a text written by two authors, to which both doctor and patient contribute.

This is why the doctor must train themselves to listen and investigate the aspects of the patient's life that are essential to explain what is happening and to make a decision.

Understanding is the key word here. Understanding before judging is the *right* attitude while understanding before acting is the *prudent* attitude.

For this, it is necessary to train oneself in listening and reading the text of the disease.

That is already therapeutic.

The patient who knows they are being heard is a patient who feels relieved.

The patient who understands that the best treatment has been selected according to their requirements tends to follow those treatments better.

The patient who has realistic expectations regarding the efficacy of the treatment suffers less disappointment than the one who feels deceived or deluded regarding the success.

The doctor who feels that they are acting after having listened to their patient feels more secure.

The doctor who selects the treatment considering the disease and respecting the patient's values applies the most scientific and humane medicine.

Training in this discipline is ongoing throughout our professional life and should ideally begin in medical school [42, 67–73].

This path begins when the doctor is genuinely interested in listening and learning from the patient and assessing the narrative of each patient's life.

For this, we must remember that patient care is our main objective and the reason for our vocation; therefore, the patient is the last and most important evaluator of medical quality.

4.4.2   The Patient as Evaluator of Medical Quality

We began this chapter by analyzing the models of the doctor–patient relationship, and we have seen how the figure of the paternalistic doctor and the patient, silent and obedient, changed throughout the twentieth century and how this was, to a great extent, measured mostly by loss of medical authority due to several medical atrocities committed by doctors.

We have analyzed the complexity of medical language, which incorporates 55,000 new terms into the language we speak, and the need for the doctor to translate this information to the patient.

We have seen how, since the beginning of this century, the patient's narrative has become a key element for decision-making from the scientific and ethical point of view.

How the hermeneutics of the biographical condition of the patient requires training in order to listen and understand the context in which the disease or illness develops.

Now we come to the last point.

The patient as judge.

Quality assessment is an idea that arose in the middle of the last century in companies producing goods, but it has spread to companies providing services and academic fields.

Among its most prominent principles is that every task can be defined within a process and that in every process there is an internal or external "client" who receives the fruit of a job and who judges whether it is appropriate or not.

If for some reason the product or service is inadequate, in the traditional way of production it was considered an error and someone responsible was sought. In a quality-based system, on the other hand, the inadequacy is seen as an opportunity for improvement, looking for ways to modify the process so that this inadequacy does not occur.

In this way, a virtuous circle is generated in which each difficulty is also a stimulus to improve.

This spirit of quality is also applied in the field of health.

In the first place, other members of the health team were given a voice, constituting the so-called committees, "patient safety committee," "infection control committee," "ethics committee," and "research committee." In these spaces, the voice of the doctor is one of many and all those who participate contribute their vision in analyzing any difficulties and solutions that may arise.

Starting in the 1970s, the voice of patients was incorporated into many of these committees, beginning with the ethics committees, but this soon expanded into many areas of decision-making.

One of the first aspects in which the patient's voice had priority was in the evaluation of the patient's quality of life and autonomy [74, 75].

The concept of quality of life is easy to understand but difficult to standardize. Each of us considers that they have a good or bad quality of life, but it is very unlikely that we agree on what makes good or bad quality of life beyond the first four or five points.

An attempt was made to objectively establish a scale to measure the impact of pain on a person's life, called a pain scale or algometer.

For physical pain, especially somatic pain (affecting the skin, muscles, joints, and bones), measurement instruments were designed based on numerical scales (0 = no pain to 10 = severe pain), word scales, or semantic determinants (painless to severe pain) or visual analogs such as along a line, color changes (painless blue to severe pain red), and for illiterate or pediatric patients faces ranging from smiling to hurt or fruit scales. These instruments proved less useful for visceral, neuropathic, or incidental pain, but continued to be used for lack of better alternatives [76, 77].

If we try to assess emotional pain, these instruments are less valid. No one doubts that we all probably agree that one of the most serious emotional pains is the death of a child. Even assuming we all agree that this may be the most appalling loss a person can suffer, it may not be the same if they were the only child; if they died before birth after they were born; if they died as a newborn or as a young man; whether it was due to an acute or chronic illness; whether it was a violent or peaceful death; if they committed suicide or were killed; etc.

When it comes to pain, we can see that trying to quantify emotional pain, which does not really respond to analgesics or other drugs, the complexity of establishing any kind of objective scale.

What this means is that in these circumstances we can only attempt to objectify the subjective: all these scales have the same validity as asking the patient, how much do you think this situation affects you in your life?

The only element that we can rely on is the patient's word, their response is the only way we have to assess the impact of the disease and treatments on their quality of life.

This is so important that the most recent clinical trials have incorporated the patient-reported outcome (PRO) as one of the methods used to comprehensively evaluate the usefulness of the treatments since the placebo and nocebo effects of the different therapies can modify the symptoms that affect the patient and the activities that are carried out in daily life.

The latter has been greatly facilitated by the possibility of real-time recording of symptoms, vital parameters, and physical activity recorded on a person's smartwatch or cell phone.

This prevalence of subjectivity that we find when measuring quality of life and the patient's condition, which is central in palliative medicine and provides so much information, was further extended to patient safety.

In patient safety studies, their education and participation in the design and implementation of safety protocols have been very useful [78–83].

But in addition to evaluating the quality of life and safety, the patient can help us improve the entire health system by getting rid of the "complaints" that normally underestimate poor performance or the thank you letters that overestimate good performance [84] and instead evaluating the way in which they have felt cared to, listened to, understood, and treated, with the greatest objectivity and rigor possible [85–89].

As different patients provide their information, it is possible to have a more accurate vision of the health team's performance. We must incorporate the voices and advice of patients if we truly want to offer the best healthcare possible.

A final and fundamental function of the patients' narrative is their role as teachers.

Nothing helps us incorporate a concept more clearly than when it is tied to a patient's positive or negative experience [90–92].

It is in this encounter between the student and a patient that the abstract becomes concrete and where success or error acquires a human face.

Listening allows you to truly understand what patients and their families consider important and try to meet those needs [93–96].

In order to implement this, we must begin by understanding the enormous difference that exists between information and communication, a topic that we will develop in the next chapter.

4.4.3 Teaching Exercises

1. Individual

    (a) Can you identify the different models of the doctor–patient relationship?
    (b) Do you think that paternalism is still valid today?
    (c) Do you think that the medical word is less valued today than it was before?
    (d) Did you know of any of the unethical investigations that we mentioned in this chapter? Or perhaps others we did not?
    (e) Which of them did you find most scandalous?
    (f) Were you surprised by the etymological origin of any medical term? If so, why?
    (g) Do you use abbreviations in your clinical records?
    (h) What do you think is the most difficult thing to translate into a language the patient can understand?
    (i) What value do you place on the patient's narrative?
    (j) Do you think that the health system should incorporate the evaluation of patients in its quality system?

2. Group

    (a) Discuss each of the doctor–patient relationship metaphors.
    (b) Under what conditions, if any, do you think a doctor should act paternalistically? Give examples and open the discussion.
    (c) Do you think that the results of unethical research should be used in medical practice or should they be discarded until they are properly obtained? Do you think that using the results obtained immorally "justifies" the experiments carried out to obtain them?

(d) Do you think that a doctor should always tell the truth?

(e) In which cases would you consider it reasonable not to tell the truth?

(f) What value does the patient's narrative have to you? What attitude do you take if something that is wrong makes sense to the patient (e.g., that he is responsible for the disease he suffers)?

(g) How would you react if the patient discovered an error in the diagnosis or treatment?

(h) What do you think is the role of the patient in the quality assessment process of healthcare systems?

(i) What do you think of the patient as a teacher?

References

1. Childress JF, Siegler M. Metaphors and models of doctor-patient realtionship: their implications for autonomy. Theor Med. 1984;5:17–30.
2. Szasz TS, Hollender MH. A contribution to the philosophy of medicine: the basic models of the doctor-patient relationship. AMA Arch Intern Med. 1956;97(5):585. https://doi.org/10.1001/archinte.1956.00250230079008.
3. Izmailova ES, Ellis RD. When work hits home: the cancer-treatment journey of a clinical scientist driving digital medicine. JCO Clin Cancer Inform. 2023;6:e2200033. https://doi.org/10.1200/CCI.22.
4. Savater F. Philosophical dictionary. Planet Publishing House; 1995.
5. Deza G. E. Truth vs. E. Verdict. New York: Macchi Publishing House; 2000.
6. Zambito Marsala S, Gioulis M, Pistacchi M. Cerebrospinal fluid and lumbar puncture: the history of a necessary procedure in the history of medicine. Neurol Sci. 2015;36(6):1011–5. https://doi.org/10.1007/s10072-015-2104-6.
7. Tampa M, Sarbu I, Matei C, Benea V, Georgescu SR. Brief history of syphilis. J Med Life. 2014;7(1):4.
8. Lerner BH. Sins of omission—cancer research without informed consent. N Eng J Med. 2004;351(7):628. https://doi.org/10.1056/nejmp048108.
9. Sobel RK. MSL medicine as second language. N Engl J Med. 2005;352(19):1945–6.
10. Adlan AA, ten Have HAMJ. The dilemma of revealing sensitive information on paternity status in Arabian social and cultural contexts: telling the truth about paternity in Saudi Arabia. J Bioeth Inq. 2012;9(4):403–9. https://doi.org/10.1007/s11673-012-9390-y.
11. Cascio A, Ferrand A, Racine E, et al. Discussing brain magnetic resonance imaging results for neonates with hypoxic-ischemic encephalopathy treated with hypothermia: a challenge for clinicians and parents. eNeurologicalSci. 2022;29:100424. https://doi.org/10.1016/j.ensci.2022.100424.
12. Goldie J, Schwartz L, Morrison J. Whose information is it anyway? Informing a 12-year-old patient of her terminal prognosis. J Med Ethics. 2005;31(7):427–34. https://doi.org/10.1136/jme.2004.009886.
13. Borden BA, Lee SM, Danahey K, et al. Patient-provider communications about pharmacogenomic results increase patient recall of medication changes. Pharmacog J. 2019;19(6):528–37. https://doi.org/10.1038/s41397-019-0076-2.
14. Zahedi F. The challenge of truth telling across cultures: a case study. J Med Ethics Hist Med. 2011;4:11. http://journals.tums.ac.ir/abs/20244.
15. Tang WR, Fang JT, Fang CK, Fujimori M. Truth telling in medical practice: students' opinions versus their observations of attending physicians' clinical practice. Psychooncology. 2013;22(7):1605–10. https://doi.org/10.1002/pon.3174.

16. Tuckett AG. Truth-telling in clinical practice and the arguments for and against: a review of the literature. Nurs Ethics. 2004;11(5):500–13. https://doi.org/10.1191/0969733004ne728oa.
17. Sisk B, Frankel R, Kodish E, Isaacson JH. The truth about truth-telling in American medicine: a brief history. Perm J. 2016;20(3):74–7.
18. Surbone A. Telling the truth to patients with cancer: what is the truth? Lancet Oncol. 2006;7(11):944–50. https://doi.org/10.1016/S1470-2045(06)70941-X.
19. Rich BA. Prognosis terminal: truth-telling in the context of end-of-life care. Camb Q Healthc Ethics. 2014;23(2):209–19. https://doi.org/10.1017/S0963180113000741.
20. Rosner F. Informing the patient about a fatal disease: from paternalism to autonomy-The Jewish view. Cancer Invest. 2004;22:949. www.dekker.com.
21. Alsirafy SA, Hadeer Abdel-Aziz I, Abdel-Aal HH, El-Sherief WA, Farag DE. Not telling patients their cancer diagnosis in Egypt: Is it associated with less anxiety and depression and better quality of life? JCO Glob Oncol. 2022;8:e2200080. https://doi.org/10.1200/GO.22.00080.
22. Tang WR, Chen KY, Hsu SH, et al. Effectiveness of Japanese SHARE model in improving Taiwanese healthcare personnel's preference for cancer truth telling. Psychooncology. 2014;23(3):259–65. https://doi.org/10.1002/pon.3413.
23. Shahidi J. Not telling the truth: circumstances leading to concealment of diagnosis and prognosis from cancer patients. Eur J Cancer Care (Engl). 2010;19(5):589–93. https://doi.org/10.1111/j.1365-2354.2009.01100.x.
24. de Pentheny O'KC, Urch C, Brown EA. The impact of culture and religion on truth telling at the end of life. Nephrol Dial Transplant. 2011;26(12):3838–42. https://doi.org/10.1093/ndt/gfr630.
25. Seki Y, Yamazaki Y, Mizota Y, Inoue Y. How families in Japan view the disclosure of terminal illness: a study of iatrogenic HIV infection. AIDS Care. 2009;21(4):422–30. https://doi.org/10.1080/09540120802282578.
26. Surbone A, Ritossa C, Spagnolo AG. Evolution of truth-telling attitudes and practices in Italy. Crit Rev Oncol Hematol. 2004;52(3):165–72. https://doi.org/10.1016/j.critrevonc.2004.09.002.
27. Rigatos GA. Cancer and truth-telling in Greece historical, statistical, and clinical data. Ann N Y Acad Sci. 1997;809:382.
28. Wu J, Wang Y, Jiao X, Wang J, Ye X, Wang B. Differences in practice and preferences associated with truth-telling to cancer patients. Nurs Ethics. 2021;28(2):272–81. https://doi.org/10.1177/0969733020945754.
29. Abdulhameed HE, Hammami MM, Hameed Mohamed EA. Disclosure of terminal illness to patients and families: diversity of governing codes in 14 Islamic countries. J Med Ethics. 2011;37(8):472–5. https://doi.org/10.1136/jme.2010.038497.
30. Pergert P, Lützén K. Balancing truth-telling in the preservation of hope: a relational ethics approach. Nurs Ethics. 2012;19(1):21–9. https://doi.org/10.1177/0969733011418551.
31. Pittarello A, Conte B, Caserotti M, Scrimin S, Rubaltelli E. Emotional intelligence buffers the effect of physiological arousal on dishonesty. Psychon Bull Rev. 2018;25(1):440–6. https://doi.org/10.3758/s13423-017-1285-9.
32. Dugdale LS, Siegler M, Rubin DT. Medical professionalism and the doctor-patient relationship. Perspect Biol Med. 2008;51(4):547–53. https://doi.org/10.1353/pbm.0.0054.
33. Kreitmair KV. Medical ethics, moral courage, and the embrace of fallibility. Acad Med. 2021;96(12):1630–3. https://doi.org/10.1097/ACM.0000000000004420.
34. Boissy A, Windover AK, Bokar D, et al. Communication skills training for physicians improves patient satisfaction. J Gen Intern Med. 2016;31(7):755–61. https://doi.org/10.1007/s11606-016-3597-2.
35. Funer F. The deception of certainty: how non-interpretable machine learning outcomes challenge the epistemic Authority of Physicians. A deliberative-relational approach. Med Health Care Philos. 2022;25(2):167–78. https://doi.org/10.1007/s11019-022-10076-1.
36. Kaptein AA. Novels as data: health humanities and health psychology. J Health Psychol. 2022;27(7):1615–25. https://doi.org/10.1177/1359105321999107.

37. Siegler M. Falling off the pedestal: what is happening to the traditional doctor-patient relationship? Mayo Clin Proc. 1993;68(5):461–7. https://doi.org/10.1016/S0025-6196(12)60195-5.
38. Kirklin D. Truth telling, autonomy and the role of metaphor. J Med Ethics. 2007;33(1):11–4. https://doi.org/10.1136/jme.2005.014993.
39. Nakazawa E, Yamamoto K, Ozeki-Hayashi R, Shaw MH, Akabayashi A. Is it worth knowing that you might die tomorrow? Revisiting the ethics of prognosis disclosure. Clin Pract. 2022;12(5):803–8. https://doi.org/10.3390/clinpract12050084.
40. Greene JA. Prescribing by numbers: drugs and the definition of disease. Soc History Med. 2006;20(3):613–5. https://doi.org/10.1093/shm/hkm083.
41. Bernardo MO, Cecílio-Fernandes D, Costa P, Quince TA, Costa MJ, Carvalho-Filho MA. Physicians' self-assessed empathy levels do not correlate with patients' assessments. PLoS One. 2018;13(5):e0198488. https://doi.org/10.1371/journal.pone.0198488.
42. Karnieli-Miller O, Palombo M, Meitar D. See, reflect, learn more: qualitative analysis of breaking bad news reflective narratives. Med Educ. 2018;52(5):497–512. https://doi.org/10.1111/medu.13582.
43. DeMartino ES, Dudzinski DM, Doyle CK, et al. Who decides when a patient Can't? Statutes on alternate decision makers. N Engl J Med. 2017;376(15):1478–82. https://doi.org/10.1056/nejmms1611497.
44. Cox C, Fritz Z. Presenting complaint: use of language that disempowers patients. BMJ. 2022;377:e066720. https://doi.org/10.1136/bmj-2021-066720.
45. Bakhurst Queen D. On lying and deceiving. J Med Ethics. 1992;18:63.
46. Madder H, Radcliffe J. Existential autonomy: why patients should make their own. Choices. 1997;23:221.
47. Gundersen T, Bærøe K. The future ethics of artificial intelligence in medicine: making sense of collaborative models. Sci Eng Ethics. 2022;28(2):17. https://doi.org/10.1007/s11948-022-00369-2.
48. Charon R. What narrative competence is for. Am J Bioethics. 2001;1(1):62. https://doi.org/10.1162/152651601750079186.
49. Charon R. Narrative medicine: Caring for the sick is a work of art. J Am Acad Physician Assist. 2013;26(12):8. https://doi.org/10.1097/01.JAA.0000437751.53994.94.
50. Charon R. Narrative medicine in the international education of physicians. Presse Med. 2013;42(1):3. https://doi.org/10.1016/j.lpm.2012.10.015.
51. Charon R, Wyer P, NEBM Working Group. Narrative evidence based medicine. Lancet. 2008;371(9609):296. https://doi.org/10.1016/S0140-6736(08)60156-7.
52. Charon R. Doctor-patent/reader-writer: learning to find the text. Soundings. 1989;72(1):137.
53. Charon R. Narrative medicine: attention, representation, affiliation. Narrative. 2005;13(3):261. https://doi.org/10.1353/nar.2005.0017.
54. Charon R. What to do with stories: the sciences of narrative medicine. Can Fam Phys. 2007;53(8):1265.
55. Charon R. Knowing, seeing, and telling in medicine. Lancet. 2021;398(10316):2068. https://doi.org/10.1016/S0140-6736(21)02656-8.
56. Heller EA, Heller FE. Narrative medicine: a practical application for using writing as a clinical intervention with cancer patients, caregivers and the clinicians that care for them. Psychooncology. 2016;25:4381.
57. Selzer R, Charon R. Stories for a humanistic medicine. J Assoc Am Med Coll. 1999;74(1):42–4. https://doi.org/10.1097/00001888-199901000-00016.
58. Hanlon V. A place for humanities in medical education. Can Med Assoc J. 2015;187(10):E328. https://doi.org/10.1503/cmaj.140532.
59. San Julian Mark M, Todd K, Todd D. The language of illness: the art of telling, listening, and self-care through narrative medicine (TH314). J Pain Symptom Manage. 2017;53(2):P321. https://doi.org/10.1016/j.jpainsymman.2016.12.040.
60. Courteau C, Laneuville L. Reading patients: our story of narrative medicine. Int J Whole Person Care. 2020;7(1):44. https://doi.org/10.26443/ijwpc.v7i1.232.

61. Silistraru I. Narrative Medicine—the methodology of doctor-patient communication analysis. Social Change Rev. 2017;15(1–2):105. https://doi.org/10.1515/scr-2017-0005.
62. Grant A. Pain, suffering and the vulnerability of the empath. J Aust Trad Med Soc. 2018;24(3):144.
63. Zaharias G. Learning narrative-based medicine skills narrative-based medicine 3. Can Fam Phys. 2018;64(5):352.
64. Zaharias G. Narrative-based medicine and the general practice consultation: narrative-based medicine 2. Can Fam Phys. 2018;64(4):286.
65. Zaharias G. What is narrative-based medicine?: narrative-based medicine 1. Can Fam Phys. 2018;64(3):176.
66. Charon R. Narrative medicine: honoring the stories of illness. Ann Intern Med. 2007;146(2):1. https://doi.org/10.7326/0003-4819-146-2-200701160-00021.
67. Campbell BH, Treat R, Johnson B, Derse AR. Creating reflective space for reflective and "unreflective" medical students: exploring seminal moments in a large-group writing session. Acad Med. 2020;95(6):882–7. https://doi.org/10.1097/ACM.0000000000003241.
68. Dasgupta S, Charon R. Personal illness narratives: using reflective writing to teach empathy teaching empathy through reflection. Acad Med. 2004;79:351.
69. Dressler JA, Ryder BA, Connolly M, Blais MD, Miner TJ, Harrington DT. "Tweet"-format writing is an effective tool for medical student reflection. J Surg Educ. 2018;75(5):1206–10. https://doi.org/10.1016/j.jsurg.2018.03.002.
70. Wen CC, Lin MJ, Lin CW, Chu SY. Exploratory study of the characteristics of feedback in the reflective dialogue group given to medical students in a clinical clerkship. Med Educ. 2015;20(1):25965. https://doi.org/10.3402/meo.v20.25965.
71. Toivonen AK, Lindblom-Ylänne S, Louhiala P, Pyörälä E. Medical students' reflections on emotions concerning breaking bad news. Patient Educ Couns. 2017;100(10):1903–9. https://doi.org/10.1016/j.pec.2017.05.036.
72. Campbell BH, Havas N, Derse AR, Holloway RL. Creating a residency application personal statement writers workshop: fostering narrative, teamwork, and insight at a time of stress. Acad Med. 2016;91:371–5. https://doi.org/10.1097/ACM.0000000000000863.
73. Lin CW, Lin MJ, Wen CC, Chu SY. A word-count approach to analyze linguistic patterns in the reflective writings of medical students. Med Educ. 2016;21(1):29522. https://doi.org/10.3402/meo.v21.29522.
74. Chow R, Bruera E, Temel JS, Krishnan M, Im J, Lock M. Inter-rater reliability in performance status assessment among healthcare professionals: an updated systematic review and meta-analysis. Support Care Cancer. 2020;28(5):2071–8. https://doi.org/10.1007/s00520-019-05261-7.
75. Chow R, Zimmermann C, Bruera E, Temel J, Im J, Lock M. Inter-rater reliability in performance status assessment between clinicians and patients: a systematic review and meta-analysis. BMJ Support Palliat Care. 2020;10(2):129–35. https://doi.org/10.1136/bmjspcare-2019-002080.
76. Borelli E, Bigi S, Potenza L, et al. Different semantic and affective meaning of the words associated to physical and social pain in cancer patients on early palliative/ supportive care and in healthy, pain-free individuals. PLoS One. 2021;16(3 March 2021):1–17. https://doi.org/10.1371/journal.pone.0248755.
77. Pauff SM, Miller SC. The lack of standard definitions in the supportive and palliative oncology literature David. Bone. 2012;78(2):711–6. https://doi.org/10.1016/j.jpainsymman.2011.04.016.
78. Anel Rodriguez RM, Aibar Remon C, Martin Rodriguez MD. Patient participation in its own safety. Athens Primary. 2021;53:102215. https://doi.org/10.1016/j.april.2021.102215.
79. Longtin Y, Sax H, Leape LL, Sheridan SE, Donaldson L, Pittet D. Patient participation: current knowledge and applicability to patient safety. Mayo Clin Proc. 2010;85(1):53. https://doi.org/10.4065/mcp.2009.0248.

80. Sahlström M, Partanen P, Rathert C, Turunen H. Patient participation in patient safety still missing: patient safety experts' views. Int J Nurs Pract. 2016;22(5):461. https://doi.org/10.1111/ijn.12476.

81. Davis RE, Jacklin R, Sevdalis N, Vincent CA. Patient involvement in patient safety: what factors influence patient participation and engagement? Health Expect. 2007;10(3):259. https://doi.org/10.1111/j.1369-7625.2007.00450.x.

82. Hwang JI, Kim SW, Chin HJ. Patient participation in patient safety and its relationships with nurses' patient-centered care competency, teamwork, and safety climate. Asian Nurs Res (Korean Soc Nurs Sci). 2019;13(2):130. https://doi.org/10.1016/j.anr.2019.03.001.

83. Kim YS, Kim HA, Kim MS, et al. How to improve patient safety literacy? Int J Environ Res Public Health. 2020;17(19):7308. https://doi.org/10.3390/ijerph17197308.

84. Miron-Shatz T, Becker S, Zaromb F, Mertens A, Tsafrir A. "A Phenomenal person and doctor": thank you letters to medical care providers. Interact J Med Res. 2017;6(2):e22. https://doi.org/10.2196/ijmr.7107.

85. Wang X, Chen J, Yang Y, Burström B, Burström K. Validation of the patient-reported experience measure for care in Chinese hospitals (PREM-CCH). Int J Equity Health. 2021;20(1):25. https://doi.org/10.1186/s12939-020-01370-6.

86. Verulava T, Jorbenadze R, Karimi L, Dangadze B, Barkalaia T. Evaluation of patient satisfaction with cardiology services. Open Public Health J. 2018;11(1):201. https://doi.org/10.2174/1874944501811010201.

87. Baines R, Regan De Bere S, Stevens S, et al. The impact of patient feedback on the medical performance of qualified doctors: a systematic review. BMC Med Educ. 2018;18(1):173. https://doi.org/10.1186/s12909-018-1277-0.

88. Pękacz A, Kądalska E, Skoczylas A, Targowski T. Patient satisfaction as an element of healthcare quality—a single-center polish survey. Rheumatology. 2019;57(3):135. https://doi.org/10.5114/reum.2019.86423.

89. Miller M, Supranowicz P, Gebska-Kuczerowska A, Car J. Evaluation of medical service quality by hospitalized patients. Rev Epidemiol. 2008;62(3):643.

90. Baylor C, Burns M, McDonough K, Mach H, Yorkston K. Teaching medical students skills for effective communication with patients who have communication disorders. Am J Speech Lang Pathol. 2019;28(1):155. https://doi.org/10.1044/2018_AJSLP-18-0130.

91. Kirkman MA, Sevdalis N, Arora S, Baker P, Vincent C, Ahmed M. The outcomes of recent patient safety education interventions for trainee physicians and medical students: a systematic review. BMJ Open. 2015;5(5):e007705. https://doi.org/10.1136/bmjopen-2015-007705.

92. Dijk SW, Duijzer EJ, Wienold M. Role of active patient involvement in undergraduate medical education: a systematic review. BMJ Open. 2020;10(7):e037217. https://doi.org/10.1136/bmjopen-2020-037217.

93. Auriemma CL, Harhay MO, Haines KJ, Barg FK, Halpern SD, Lyon SM. What matters to patients and their families during and after critical illness: a qualitative study. Am J Critical Care. 2021;30(1):11. https://doi.org/10.4037/ajcc2021398.

94. Walkey AJ, Barnato AE, Wiener RS, Nallamothu BK. Accounting for patient preferences regarding life-sustaining treatment in evaluations of medical effectiveness and quality. Am J Respir Crit Care Med. 2017;196(8):958. https://doi.org/10.1164/rccm.201701-0165CP.

95. Kagan I, Porat N, Barnoy S. The quality and safety culture in general hospitals: Patients', physicians' and nurses' evaluation of its effect on patient satisfaction. Int J Quality Health Care. 2019;31(4):261. https://doi.org/10.1093/intqhc/mzy138.

96. Pannick S, Archer S, Long SJ, Husson F, Athanasiou T, Sevdalis N. What matters to medical ward patients, and do we measure it? A qualitative comparison of patient priorities and current practice in quality measurement, on UK NHS medical wards. BMJ Open. 2019;9(3):e024058. https://doi.org/10.1136/bmjopen-2018-024058.

Chapter 5
Information Versus Communication

5.1 A Misunderstanding of Terms

We live in the so-called "communication era," "to exist is to communicate," and "information is at your fingertips." These are some of the slogans that seek to define we have all heard regarding the twenty-first century and our place in it.If we were to count the evolution of information in the manner of Philomena Cunk (a character played by Diane Morgan, who makes wonderful Mockumentaries, which are fictional stories that are presented in the format of documentaries), we would begin by saying: clearly today we have more information in 1 min than many of our ancestors had in their entire life.

Our ancestors began by communicating nonverbally, and the information they possessed was only that which they could perceive with their senses. Their companions were close, night ruled over day, and stories were ephemeral.

Then the spoken word was added to the mix, and they could share their experiences, memories, and feelings. The fire became a home, and the stories became stories in the night.

Later still, paintings were added and we had the first nonspoken record of their stories (Cunk would say they were boring and repetitive).

These drawings later became hieroglyphics, meaning stories could now be recorded on stone, parchment, or papyrus (which were difficult to transport and keep in good condition).

These hieroglyphics would evolve and change into letters and thus the most formidable invention of humanity was produced: the alphabet. And with it, stories became history (Cunk would say that we finally had something translatable).

The alphabet made it possible to not only express ideas, but to create them, model them, shape them, and mix them. Culture became language.

© The Author(s), under exclusive license to Springer Nature
Switzerland AG 2024

E. Gil Deza, *Improving Clinical Communication*,
https://doi.org/10.1007/978-3-031-62446-9_5

Language elevated letters to poetry and algebra pushed mathematics to the limit when the concept of zero was born.

Culture became universal. Everyone contributed something; Greeks, Romans, Jews, Arabs, Chinese, Japanese, Korean, English, French, German, all of them and more live in each and every language. There is no dictionary today that can explain the world in words born of a single language (Cunk would say that monogamy does not exist for ideas).

The printing press gave these words wings, and ideas became easily transportable, libertarian, and revolutionary. Books left the libraries, proliferated, and began to inhabit the houses of many people.

Electricity gave us light to keep the night away and speed to close distances. Ideas began to be transmitted by cables at a speed that had never been seen before. First with words and then with images, distant events became closer and closer.

With the advent of mass media, our compatriots became a distant, anonymous, invisible, and influenceable spectator. Propaganda became the government and fear became a source of power.

Machines became so powerful that it took another machine to beat them. And this did not happen in some science fiction publication; it happened in the 1940s in England at Bletchley park.

The digital revolution transformed letters and shapes into numbers and put the world in the palm of your hand. No language is untranslatable, no secret can be hidden for long, and almost no barrier is insurmountable.

The truth became fluid, malleable, adaptable, and debatable. Reality integrated the virtual space and knowledge became incomprehensible.

Today, more than in Socrates' times, we know that we do not know anything ... but if it exists, it is on the Internet and surely there is a video on YouTube that explains how to do it.

That is the difference between information and communication.

Information is everything that is broadcast, everything that has been broadcast, and everything that can be broadcast and perceived by someone at any time.

We will see later that communication theories have been modifying their approaches to this problem, but we must remember that the sender is the most vital element when it comes to information.

This is because information is poured. While the effectiveness of any information will be evaluated on several levels: whether or not someone receives it, understands it, interprets it properly, and carries out what is requested, even if no one sees it, the information is there, in one way or another.

Even if no one goes to the theater, the "Exit"signs continue to indicate where to exit and even if there are no passengers on a flight, the instruction booklet will still explain what should be done in the event of a "sudden decompression."

That is information.

Communication, on the other hand, is based on the receiver.

5.2 Communication Theories

Communication theories try to explain the influence of interactions between living beings, more specifically between people.

From this perspective, it is a very old discipline since it was explicitly analyzed by Aristotle in his texts on rhetoric and dialectic [1–3], especially in the book of topics. In Greece, the cradle of democracy, these ideas were extremely important because political issues were publicly debated and citizens had to explain their points of view to their peers. Hence, they hired sophists (teachers) to train them in the art of rhetoric.

However, even though communication theories can be traced back to such remote times, it is also, paradoxically, a relatively new discipline.

Communication theory is understood as the multidisciplinary field of study (different disciplines make it up: philosophy, psychology, sociology, biology, engineering, politics, and communication) that analyzes how information is transmitted, received, and processed between different individuals, groups, and/or cultures [4–6].

The first systematic studies on communication theory were carried out throughout the twentieth century by studying the influence of mass media (newspapers, radio, television, and the Internet) on the general public's opinion regarding different topics.

Each of these theories or models of social communication can explain certain conditions of interpersonal communication.

For example, Harold Laswell's "Hypodermic Needle" theory, which is a theory from the early twentieth century aimed at explaining political propaganda in Europe and the United States, applies the same kind of language we can find in classrooms, in public dissertations, or at a doctor's office [7].

Assertive, unidirectional language, where the truth is clearly delimited and has no controversies or flexibility, is the main characteristic of this type of communication.

This can also be seen in professionals who relate with the patient in a teacher–student perspective. They show great confidence in their decision-making and only following their proposed path ensures success, any other alternative is suboptimal.

This type of communication is rarely desirable, with the notable exception of disaster relief, where singular, centralized, and command-based communication saves more lives overall, but in all other cases deliberative communication is more desirable.

Even though propaganda has a limited effect on interpersonal communication, it has a much more important effect on the selection of issues and policies, which is called "agenda setting," and was extensively studied by Bernard Cohen in the 1960's [8].

This is sometimes achieved by resorting to satire or humor [9].

How does this influence interpersonal relationships then? By establishing which topics and themes are considered appropriate. For example, today we live in societies that are essentially medicalized. They assume that there must be a medical solution for every problem, whether personal or social, and this has in turn changed the way we see medicine and what role a doctor fulfills [10].

If we were to analyze society's overall feelings regarding topics such as abortion, euthanasia, homosexuality, gender fluidity, assisted reproduction, experimentation with embryos, drug costs, patients' rights, the availability of medical information, or the use artificial intelligence in medicine, we would see that it is the positions presented by politicians and "influencers" that have the biggest impact, whether for or against.

This means that this public agenda is also present many times in the doctor–patient relationship and in doctor–patient communication, not only in the subject matter but also in the way of approaching it and the terms used when discussing it.

Of all the theories of social communication, the one that in my opinion has the greatest importance in the medical field is that of Charles Berger [11].

Clearly one of the main objectives of interpersonal communication is the reduction of uncertainty.

This uncertainty has two dimensions: the first is given by the distance between the patient's knowledge about his condition and the doctor's knowledge about what affects the patient. This distance is similar to that we can see between citizen and politician, parishioner and priest, student and teacher. We can shorten this distance with information [12–15].

The second aspect of uncertainty is given by the distance between the present and the future, which is common to both parties. Since it is shared by both, it cannot be filled with information. What can we fill it with, then? With confidence born out of experience and with imagination of possible futures.

How can you apply this knowledge in doctor–patient communication?

The patient–doctor communication theory that best explains the therapeutic value of the medical word is the "Patient-Centered Care Theory," in which the emphasis is placed on understanding the patient's perspective, their needs, and their preferences in medical care.

Ideally, physician and patient should establish a collaborative relationship to deliberate and find the optimal course of action for each patient.

To do this, the doctor must

1. Respect the patient's preferences. The doctor is the expert on the ailment, but the patient is the expert on their own life.
2. Coordinate and integrate patient care so that the patient can develop their life with the greatest well-being and freedom.
3. Inform and educate the patient in a truthful and understandable way.
4. Provide emotional support throughout the entire disease and treatments.

Following these steps has shown to increase patient satisfaction, improve adherence to treatments, as well as improve treatment efficiency and reduce doctor burnout [16–24].

We must emphasize that the first meeting with the patient is crucial to build the confidence necessary for the patient to talk about what is happening to them, the reasons why they believe it is happening, the expectations they have regarding the disease's evolution and the success of the treatments, and the reasons why you expect a favorable evolution.

What is the first step to building that trust?

Let the patient feel like they are being listened to.

How does the patient know that we listen to him?

First of all, from our attitude: make sure you will not be interrupted (especially by telephone), invite the patient to talk about what is happening to them and what questions they expect you to answer first, and then write.

Most patients are interrupted within 18 s of starting to speak; try to avoid this, let the patient speak.

I prefer to write down what the patient says by hand; that way I can look at them while they speak, "listening" with my eyes. This is something that allows us to discover the points of discomfort or certainty in what the patient expresses.

At the end, I register the questions.

Then I tell the patient: "Let me read what I understood to see if there are any errors," and I read them what I understood, allowing them to correct any errors.

Finally, I read the questions they asked me for this consultation.

What does all this achieve?

That the patient perceives themselves to have been listened to and understood.

Gregorio Marañón once said that the most important instrument in medicine is the chair (https://elpais.com/elpais/2018/10/05/planeta_futuro/1538764994_443426.html), showing that the doctor's listening attitude and the time we dedicate to observing the patient is what allows for the best diagnoses and the best therapies, which are those that adapt to the values and desires of the patient.

An additional tool to help us understand in greater depth what the patient believes and expects is the "Health belief Model," which is a communication theory that proposes that an individual's behaviors when it comes to health are influenced by their own beliefs and attitudes regarding health and disease.

This can be seen in the four key factors of this model:

1. Susceptibility perception: the individual perception of the probability they will develop the disease.
2. Perception of severity: the individual perception of the severity and possible consequences of an ailment.
3. Perception of benefit: the individual perception of the probability that they will benefit from a given behavioral change.
4. Barriers: the individual perception of the difficulties or challenges of changing a certain behavior.

This individual perception of risk, severity, benefits, and difficulties are the ones that have the greatest impact on the behavior of the person regarding their health.

Understanding this is crucial to the acquisition of healthy habits, disease prevention, and patient safety [25–40].

This also explains the patient's "surprise" when faced with the diagnosis of a certain disease where the most probable cause is a toxic habit such as smoking: the patient, like all of us, believes that he is going to be an exception to the rule. It is other people who develop lung cancer, contract AIDS, or become dependent on a drug. That exceptionalism is what often leads us to take excessive risks in our lives.

The first interview allows us to explore the patient's beliefs and demystify some misconceptions. This is very common, for example, in cancer patients who must start chemotherapy treatment, who frequently have exaggerated ideas about toxicity and erroneous ideas about efficacy.

A large part of these ideas come from the enormous supply of information, of very varied quality, offered by the Internet and social networks.

This supply of information is so overwhelming that the act of processing it correctly has been analyzed in great depth, leading to terms such as "information overload" or "Infodemic," "Infoxication," or "Infosaturation." [41–44]

We will address these topics in the next section.

5.3   Overinformation and Lack of Communication

Today we do not simply live in the information age, but also an age of information overload, misinformation, and fake news, that is, lies, inventions, and falsehoods.

The problem is that the oversupply of information leaves us dissatisfied and anguished, as evidenced by the American psychologist Barry Schwartz and his studies regarding consumer goods [45–48].

Therefore, we have several problems that we must solve:

(a) How to deal with the volume of accessible information: that is, what do we want to know and where are we going to look for the answer?
(b) How to distinguish true from false information.
(c) How to organize information so that the message is clearly emitted or understood.
(d) How to organize information to make a decision.

We will begin to analyze these four topics.

5.3.1   *How to Deal with the Volume of Information Available*

Today we have a large amount of information within reach at any time of the day and almost anywhere.

The first thing we have to understand is that we cannot access all the information available.

There is necessarily information that we will have to leave aside, either because of the language barrier, because of its sheer volume, or because we do not have enough time to properly analyze it.

Therefore, we dive into the enormous library represented by the Internet; we must be clear about at least the following points:

1. **What question do we want to ask**? It is important to understand that we must make a choice between searching with a **general** query that allows us to cover the topic exhaustively and a very **specific** query that allows us to find the answer we are looking for.
2. **Where do we want to find the information**? When it comes to health, there are online libraries in the United States, the United Kingdom, Canada, Europe, or Latin America that are very serious and have very good quality information for patients. Unfortunately, not all of them are written following the rules of clear language and reading comprehension, so the material for patients sometimes requires a high degree of comprehension in the language of health or "health literacy."
3. **Refine search,** so that we obtain a manageable volume of information.

5.3.2 How to Distinguish Between True and False Information

The most dubious type of information is **testimonial**, not because it is necessarily false but because we usually do not know its full context, and sometimes important details of both diagnosis and treatment are omitted.

It is important to understand that honesty, truthfulness, and truth are not synonymous. Many witnesses are honest, that is, they say what they believe or think (but they may be wrong) and they are truthful, that is, they are convinced that what they observed or heard is what they faithfully repeat, but it is not necessarily the truth, which means that it is a genuine reflection of exactly what happened [49].

The second type of information that we must doubt is that **provided for commercial purposes**, or whose authors are subsidized by the manufacturer of a product, since the information they provide is usually biased and exaggerates the benefits and minimizes the damages [50–63].

The third piece of information we should be skeptical of is information that **has not been independently confirmed** or the results of which have not been independently reviewed.

The scientific method is not based only on experimentation but above all on the independent confirmation of results.

This does not assure us that the result we obtain is true, but it assures us that we have taken the necessary precautions so as not to be deceived.

5.3.3   How to Organize Information so that the Message Is Clearly Delivered or Understood

A method that I find very useful is the following:

1. First, select the answers to the most important questions (curability, survival, quality of life).
2. From the answers, I take the results that have been confirmed (sadly, fewer and fewer studies are independently confirmed).
3. I evaluate these answers according to the way in which they were obtained (e.g., by rating double-blind randomized studies higher).
4. Finally, I order the results from highest to lowest by the number of patients included (sadly, there are more and more studies with fewer patients).

5.3.4   How to Organize Information to Make a Decision

From a practical point of view, I take the previous table and give the highest score to the **most effective treatments** (greater survival, greater responses, longer duration of response), that are **less toxic** (fewer patients drop out, are hospitalized or die from treatment), **more practical** (oral vs. intravenous; every three to 4 weeks vs. weekly; bolus intravenous vs. continuous infusion), and **affordable** (administered at the hospital close to home and covered by my health system).

From there I go down the rating.

This does go against what most methodologists say, which is that you should not compare the results of different clinical studies against each other. However, in order to choose one over the other, both doctors and patients end up comparing their results whether the experts like it or not.

This process ensures that I have realistic and accessible expectations to analyze.

I always select pessimistically: I mentally subtract 20% from maximum efficacy and add 20% from maximum toxicity.

I keep this material on my computer, and when a "new" study appears I update the computer and mental file since this will be my tool when interacting with a patient.

At that point there are two additional steps I take.

First of all, I try to limit the available options to no less than three and no more than five.

This allows you to have a limited number of representative options to choose from comfortably. (Very rarely are there more than five or less than three options.)

Secondly, I transform statistical mathematics into a human language.

This involves rounding numbers to understandable figures.

Usually I transform percentages into proportions. For example, 12.8% becomes one in ten; 2.7% becomes three in one hundred, while 0.17% becomes two in a thousand. A 20% difference is one in five.

I also humanize the times to values that make sense. Eleven-month median survival is about 1 year and 13 months as well (I treat adult cancer patients and while it is true that a two-month difference in survival is *statistically* significant, it is not *practically* significant for most patients).

Of course, the patient has the right to choose to receive a treatment no matter how small the difference between that and any other treatment for their ailment is.

What I explain to my patients is that these small differences, which require a large number of patients to demonstrate that they exist, are realistic when the treatment in question lacks toxicity. But when treatments are toxic, these differences in efficacy are unlikely to be seen in the real world because patients selected for clinical trials tend to tolerate treatments better than patients in the office.

I always *choose* with optimism: once I have made a decision I think it is the best possible choice and it is going to be the most beneficial.

5.4 Selecting and Organizing the Message

How do we organize all this information to present it to the patient? From a practical point of view, I first answer the questions that interest my patient, so before writing what the patient tells me about his ailment, I ask him what they hope to obtain in this consultation? What are their most important doubts? If they are asking me for advice to make a decision, what is the decision they have to make?

I let the patient speak while I make a mental note of the way in which they tell me what has happened to them: when do they pause, what topics do they find difficult to discuss. I write everything down on paper, because although I will then have to upload it to the Electronic Medical Record, paper allows me to do two things: (a) it lets me write things down as I listen and allows me to look at the patient and (b) it allows me to write things down in the order in which I am later going to repeat it.

When the patient finishes speaking, I tell him: "Now I am going to read back to you what I understood, so that if there is something that we should correct because I misunderstood, we can do it." While it is true that one of my aims is to correct errors, the primary objective of this gesture is for the patient to perceive that they were heard and that what they said was adequately understood [64–67].

In other words, the first communication gesture with my patient is to give them time to tell us what is happening to them and what worries them, and the second is for the patient to know that they have been heard.

These two points have the highest priority in the communication hierarchy of the clinical message.

Only then do I see any biopsy results, then laboratory studies, and finally any images (I always read the studies first, and then read the reports, that way I can better review the studies). What is the purpose of this sequence, you may ask? (a) To certify that what the patient informed me is corroborated in the biopsy; (b) to evaluate if the clinician sees the same things as the imagenologist or if there are any differences; and (c) to analyze which of the findings described in the complimentary studies I can find in the clinical examination. After doing all this, I carry out the medical examination.

Why did I leave the clinical exam for last?

Because this step is, for me, the most important one within doctor–patient communication and the encounter with the patient.

The clinical examination, which has been widely defended by many, including Dr. Abraham Verghese, an eminent clinician and teacher currently working in California, is a moment of intimate knowledge between doctor and patient. It is also a moment of contact that consolidates the impressions that the doctor has been having up to that moment, which makes the patient loyal to the doctor and is also a moment of serene reflection due to the ritualistic nature of the gestures [68–87].

The doctor's first gesture of respect is to ask permission to examine the patient; this certifies the care you have for the person, their privacy, and their rights.

The second gesture is the warmth in the maneuvers; I personally begin by examining my patients by their feet, which means that with many of them, especially the elderly, I frequently help them remove their socks, which creates another moment of relaxation.

I start with the feet not only because it makes it easy to not forget them, but also because it allows me to see the state of their toenails, which not only serves to ascertain their nutritional status but also the kind of care that is being given to a patient: a patient whose toenails are properly cut, especially if they are hospitalized, indicates excellent nursing care.

It also allows me to check for temperature, edema, the state of the soles, and the state of the arterial, venous, and skin systems, which I will also find (and examine) in the rest of my patient's body.

Afterward, I examine the ganglionic regions, the organs and systems, leaving the gynecological examination or rectal examination for the end, and I only do them if I deem it necessary.

Clinical examination time rarely exceeds 20 min. But it is a time where I am communicating to the patient what I am doing as I am doing it, and I share any outstanding findings I come across.

Subsequently, I tell the patient to get dressed. I usually leave the office at that time in order to wash my hands and digitize the documents that I will incorporate into the Medical Record.

Upon my return to the office, I resume the dialogue with my patient.

With all the integrated knowledge of what he told me, what was found in the complementary studies and what I was able to find in the physical examination, I am in a position to begin to answer what the patient wants to know "about themselves and their possible fate," as my teacher Don Carlos Landa used to say. It is very important to answer in a prudent, affectionate, and respectful way.

The questions and answers that appear at this stage are almost always very similar to those that appear in a recent interview I had with Alejandro Borgo published on April 13, 2023, in *Skeptical Inquirer*, which you can find at https://skepticalin-quirer.org/exclusive/twenty-common-questions-and-answers-about-cancer/.

I transcribe only one of them below:

In this day and age, how likely is a person to die of cancer?

There are several possible answers to this question. It depends on the type of cancer; there are highly curable cancers (germ tumors, testicular tumors, pediatric tumors, lymphomas, some leukemias) that have high curability rates (greater than 90 percent) even when disseminated are diagnosed.

It also depends on the stage of the disease; in the most common tumors, the cure rate depends on the size of the primary tumor, whether or not regional lymph nodes are involved, or whether they are disseminated (breast, colon, lung). Small tumors without lymph node involvement are cured in more than 70 percent of the cases while disseminated tumors (with metastases) are very rarely cured.

It depends on the patient (age, comorbidities, immunocompetence, and general condition). The younger, healthier, and better general condition you are, the more likely you are to tolerate treatment and heal.

It depends on the doctor; when the doctor is not well trained or acts recklessly or indifferently, the patient's life is at serious risk. Cancer treatments are among the most toxic in medicine.

Lastly, it depends on the environment in which the patient lives and is brought. Those assisted in developed societies are cured around for seven out of ten patients; while in countries with fewer resources five out of ten patients are cured. This gap is related to education, technology, and the experience of services.

The interesting thing to note when one reviews a report is that we tend to value the answers, when what is really important are the questions. The answers are transitory but the questions are permanent.

We will now analyze the value of these questions.

5.5   The Value of Questions

In communication and philosophy, questions are much more important than answers.

Questions open doors, allow us to glimpse who the other person is by showing us what interests they have, what concerns they express, and the order in which they ask these questions. They allow us to see the reasons why someone is interested in knowing a certain answer.

Listening and recording the patient's questions is a very practical way of getting to know them.

I encourage patients to write their questions down and send them to me if want to. In fact, I keep many of them, such as those from a patient who wrote 42 questions before starting chemotherapy.

Most of these questions are related to toxicity or tolerance to the treatments: Will my hair fall out? Will I lose my appetite? Does it cause a lot of nausea?

Other questions are very age specific: Can I become sterile? Should I preserve my eggs (young women with breast cancer or other neoplasms) or sperm (young men with testicular tumors or other tumors)?

Some others are related to sports or other interests: Will I be able to play football? Is it better if I do not go to concerts?

Some are about the prognosis: Is it curable? How long do I have left to live? Will I get to see my grandson graduate?

Finally, there are some unexpected questions. Once one of my patients asked me if they could go skydiving.

While I was thinking about the answer: extreme sports, toxicity from chemotherapy, [88, 89]decreased platelets, possibility of trauma and eventual bleeding, and so forth, it occurred to me to ask him how long he had been skydiving.

He replied that he had never actually gone skydiving, he just wanted to know if he would be able to do it, should he want to.

I replied that it seemed like a risky activity and it was preferable to wait until after chemotherapy since the chance of accidents or errors in beginners is greater than in the experts.

It must be understood that I do not tell this story to make a joke, but rather to show that the patient is aware of their vulnerability and the choices or activities that they have postponed or will have to avoid due to the diagnosis.

We can safely say that most people will give up moments of happiness in the present so that they may experience happiness in the future.

The diagnosis, treatments, and prognosis of the disease make them aware that the distant future could be unattainable and therefore these options must be reconsidered.

Every question a patient asks opens a door. What are their interests and concerns? Why is that question important to your life right now? What decision would you make for each answer? Listening, inquiring, being interested in the other consolidates a relationship based on trust and makes each patient truly unique [88, 89].

I have a personal difficulty in putting names to faces or medical history. I need at least three or four meetings so that I can accurately remember the patient's name and what condition they have. That is why I tend to establish some unique characteristic that makes that patient unmistakable. Many times that characteristic arises from the questions that he asks me (such as Mr. Skydiving). There are some patients who ask absolutely original questions, and that is usually a moment of great joy in the consultation.

5.6   Writing and Drawing for the Patient

One of the most important advances in medicine was the incorporation of art, especially drawing, such as Vesalius and Jan Calcar, whose illustrated dissections in the book *De Humani Corporis Fabrica* revolutionized the history of medicine due to the impact they had on the study of human anatomy [90].

In more recent times, Testut's [91, 92] anatomy text and Frank Netter 's illustrations [93], authentic works of art, have helped all of us who studied medicine in the last century.

The usefulness of drawing for patients in terms of therapy, both pediatric and adult, has also been widely explained [94–96].

Today in some universities medical students have gone back to drawing by hand (https://penntoday.upenn.edu/news/when-words-arent-enough-medical-students-go-back-drawing-board), and a curriculum on drawing in medical education to improve students' comprehension and communication is being developed [97–100].

Therefore, the usefulness of drawing for the understanding and transmission of information is unquestionable.

Is drawing useful in daily practical consultation for those of us who are not gifted in art?

Yes, it is extremely useful.

Many doctors draw and design diagrams in the office in order to clarify our ideas and help the patient understand what it is we are saying, or planning to do [101–108].

The drawing of a statistical curve so that the patient understands the usefulness of an adjuvant treatment in oncology is something that I use very frequently, and we can see an example of it in Fig. 5.1.

Or the use of drawings to explain the risks and benefits of different treatments as in Fig. 5.2, showing the results of mastectomy with axillary dissection, quadrantectomy with axillary dissection, or lumpectomy with sentinel node in early breast cancer (Fig. 5.2).

I also use list making in addition to drawings (Fig. 5.3); took this idea from Jon Kabat Zinn's book *Full Catastrophe Living.* [109]

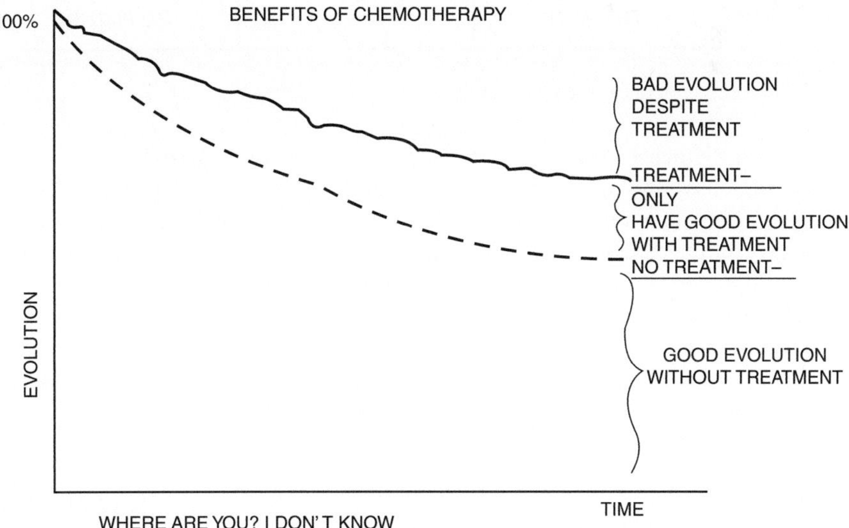

Fig. 5.1 Theoretical benefits of adjuvant chemotherapy

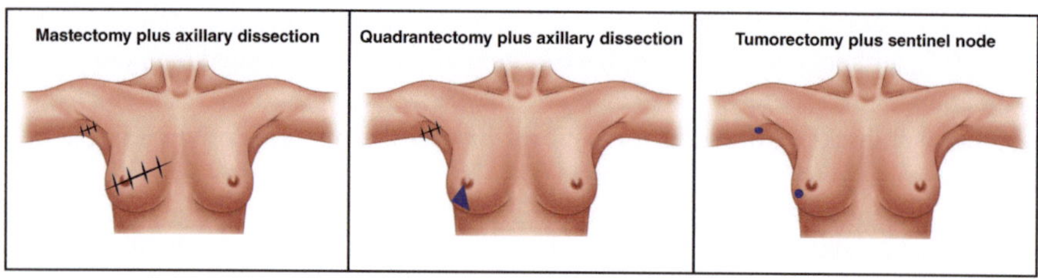

Fig. 5.2 Differences between three types of breast surgeries for the treatment of early breast cancer

Fig. 5.3 List exercise to focus on the present

All these elements have two purposes: one is to draw them in front of the patient so that they have the opportunity to reflect as we build them and that if there is something they do not understand, we can talk about it in that moment. The second purpose is for the patient to take them, those are *their* drawings, they represent *their* case. In short, we personalize the situation to each particular case.

Carrying out an activity together with the patient, when possible, is an experience that expresses in a simple and unequivocal way the empathy we feel for them.

This will be the theme that we will develop in the next chapter and will allow us to understand the multidimensionality of the medical act.

5.7   Teaching Exercises

1. Individual

    (a) Do you consider that information is more important than communication or, on the contrary, do you think they are equally important?
    (b) How do you welcome the patient and what precautions do you take in the anamnesis?
    (c) How many of your patients come to you with information acquired on the Internet?
    (d) What is your information search strategy and how do you organize it?
    (e) Do you record your patient's questions?
    (f) How do you prioritize information when talking with your patient?
    (g) Do you use drawings or diagrams?

2. Group

    (a) Which of the communication theories do you think is more valid for the current doctor–patient relationship?
    (b) What is the experience of each of the group members with respect to information overload?
    (c) What criteria do they use to consider how truthful the information they receive is?
    (d) Do you think medical study reports could use clearer and more understandable language? If you do, take a real report and rewrite it the way you think it could be improved.
    (e) Select a topic such as how to advice a patient to quit smoking. Each member of the group should then draw a diagram, a table, or a graph that exemplifies the core of the message that they want to communicate and the patient can take home.

References

1. Rubinelli S. Aristotle's topics. In: Argumentation library, vol. 15. Dordrecht: Springer; 2009. https://doi.org/10.1007/978-1-4020-9549-8_1.
2. Dow J. Dialectic, persuasion, and science in Aristotle. Proc Boston Area Colloquium Ancient Philos. 2021;36(1):1. https://doi.org/10.1163/22134417-00361P02.
3. Aristotle. Rhetoric; 2010. https://doi.org/10.1017/cbo9780511707445.
4. O'Boyle N. Communication theory for humans. Cham: Springer; 2022. https://doi.org/10.1007/978-3-031-02450-4.
5. McQuail D, Golding P, de Bens E. Communication theory and research. New Delhi: SAGE; 2012. https://doi.org/10.4135/9780857024374.
6. Hardt H. Critical communication studies: communication, history and theory in America. London: Routledge; 2012.
7. Uspayanti R. Assertive and expressive speech act used by English teachers and its implications. LETS. 2020;2(1):1.

8. Gilardi F, Gessler T, Kubli M, Müller S. Social media and political agenda setting. Polit Commun. 2022;39(1):39. https://doi.org/10.1080/10584609.2021.1910390.

9. Boukes M. Agenda-setting with satire: how political satire increased TTIP's saliency on the public, media, and political agenda. Polit Commun. 2019;36(3):426. https://doi.org/10.1080/10584609.2018.1498816.

10. Clark J. Medicalization of global health 1: has the global health agenda become too medicalized? Glob Health Action. 2014;7(SUPP.1):23998. https://doi.org/10.3402/gha.v7.23998.

11. Berger CR. Interpersonal communication: theoretical perspectives, future prospects. J Commun. 2005;55(3):415. https://doi.org/10.1093/joc/55.3.415.

12. Berger CR, Chaffee SH. On bridging the communication gap. Hum Commun Res. 1988;15(2):311. https://doi.org/10.1111/j.1468-2958.1988.tb00187.x.

13. Berger CR, Roloff ME, Roskos-Ewoldsen DR. What is communication science? In: The handbook of communication science. New Delhi: Sage; 2010. https://doi.org/10.4135/9781412982818.n1.

14. Berger CR. Producing messages under uncertainty. In: Message production: advances in communication theory. London: Routledge; 2013. https://doi.org/10.4324/9780203810996-18.

15. Berger CR, Knowlton SW, Abrahams MF. The hierarchy principle in strategic communication. Commun Theory. 1996;6(2):111. https://doi.org/10.1111/j.1468-2885.1996.tb00123.x.

16. Baker SC, Watson BM, Jamieson B, Jamieson R. How do patients define satisfaction? The role of patient perceptions of their participation and health provider emotional expression. Health Commun. 2021;36(14):1970. https://doi.org/10.1080/10410236.2020.1808409.

17. Gorman JR, Drizin JH, Smith E, Flores-Sanchez Y, Harvey SM. Patient-centered communication to address young adult breast cancer survivors' reproductive and sexual health concerns. Health Commun. 2021;36(13):1743. https://doi.org/10.1080/10410236.2020.1794550.

18. Clayton MF, Dudley WN, Musters A. Communication with breast cancer survivors. Health Commun. 2008;23(3):207. https://doi.org/10.1080/10410230701808376.

19. Bensing J. Bridging the gap: the separate worlds of evidence-based medicine and patient-centered medicine. Patient Educ Couns. 2000;39(1):17. https://doi.org/10.1016/S0738-3991(99)00087-7.

20. Elwyn G, Lloyd A, May C, et al. Collaborative deliberation: a model for patient care. Patient Educ Couns. 2014;97(2):158. https://doi.org/10.1016/j.pec.2014.07.027.

21. Mallinger JB, Griggs JJ, Shields CG. Patient-centered care and breast cancer survivors' satisfaction with information. Patient Educ Couns. 2005;57(3):342. https://doi.org/10.1016/j.pec.2004.09.009.

22. McCormack LA, Treiman K, Rupert D, et al. Measuring patient-centered communication in cancer care: a literature review and the development of a systematic approach. Soc Sci Med. 2011;72(7):1085. https://doi.org/10.1016/j.socscimed.2011.01.020.

23. Thom DH, Campbell B. Patient-physician trust: an exploratory study. J Fam Pract. 1997;44(2):169.

24. Greenhalgh J. The applications of PROs in clinical practice: what are they, do they work, and why? Qual Life Res. 2009;18(1):115. https://doi.org/10.1007/s11136-008-9430-6.

25. Wang T, Wang H, Zeng Y, Cai X, Xie L. Health beliefs associated with preventive behaviors against noncommunicable diseases. Patient Educ Couns. 2022;105(1):173. https://doi.org/10.1016/j.pec.2021.05.024.

26. Sohail A, Akritidis J, McGuinness S, Leder K. Perceptions of travel-related health risks and pre-travel health-seeking behaviour among students: a qualitative analysis. Travel Med Infect Dis. 2023;52:52. https://doi.org/10.1016/j.tmaid.2022.102532.

27. Bishop AC, Baker GR, Boyle TA, MacKinnon NJ. Using the health belief model to explain patient involvement in patient safety. Health Expect. 2015;18(6):3019. https://doi.org/10.1111/hex.12286.

28. Wang Z, Feng T, Lau JTF, Kim Y. Acceptability of voluntary medical male circumcision (VMMC) among male sexually transmitted diseases patients (MSTDP) in China. PLoS One. 2016;11(2):e0149801. https://doi.org/10.1371/journal.pone.0149801.

29. Sadeghian Motavali Z, Abedi H, Davaridolatabadi E. Self-medication and its effective modifiable factors among elderly referred health care centers in Shahr-e-Kord in 2015. Electron Physician. 2016;8(11):3205. https://doi.org/10.19082/3205.

30. Watanabe N, Kaneko A, Yamar S, et al. Determinants of the use of insecticide-treated bed nets on islands of pre-and post-malaria elimination: an application of the health belief model in Vanuatu. Malar J. 2014;13(1):441. https://doi.org/10.1186/1475-2875-13-441.

31. Krawczyk A, Knäuper B, Gilca V, et al. Parents' decision-making about the human papillomavirus vaccine for their daughters: I. Quantitative results. Hum Vaccin Immunother. 2015;11(2):322. https://doi.org/10.1080/21645515.2014.1004030.

32. Batista A, Mouttapa M, Wallace S, McMahan S. Empieza con Fuerza Tu Día (kick start your day). Calif J Health Promot. 2014;12(2):99. https://doi.org/10.32398/cjhp.v12i2.2154.

33. Soleymanian A, Niknami S, Hajizadeh E, Shojaeizadeh D, Montazeri A. Development and validation of a health belief model based instrument for measuring factors influencing exercise behaviors to prevent osteoporosis in pre-menopausal women (HOPE). BMC Musculoskelet Disord. 2014;15(1):1. https://doi.org/10.1186/1471-2474-15-61.

34. Chen J, Liao Y, Li Z, et al. Determinants of salt-restriction-spoon using behavior in China: application of the health belief model. PLoS One. 2013;8(12):e83262. https://doi.org/10.1371/journal.pone.0083262.

35. Quick BL, LaVoie NR, Stone AM. An examination of organ donation in the news: a content analysis from 2005–2010 of the barriers to becoming an organ donor. In: Organ donation and transplantation—public policy and clinical perspectives. London: IntechOpen; 2012. https://doi.org/10.5772/32665.

36. Zhao J, Song F, Ren S, et al. Predictors of condom use behaviors based on the health belief model (HBM) among female sex workers: a cross-sectional study in Hubei Province, China. PLoS One. 2012;7(11):e49542. https://doi.org/10.1371/journal.pone.0049542.

37. Katz DA, Graber M, Birrer E, et al. Health beliefs toward cardiovascular risk reduction in patients admitted to chest pain observation units. Acad Emerg Med. 2009;16(5):379. https://doi.org/10.1111/j.1553-2712.2009.00383.x.

38. Soto Mas F, Lacoste Marín JA, Papenfuss RL, Gutiérrez LA. The health belief model. A theoretical approach to AIDS prevention. Rev Esp Public Health. 1997;71(4):335. https://doi.org/10.1590/s1135-57271997000400002.

39. Deshpande S, Basil MD, Basil DZ. Factors influencing healthy eating habits among college students: an application of the health belief model. Health Mark Q. 2009;26(2):145. https://doi.org/10.1080/07359680802619834.

40. Ahadzadeh AS, Pahlevan Sharif S, Ong FS, Khong KW. Integrating health belief model and technology acceptance model: an investigation of health-related internet use. J Med Internet Res. 2015;17(2):e45. https://doi.org/10.2196/jmir.3564.

41. Diaz AFC. Technology vs. infoxication—The challenges of obtaining intelligence from the buzz. New York: IEEE; 2011. https://doi.org/10.1109/eisic.2011.74.

42. Fernández PC. Effects of information overload on news consumer behavior. The doomscrolling. VISUAL review international visual culture review. Rev Int Cult. 2023;10(3):1. https://doi.org/10.37467/revvisual.v10.4592.

43. From DP. "Infoxication" to " infosaturation ": a theoretical overview of the cognitive and social effects of digital immersion. Scopes Magazine Int Commun. 2014;2014:24.

44. Veneroni FL. From pandemic to Infodemic: the virus of Infoxication. Rev Mex Cienc Polit Soc. 2021;66(242):1.

45. Bawden D, Robinson L. The dark side of information: overload, anxiety and other paradoxes and pathologies. J Inf Sci. 2009;35(2):180. https://doi.org/10.1177/0165551508095781.

46. Fernandez C. The paradox of choice: why more is less. Vikalpa. 2017;42(4):265. https://doi.org/10.1177/0256090917732442.

47. Caldwell C. Select all: can you have too many choices? New Yorker. 2004;80(2):1.

48. Marck M. Barry Schwartz the paradox of choice, why more is less. Int J Mark Res. 2010;52(5):699. https://doi.org/10.2501/S1470785310201594.

49. Abad CS. The first fake news of history. Hist Comun Soc. 2019;24(2):411. https://doi.org/10.5209/hics.66268.
50. Naci H, Dias S, Ades AE. Industry sponsorship bias in research findings: a network meta-analysis of LDL cholesterol reduction in randomised trials of statins. BMJ (Online). 2014;349:349. https://doi.org/10.1136/bmj.g5741.
51. Leefmann J. How to assess the epistemic wrongness of sponsorship bias? The case of manufactured certainty. Front Res Metr Anal. 2021;6:6. https://doi.org/10.3389/frma.2021.599909.
52. Sismondo S. Ghost management: how much of the medical literature is shaped behind the scenes by the pharmaceutical industry? PLoS Med. 2007;4(9):1429–33. https://doi.org/10.1371/journal.pmed.0040286.
53. Barton S, Peckitt C, Sclafani F, Cunningham D, Chau I. The influence of industry sponsorship on the reporting of subgroup analyses within phase III randomised controlled trials in gastrointestinal oncology. Eur J Cancer. 2015;51(18):2732–9. https://doi.org/10.1016/j.ejca.2015.08.030.
54. Addeo A, Weiss GJ, Gyawali B. Association of industry and academic sponsorship with negative phase 3 oncology trials and reported outcomes on participant survival a pooled analysis. JAMA Netw Open. 2019;2(5):e193684. https://doi.org/10.1001/jamanetworkopen.2019.3684.
55. Wells JC, Sharma S, Del Paggio JC, et al. An analysis of contemporary oncology randomized clinical trials from low/middle-income vs high-income countries. JAMA Oncol. 2021;7(3):379–85. https://doi.org/10.1001/jamaoncol.2020.7478.
56. Rubagumya F, Hopman WM, Gyawali B, et al. Participation of lower and upper middle-income countries in clinical trials led by high-income countries. JAMA Netw Open. 2022;5(8):E2227252. https://doi.org/10.1001/jamanetworkopen.2022.27252.
57. Del Paggio JC, Berry JS, Hopman WM, et al. Evolution of the randomized clinical trial in the era of precision oncology. JAMA Oncol. 2021;7(5):728–34. https://doi.org/10.1001/jamaoncol.2021.0379.
58. Fundytus A, Wells JC, Sharma S, et al. Industry funding of oncology randomised controlled trials: implications for design, results and interpretation. Clin Oncol. 2022;34(1):28–35. https://doi.org/10.1016/j.clon.2021.08.003.
59. Gazendam AM, Slawaska-Eng D, Nucci N, Bhatt O, Ghert M. The impact of industry funding on randomized controlled trials of biologic therapies. Medicines. 2022;9(3):18. https://doi.org/10.3390/medicines9030018.
60. Buchkowsky SS, Jewesson PJ. Industry sponsorship and authorship of clinical trials over 20 years. Ann Pharmacother. 2004;38(4):579–85. https://doi.org/10.1345/aph.1D267.
61. Sismondo S. How pharmaceutical industry funding affects trial outcomes: causal structures and responses. Soc Sci Med. 2008;66(9):1909–14. https://doi.org/10.1016/j.socscimed.2008.01.010.
62. Doucet M, Sismondo S. Evaluating solutions to sponsorship bias. J Med Ethics. 2008;34(8):627–30. https://doi.org/10.1136/jme.2007.022467.
63. Smith T. Doctors should admit their mistakes. Int J Risk Safe Med. 1990;1(1):45.
64. Back A, Arnold R, Tulsky J. Mastering communication with seriously Ill patients: balancing honesty with empathy and hope. Cambridge: Cambridge University Press; 2009. https://doi.org/10.1017/CBO9780511576454.
65. Ciarlo G, Rudolph I, Keinki C, Micke O, Huebner J. Information needs in cancer care—a comparison of patients' and professionals' needs. Trace Elements Electrolytes. 2018;35(07):109. https://doi.org/10.5414/tex01529.
66. Joolaee S, Joolaei A, Tschudin V, Bahrani N, Nasrabadi N. Caring relationship: the core component of patients' rights practice as experienced by patients and their companions. J Med Ethics Hist Med. 2010;3:4.
67. Chen A. A conversation analysis of sensitive talk in clinic interaction. Int J Front Sociology. 2021;3(13):91. https://doi.org/10.25236/ijfs.2021.031306.

68. Elder AT, Mcmanus C, Patrick A, Nair K, Vaughan L, Dacre J. The value of the physical examination in clinical practice: an international survey. Clin Med. 2017;17(6):490–8.
69. Garibaldi BT, Elder A. Seven reasons why the physical examination remains important. J Royal Coll Phys Edinburgh. 2021;51(3):211–4. https://doi.org/10.4997/JRCPE.2021.301.
70. Garibaldi BT, Olson APJ. The hypothesis-driven physical examination. Med Clin North Am. 2018;102(3):433–42. https://doi.org/10.1016/j.mcna.2017.12.005.
71. Zaman JAB. The enduring value of the physical examination. Med Clin North Am. 2018;102(3):417–23. https://doi.org/10.1016/j.mcna.2017.12.003.
72. Artandi MK, Stewart RW. The outpatient physical examination. Med Clin North Am. 2018;102(3):465–73. https://doi.org/10.1016/j.mcna.2017.12.008.
73. Verghese A, Charlton B, Kassirer JP, Ramsey M, Ioannidis JPA. Inadequacies of physical examination as a cause of medical errors and adverse events: a collection of vignettes. Am J Med. 2015;128(12):1322. https://doi.org/10.1016/j.amjmed.2015.06.004.
74. Brown-Johnson C, Schwartz R, Maitra A, et al. What is clinician presence? A qualitative interview study comparing physician and non-physician insights about practices of human connection. BMJ Open. 2019;9(11):e030831. https://doi.org/10.1136/bmjopen-2019-030831.
75. Zaman J, Verghese A, Elder A. The value of physical examination: a new conceptual framework. South Med J. 2016;109(12):754. https://doi.org/10.14423/SMJ.0000000000000573.
76. Verghese A, Brady E, Kapur CC, Horwitz RI. The bedside evaluation: ritual and reason. Ann Intern Med. 2011;155(8):550. https://doi.org/10.7326/0003-4819-155-8-201110180-00013.
77. Rosenthal DI, Verghese A. Meaning and the nature of physicians' work. N Engl J Med. 2016;375(19):1813. https://doi.org/10.1056/nejmp1609055.
78. Costanzo C, Verghese A. The physical examination as ritual: social sciences and embodiment in the context of the physical examination. Med Clin North Am. 2018;102(3):425. https://doi.org/10.1016/j.mcna.2017.12.004.
79. Verghese A, Charlton B, Cotter B, Kugler J. A history of physical examination texts and the conception of bedside diagnosis. Trans Am Clin Climatol Assoc. 2011;122:290.
80. Verghese A, Horwitz RI. In praise of the physical examination. BMJ. 2009;339(7735):339. https://doi.org/10.1136/bmj.b5448.
81. Maitra A, Verghese A. Diagnosis and the illness experience: ways of knowing. JAMA. 2021;326(19):1907. https://doi.org/10.1001/jama.2021.19496.
82. Russell SW, Garibaldi BT, Elder A, Verghese A. The power of touch. Lancet. 2020;395(10230):57. https://doi.org/10.1016/S0140-6736(20)30170-7.
83. Verghese A. A doctor's touch. TED Talk.
84. Florindez J, Vazquez Guillamet R, Vazquez Guillamet C, Manthous C, Lighthall J. Physicians perceptions of the utility of physical exam in the intensive care unit. A qualitative study. New York: American Thoracic Society; 2012. https://doi.org/10.1164/ajrccm-conference.2012.185.1_meetingabstracts.a1661.
85. Wu EH, Fagan MJ, Reinert SE, Diaz JA. Self-confidence in and perceived utility of the physical examination: a comparison of medical students, residents, and faculty internists. J Gen Intern Med. 2007;22(12):1725. https://doi.org/10.1007/s11606-007-0409-8.
86. Hashim MM, Edgeworth DM, Saunders JA, Harmon DC. Patient's perceptions of physical examination in the setting of chronic pain. Ir J Med Sci. 2021;190(1):313. https://doi.org/10.1007/s11845-020-02250-2.
87. Ramani S. Twelve tips for excellent physical examination teaching. Med Teach. 2008;30(9–10):851. https://doi.org/10.1080/01421590802206747.
88. Yin K, Jung J, Coiera E, et al. Patient work and their contexts: scoping review. J Med Internet Res. 2020;22(6):e16656. https://doi.org/10.2196/16656.
89. Howe LC, Leibowitz KA, Crum AJ. When your doctor "gets it" and "gets you": the critical role of competence and warmth in the patient-provider interaction. Front Psychiatry. 2019;10:10. https://doi.org/10.3389/fpsyt.2019.00475.
90. Porzionato A, Macchi V, Stecco C, Parenti A, De Caro R. The anatomical school of Padua. Anat Rec. 2012;295(6):902. https://doi.org/10.1002/ar.22460.

91. Fessy MH, Carret JP, Viste A. The history of anatomy teaching in Lyon University: in the footsteps of Rabelais, petit, Lisfranc, Testut and Latarjet, and many others. Surg Radiol Anat. 2019;41(10):1129. https://doi.org/10.1007/s00276-019-02321-9.

92. Romero R. In: Acquatella Monserratte H, Briceño-Iragorry L, editors. The Testut- Latarjet Human Anatomy treatise , more than 100 years of application in Venezuela for teaching and apre, vol. XVIII. Collection Razzetti; 2016.

93. Shivakumar N, Hammad AY, Gamblin TC. Frank netter: a man of art and science. Am Surg. 2016;82(5):377. https://doi.org/10.1177/000313481608200508.

94. Aguilar BA. The efficacy of art therapy in pediatric oncology patients: an integrative literature review. J Pediatr Nurs. 2017;36:36. https://doi.org/10.1016/j.pedn.2017.06.015.

95. Zhang K, Ma J, Chen J, Xu L, Gu C. Effects of drawing therapy on pediatric oncology patients: a systematic review. Cancer Nurs. 2022;45(2):E397. https://doi.org/10.1097/NCC.0000000000000929.

96. Timberlake JK. In-session sketching: an adjunctive technique for brief dynamic therapies. Prof Psychol Res Pr. 2014;45(4):291. https://doi.org/10.1037/a0037218.

97. Card EB, Lejbman J, Trueblood E, et al. Drawing for visual communication in medicine: a novel pilot course for senior medical students. J Surg Educ. 2022;79(2):389. https://doi.org/10.1016/j.jsurg.2021.09.006.

98. Fahrenfort M. Patient education in Dutch hospitals: the fruits of a decade of endeavors. Patient Educ Couns. 1990;15(2):139. https://doi.org/10.1016/0738-3991(90)90057-R.

99. Cheung MMY, Saini B, Smith L. Integrating drawings into health curricula: university educators' perspectives. Med Humanit. 2020;46(4):394. https://doi.org/10.1136/medhum-2019-011775.

100. Ronan LK, Czerwiec MK. A novel graphic medicine curriculum for resident physicians: boosting empathy and communication through comics. J Med Humanit. 2020;41(4):573. https://doi.org/10.1007/s10912-020-09654-2.

101. Cox A, Li S. The medical consultation through the lenses of language and social interaction theory. Adv Health Sci Educ. 2020;25(1):241. https://doi.org/10.1007/s10459-018-09873-2.

102. Kearns C, Kearns N, Paisley AM. The art of consent: visual materials help adult patients make informed choices about surgical care. J Vis Commun Med. 2020;43(2):76. https://doi.org/10.1080/17453054.2019.1671168.

103. Laursen JB, Jensen LV, Thinggaard E. Drawing improves understanding of anatomy, operation planning and communication. Ugeskr Laeger. 2020;181(16):V03190153.

104. Shamaskin-Garroway A, DeCaporale-Ryan L, Bell K, McDaniel S. Physician communication coaching: how psychologists can elevate skills and support resident education, professionalism, and Well-being. J Clin Psychol Med Settings. 2022;29(3):608. https://doi.org/10.1007/s10880-021-09808-x.

105. Epstein RM, Street RL. Shared mind: communication, decision making, and autonomy in serious illness. Ann Fam Med. 2011;9(5):454. https://doi.org/10.1370/afm.1301.

106. van de Water LF, van Kleef JJ, Dijksterhuis WPM, et al. Communicating treatment risks and benefits to cancer patients: a systematic review of communication methods. Qual Life Res. 2020;29(7):1746. https://doi.org/10.1007/s11136-020-02503-8.

107. Kearns C, Murton S, Oldfield K, et al. Estimating the prevalence of drawing in clinical practice among kiwi doctors. J Vis Commun Med. 2022;45(4):234. https://doi.org/10.1080/17453054.2022.2106197.

108. Kearns C. Is drawing a valuable skill in surgical practice? 100 surgeons weigh in. J Vis Commun Med. 2019;42(1):4. https://doi.org/10.1080/17453054.2018.1558996.

109. Kabat-Zinn J. Full catastrophe living: using the wisdom of your body and mind to face stress, pain, and illness, 15th Anniversary Ed.; 2005.

Chapter 6
Empathy and Communication

6.1 What Is Empathy?

Empathy, as Dr. Vidal y Benito maintains [1], is a polysemic word, "nomadic" in his words, because it changes meaning depending on the context in which it is used.

Other authors have highlighted this lack of consensus and consistency in the definition of empathy while advocating for its importance during the consultation [2].

Therefore, our first challenge will be to understand what empathy means in the medical practice.

To start, we will use the definition found in the Dictionary of Medical Terms of the Royal Spanish Academy.

Empathy is the "ability to recognize and understand the feelings and thoughts of another person, just as they experience it" (https://dtme.ranm.es/buscador. aspx?NIVEL_BUS=3&LEMA_BUS=Empat%C3%ADa).

Therefore, if we dive into this definition, we see that it is a condition or ability, being able to integrate someone else's experiences into our knowledge. Or, as it was originally defined in the 1950s, "the capacity to think and feel oneself into the inner life of another person" [3].

Sixteen years later, practically an entire volume of *The Counseling Psychologist* was devoted to exploring this issue, beginning with a seminal article by Carl Rogers and another by David Aspy [4, 5]. Both authors wrote that empathy was not only a skill, but a behavior, a habit, a way of being.

This way of seeing empathy incorporates the cognitive aspect (recognizing) with the affective, evaluative (understanding), behavioral (attitudes), and relational aspects. These are the domains that work to develop empathy.

Therefore, we could accept as an operational definition that empathy is the condition of the human being who has the habit of recognizing and understanding what someone else feels and thinks, and who can communicate how they perceive reality from the perspective of the other person.

© The Author(s), under exclusive license to Springer Nature
Switzerland AG 2024
E. Gil Deza, *Improving Clinical Communication*,
https://doi.org/10.1007/978-3-031-62446-9_6

It is a different concept from *sympathy* that is having an affinity for someone, or *antipathy,* which is feeling aversion to someone. Empathy is recognizing and understanding what others feel and think, regardless of whether we like them or not.

Some see empathy as a risk of losing professional objectivity, becoming emotionally involved with the patient, and running a greater risk of professional burnout.

I believe the exact opposite: empathy allows us to understand the patient's experience in greater depth and enrich ourselves with their point of view.

This knowledge, from my perspective, is essential to adapt treatments to the patient's desires, circumstances, and values instead of doing the opposite, sometimes forcibly, like in a Procrustes bed.

Empathy has different components, which have been developed in Tan's work [2]. The authors maintain that this study, which used 14 focus groups, enjoyed several advantages: not only did it interview all members of the medical staff as well as patients, but it was also carried out in Singapore. This means that British, American, Asian, and even Confucianism sensibilities could be found in the interviewees' educational background. This cultural exchange further enriches the prospect of a comprehensive definition of empathy.

The components identified in this work in relation to clinical empathy were the following:

1. **Intrinsic feeling of empathy** by the doctor or nurse, which consists of three domains: the ability to "put oneself in the other's shoes" (imaginative); feeling what the patient is feeling (affective) and understanding the patient's perspective (cognitive).
2. **Empathetic behavior**: This means firstly a genuine concern for what is happening to the patient (empathy cares about people, not tasks or practices) and secondly communicating empathetically (which is reflected fundamentally in nonverbal communication, especially in silence and attention).
3. **Empathy as a sense of trust and bonding (connection):** This is especially true, in Tan's work, for nurses, as it is expressed as attention to small details for the comfort and care of the patient.
4. **Cultural aspects:** Even when there are great cultural differences in other subjects, when it comes of empathy there seems to be a universal need to feel genuinely appreciated and understood by those who care for our health. When these aspects are analyzed, the differences seem to arise in two ways: (a) the role of spiritual support and religious beliefs and (b) the way or style of expressing empathetic behaviors (social distance, expression of affection, gestures).

It makes sense that a complex phenomenon such as empathy would be difficult to define precisely because it requires us to listen to our right brain, as Iain McGilchrist argues in his latest text [6].

McGilchrist is a neurologist, psychiatrist, and an eminent writer [7, 8] whose most important task has been to study the asymmetric relationship between the left brain and the right brain. In summary, we can say that the left brain observes a representation of what the right brain experiences. This is why for the left brain reality is inanimate, fragmented, reified, dimensioned, segmented, classified; the left brain's purpose is to apprehend and manipulate. Meanwhile, reality for the right brain is vital, unified, holistic, multidimensional, and fluid; the right brain's purpose is to understand and know.

Cerebral asymmetry is explained as a consequence of evolution and the need to perceive reality and react quickly, which is why one hemisphere perceives the whole and another does not.

In the case of empathy, it is clearly an activity in which we use our imagination to try to learn what we believe to be our patient's experience, and that allows us to get closer to them.

For this, we must be aware of the multifaceted nature of both human beings and the doctor–patient relationship.

6.2 The Multifaceted Nature of Human Beings

At this point, we will dive deep into the concept of humanity that the Spanish philosopher Julián Marías bequeathed to us, as he is one of those who has reflected the most on this subject. We will focus on two key texts: "person" and "map of the personal world" [9, 10].

The phenomenology proposed by Marías allows us to put ourselves in the other's shoes more easily.

We will take three outstanding notes that human beings have for this author:

(a) **Presence**: The radical reality of the human being is his life. Or, to put it another way, the place where all reality occurs is his life. Sickness does not happen to someone, they *get sick*. Their whole life is turned upside down when they are affected by an illness.

   If that disease is life-threatening or, like cancer, it has a connotation death, pain, or mutilation, the person feels that their entire existence is challenged.

   Nobody, or almost nobody, goes to the doctor's office if they do not think that what they are suffering from is serious; conversely, if you go for a routine checkup it is because you think you do not have anything.

   Therefore, the first thing we have to understand is that our patient is **afraid**. It is presented in the form of restlessness, discomfort, anxiety, or explicitly as fear. But the deep reality is one of vulnerability, mortality, and injustice.

   Illness abruptly bursts into consciousness as an **undeniable and undesirable reality** in a person's existence, as Anatole Broyard argues in his book *Intoxicated by My Ilness* [11]: "Choosing a doctor is difficult because it is our first explicit confrontation of our illness. 'How Good is this man?' is simply the reverse of 'How bad am I?'" [11].

   Therefore, the first thing that doctors must understand is that what brings patients to our consultation is, fundamentally, the fear of dying and suffering from a disease that could kill them or seriously affect their current life.

The second thing we must understand is that the disease is always **surprising**; it is a surprise even for those who suspect it and go looking for it. The news might be unexpected or confirmatory, but it is always *news*.

(b) **Corporeality**: We are a body, we perceive things through our body and our senses. We relate to each other through our body. How does our body experience illness? As strangeness, betrayal, limitation, and invasion.

Strangeness, because we noticed something radically new (a nodule, stain, tremor, pain, weakness, etc.), something that either was not there or we did not perceive and that now we cannot ignore.

Betrayal, because our body is unable to do what it used to without difficulty or because it refuses to obey our orders. Without giving us prior notice, our body abruptly ceases to be our ally.

Limitation, aging is knowing that tomorrow we will be a little less free, a little less capable, a little weaker than today. Illness acts as a catalyst for that vital entropy.

Invasion, often especially in the case of infectious diseases or tumors, we feel that our body has been taken by assault, by hostile forces that have undermined our defenses and now feed on our own being to destroy it. In fact, in the case of some cancer patients, they give each tumor its own name.

Understanding what our patient is experiencing helps us select the best words or examples to explain what we think about their situation.

(c) **Worldliness.** People do not live in *a* world, but rather in *their own* world. The reality we know is a part of reality, the world we live in is a part of the world as a whole. What is that reality and what is that part?

It is the one that we make our own, that is why we live our lives in our reality, limited and personal.

This does not mean that there is no objective reality that we can share among all.

This means that from the existential point of view each one of us feels that they live better when they have control over their world and existence, even if it is not complete control.

From this perspective, illness is experienced as expropriation and injustice.

Expropriation: What does disease take away from us? Pleasure, meaning, future.

Pleasure, because in addition to not being able to do what we want, we also have no desires. Many times the disease becomes the task of our life and certain acts or encounters no longer offer us the enjoyment they once did, nor do we have the strength or desire to do them.

Sense, for many people the meaning of life is to be able to care for, protect, provide, and sustain the beings they love. Now that they are limited by their illness, it is they who must be cared and provided for, sustained, and protected by their loved ones before.

For many patients, the greatest drama of being sick is feeling that they fill their loved ones with sorrow and work, which makes it less appealing for them to continue living. This is probably the worst consequence of an illness.

As Viktor Frankl argues in his book *Man's Search for Meaning* where he recounts his experience as psychiatrist in the Nazi concentration camps: "Any attempt to restore a man's inner strength in the camp had first to succeed in showing him some future goal. Nietzsche's words, 'He who has a why to live for can bear with almost any how'" [12]. The same is true for anyone who yearns to live.

Future, the human being moves toward an uncertain but desirable future, they are a project, self-launched toward the future. That unreality is part of our reality. We imagine and desire a future as part of our daily reality. Illness cuts us off from that future. It makes our temporal nature present to us and puts the horizon of our end within our sight. Personal projects seem unrealizable and that takes away hope.

Therefore, if we summarize what we have just written, we can have a phenomenology of serious illness: it is an undeniable and undesirable reality that generates a surprising fear of dying; experienced as a betrayal or an invasion of his own body; a reality that takes away hope, meaning, pleasure, and future from a patient's life.

This is what we empathetically perceive in our patients, their personal notes make each of these aspects manifest in a different way, and there may even be other unique characteristics in each patient (punishment, guilt, and even relief or liberation) but those that we have mentioned are those that in our experience appear as the most outstanding.

6.3   The Multifaceted Nature of the Doctor–Patient Relationship

Empathy develops in an encounter, which in this case is between doctor and patient.

Empathy in that encounter allows us to measure the multiple levels of interaction that take place in that area at that moment.

If we understand the doctor–patient relationship as the encounter between a conscience (that of the doctor) and a trust (that of the patient), we can understand the nature of that encounter.

6.3.1   The Dimension of Experience

What does the experience of the doctor mean in the medical act?

The witness' knowledge.

Over time, the doctor has treasured encounters with patients and has witnessed those patients' illnesses, as we described in the previous topic: vulnerability (invasion), limitation (expropriation), ailing (punishment), suffering (anguish), and death (disappearance). The older the doctor is, the more they have seen, if they have observed carefully and respectfully.

But they have also witnessed the patient's healing process: recovery (appropriation), restoration (domain), harmony (liberation), learning (revaluation), and vitality (improvement).

Every experienced doctor has witnessed statistical extremes; those who should have evolved well and unfortunately worsened as well as those who should have evolved poorly and surprisingly evolved very well. Doctors who have not seen a "miracle" just have to wait a bit.

Biology is always amazing in some way.

That experience humanizes us because it gives us humility. One of the best works written about this phenomenon was written by Dr. Klein and published in the *Journal of Clinical Oncology* in May 2023. In it, he describes his experience as a first-year resident, 42 years ago during Christmas shift in 1981 [13].

Accumulating experience is also accumulating mistakes.

As a teacher, it is interesting to reflect on the value of errors. We never learn as much as we do from our mistakes. At the same time that we feel humiliated and gain humility. Furthermore, many of them are unforgettable; we can remember with much greater precision the moment and circumstance in which a given mistake happened.

It is remarkable if we go back to Dr. Klein's text how 40 years later he still has that day fresh in his memory, the cafeteria, probably what he was eating when the phone rang, and he was told that his patient had died. How many of us absolutely identify with that image! How many times have we fallen apart, collided with reality, our theories shattered in an instant.

I am not saying that we should be masochistic and wallow in self-mutilation as a reminder of our mistakes, but rather that we should be realistic and occasionally look at our scars with pride, knowing they are a sign that we have lived honestly.

6.3.2   *The Scientific Dimension of Medicine*

Medicine has progressed in these last 50 years more than in the 2500 years that separate us from Hippocrates. The success in rate of diagnosis, treatment, and prognosis of diseases is remarkable in all fields. This at times can translate into excessive pride (Hubris) that leads us to forget the reductionist nature of science and leads us to medical scientism, which is a common disease among professionals.

We must take advantage of scientific knowledge while making an effort not to turn a person into a body; a body into disease; disease into an ailment; the ailment into a parameter; and parameter into the measurement.

If we act in a reductionist way, the patient's suffering ends up being reduced to a parameter's altered measurement and there we end up reducing medicine to the restoration of this altered parameter instead of caring for the patient's suffering.

In curable acute diseases, it is possible that this excess of scientific pride goes unnoticed, but in the care of chronic patients and especially in the care of incurable or dying patients, this pride ends up being an insurmountable obstacle.

Empathy is the cure against scientism by allowing us to perceive the mysteries that the disease confronts us with.

6.3.3   The Magical Dimension of Medicine

When we talk about the magical dimension of medicine, the epistemology of which we analyze in Chap. 3, we must remember that it has to do with the person as an unknown.

That is, it pertains to the mysteries that are related to life both as a whole and personally. Why me? Why right now? What will happen? How much time do I have?

They are all questions for which there is no scientific answer, if there is an answer at all.

The patient may not need an answer, they may just need to hear themselves ask the question without the risk of getting an answer.

A mystery, unlike a puzzle, cannot be solved with more information, it is beyond information. The mystery is a limit, an abyss, a border. Physicians and all members of the health team work on that border between normal and abnormal, life and death, joy and pain, pleasure and suffering, hope and discouragement.

The mystery is glimpsed, registered, listened to, observed, but not answered. This is where the art of knowing how to listen and knowing how to keep quiet acquires transcendence.

6.3.4   The Artistic Dimension of the Medical Act

The artistic dimension of the medical act is strictly related to empathy.

It is the doctor's way of acting: cordiality, sympathy, careful manners, the ritual of the clinical act, thoroughness, respect, and modesty. All of these are ways that are intended to make the patient feel safe and valued.

Explaining what is happening or going to happen and sharing those findings with the patient is highly appreciated by most patients.

But above all taking care of which words and terms we use, as well as taking the time to make sure our patient understands are all things that make our consultation an experience that stands out.

The patient should leave the office a little better than they entered. That is the secret.

Even when we have to give bad news, or better yet, especially when we have to give bad news, we must do it in such a way that the patient feels that we have taken special care in delivering them.

Nothing worsens the relationship between the doctor and the patient more than indifference in treatment: "he didn't even look at me," "he didn't sit down," "he doesn't talk to me," "I'm just one more patient," "he just looks at the computer," these are some of the expressions of patients who feel that their doctor paid more attention to the case than to them; they cared more about the technical and bureaucratic aspects than the human aspect.

6.3.5 The Moral Dimension of the Medical Act

The consultation is also a moment for the patient to make decisions, not only about treatments but also about their own life.

The re-evaluation of the "here and now," showing how many times in life we postpone moments of present happiness in favor of moments of future happiness.

The re-evaluation of the family and genuine human relationships over superficial and forgettable ones.

The re-evaluation of health and life as gifts we may despise and yet they acquire a unique relevance when we are about to lose them.

It is also a time for gratitude, forgiveness, reconciliation, letting go of guilt and responsibilities, and thinking of our legacy.

Many times in the consultation we deal with existential problems where the patient is a mirror in which we also see ourselves reflected.

All of this shows our understanding of the uniqueness of the person in front of us.

6.3.6 The Human Dimension of the Medical Act

All doctors evolve in our profession based on the acquisition of skills, knowledge, and experiences.

The latter are the ones left to us by patients who *make us,* polish us, and complete our training.

They are those patients that we remember with their own names and whose words are still present in our lives.

There are patients who we find admirable for the serenity and wisdom with which they faced the end of life.

There are patients who taught us that the value of living is in the journey and not in reaching a certain goal.

There are patients who taught us that hope is built daily and laboriously, that people are more valuable than things, that relationships transcend physical death, and that alleviating is as important as curing, on many occasions.

This is the reality of the doctor–patient encounter that has as much to do with the biological as with the biographical and in which both doctor and patient are nourished by what is possible, what is desirable, and what is expected.

Now, is there evidence that medical empathy is related to the evolution of diseases?

We will see that next.

6.4   Evidence That the Evolution of Patients Is Related to the Empathy of the Doctor or the Health Team

Analyzing this topic is as important as asking ourselves how much the doctor or health team influences the treatment of a patient since I agree with Rogers: empathy is not only a way of knowing but above all a way of being [4].

This way of being is characterized above all by the ability to perceive or be interested in emotions or feelings, which is known as the inner life of the other.

In medicine, this attitude has always been seen as dangerous due to the risk of emotional commitment that ends up compromising professionalism. It is as if the relationship between doctor and patient was a tug of war between two forces: on one end, the need for empathy and understanding the patient's inner thoughts; and on the other end, the professional distance necessary to offer or make radical decisions [1, 3, 14–17].

Clearly empathy plays a key role in placing the patient at the center of decisions [18].

When Sackett described evidence-based medicine, he raised three sources that must be integrated:

(a) **The best scientific answer** to the question that we ask ourselves, which means that doctors must be trained to formulate the best question with the greatest rigor, since obtaining the best answer depends on it.
(b) **The medical experience**, which has to do with the realism of expectations, since critical vision and skepticism arise from understanding the distance between what we have been told and what really happens.
(c) **The patients' values**, in order to respect their wishes and select the best treatment for their condition.

Forgetting these precepts is what leads us to feel that the origin and meaning of evidence-based medicine have been distorted [19].

Does this condition of empathy influence the evolution of patients?

The answer is categorically yes.

There is ample evidence of the usefulness of empathy for the well-being of the patient [20–24].

Empathy is one of the foundations of trust, and that in itself is already therapeutic, as Aspy maintains: [5] when a patient feels understood and listened to, it alleviates their suffering.

Empathy makes the doctor–patient relationship more realistic, complex, and enriching, which makes both doctor and patient want to continue with it, and that builds a bond between them as they search for health [1].

It increases patient satisfaction, and therefore the patient adheres more to the treatments or recommendations [25–27].

An empathetic attitude is particularly important, especially in the face of stigmatizing diseases such as AIDS, cancer, or mental illness, since both patients and their families are afraid of rejection [28].

Even in specialties immersed in emergency and stress, such as trauma surgery, the empathy of doctors influences the favorable evolution of patients [29].

As Paracelsus maintains in his text *Spitalbuch*, the foundation of medicine is love since it has also been shown that the greater one's empathy, the greater one's mastery of the medical art, what today we call clinical competence [30].

Empathy brings us closer to the privacy of the patient. Within this privacy, one of the least explored values is religiosity, as shown by Viktor Frankl [31] and in numerous situations in the practice of oncology [32].

There is also a B side of empathy: the patient who feels a high degree of empathy toward the doctor perceives fewer medical errors [33], and this is an essential element for the patient's risk. Therefore, doctors should explain to their patients that they, and other members of the health team, should be vigilant and try to point these errors out as they can have a huge impact on the patient's life.

If one reviews the evidence on the impact of empathy on the evolution of a patient's disease, there are two challenges that we must solve:

(a) First of all, which of the variables are we going to analyze? Survival, surrogate efficacy of the treatments, adherence to therapy, patient satisfaction or reduction of litigation, or something else?
(b) Secondly, how do we measure empathy? Self-assessment by doctors or members of the health team has the drawback of bias, which Dunning and Kruger clearly described, an effect that can be seen in all the disciplines [34–38].

Therefore, the next step is to analyze how to study empathy.

6.5   How Is Empathy Studied?

In the case of a domain such as empathy, there are many ways to assess it. You can do it through direct observation or through recording the doctor–patient interaction. You can do it by evaluating the clinical records to see if there is mention of any of the topics related to what the patient feels or believes. We can even study it more quantitatively using measurement scales.

Of these, there are some general scales used in research, such as The Dymond Scale, Hogan Scale, and the Questionnaire Measure of Emotional Empathy [39–43]. But there are also specific scales used for certain professions. In the case of medicine, the most frequently used is the Jefferson scale.

The Jefferson scale has been used by both doctors, nurses, students, and professionals; in different countries of the world and in different cultural contexts [43–49].

Therefore, it is a scale that has been validated and translated into different languages, which means that it is the most useful instrument to measure empathy in medicine we have so far.

In Fig. 6.1, I have presented the first two questions of the Jefferson scale so that you have an approximate idea of what it consists of.

As you can see, it is very simple to administer and use a seven-point numerical ordinal scale to see the degree of agreement or disagreement with respect to the statement on the left.

These values are ultimately integrated to assess a person's level of empathy.

Now, there is a question that is valid to ask ourselves: What is the use of "measuring" empathy? Is it not enough to feel or perceive it?

Without falling into the scientism that reduces something complex into something simple, or the deterministic mechanism that predicts an unfailing behavior based on a given result, the value of the quantifying or at least semi-quantifying a complex phenomenon such as empathy is that it allows comparison between individuals or communities. Perhaps even more importantly, it helps to see if the person changes their level of empathy over time.

Has this comparison ever been made? If so, what are the results?

In the first place, there are very robust correlations between the level of empathy and the level of sociability of a person, which was to be expected. But studies also found a correlation with self-esteem: the higher it is, the more open they are to the feelings or values of others [50, 51].

Another interesting finding is the relationship between empathy and altruistic behaviors. Perceiving what the other feels seems to be the first step in wanting to help them [52–55].

Finally, there is a close relationship between someone's empathy and their non-violent behavior. Perceiving someone's suffering literally disarms us [56–62].

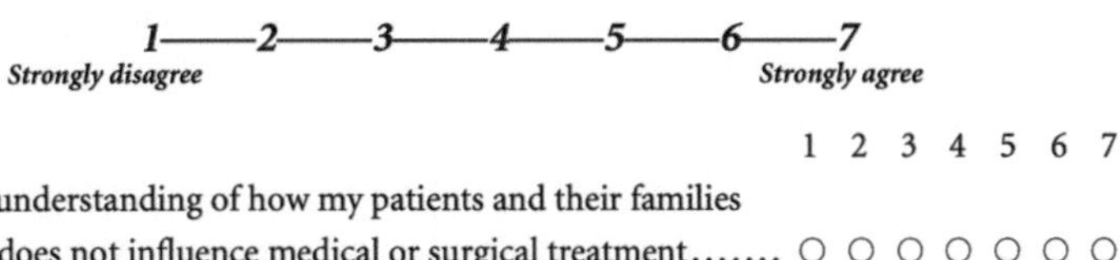

Instructions: Please indicate the extent of your agreement or disagreement with *each* of the following statements by marking the appropriate circle to the right of each statement.

Please use the following 7-point scale (*a higher number on the scale indicates more agreement*):
Mark <u>one and only one</u> response for each statement.

1——2——3——4——5——6——7
Strongly disagree   *Strongly agree*

                  1 2 3 4 5 6 7

1. My understanding of how my patients and their families feel does not influence medical or surgical treatment....... ○ ○ ○ ○ ○ ○ ○
2. My patients feel better when I understand their feelings.... ○ ○ ○ ○ ○ ○ ○

Fig. 6.1 Extract from the Jefferson scale to measure medical empathy

If we take these elements together, we see that the study of empathy and above all how to generate or improve it can help us be more supportive, peaceful, and better caretakers of the environment.

This is particularly important in early childhood education.

What else have studies on medical empathy shown?

When we compare the level of empathy during the first year and the last year of medical school, the level of empathy tends to fall and rarely remains stable [63–66].

This decrease in empathy can be explained by the stress and burnout suffered by students as they work through their subjects or by the difference between what the student imagined his work would be like and actual experience. Somehow, exposure to a painful or stressful stimulus tends to desensitize us.

In any case, what this shows is that empathy is a dynamic phenomenon, and while it can decrease, it can also increase. This of course begs the question: What do the guidelines of different scientific bodies say about empathy?

6.6 What Do the Oncology Communication Guidelines Say About Empathy?

All guidelines have either implicit or explicit recommendations regarding empathy.

For example, in the *Patient-Clinician Communication: American Society of Clinical Oncology Consensus Guideline* of 2017 [67], the text touches on many aspects closely related to empathy, like characterizing what we communicate as *devastating news* and, on the other hand, the patient's reaction of fear, anger, or denial, which may be shared by their family and friends.

Later on, the text gives an explicit recommendation when communicating bad news, which we will analyze in detail:

(a) The first strategy for an empathetic response is to "name" the emotion that we perceive in the other person.

To name something, especially an emotion, is to be able to analyze it, limit it, and evaluate its consequences in our lives. Formulating this denomination in the form of a question to the patient allows him to correct or complement our observation.

(b) An invitation to remain silent, observing and accompanying. Knowing how to shut up is an art as important as knowing how to speak. It is correct to point out that in an emotional crisis the patient is not in a position to register or process information. We have to wait. This waiting must be attentive and warm.

Once the crisis passes, *then* we can return to the dialogue and try to understand more about what our patient feels, thinks, and wants.

The guide returns, this time explicitly, to the problem of empathy in the specific discussion of end-of-life care.

There are two or three very difficult moments in the dialogues that take place in patient care: these are discussing a medical error and talking about end-of-life care.

Talking about the end of life is, in essence, also talking about the failure of previous treatments and the uselessness of any future treatments.

It is reasonable for the doctor to have this conversation, or at least a hint of it, when the patient is well. At the beginning of the doctor–patient relationship, exploring these desires is relatively easy because it is still an abstract and future topic. "In the event that the disease worsens and we do not have treatments that can cure it or prolong your life, what would you want us to do?" is a way to open the conversation at some point.

Picking up this conversation several months or even years later is easier than starting it right at the end.

It is true that the "Lazarus effect" [68–71] of new treatments in oncology makes this conversation more difficult. We should note many of these publications give an impression of normality to something that is usually quite rare. However, these unexpected evolutions are longed for both by the patient and the doctor, which ends up bringing us closer to "miracle medicine."

The problem with the "therapeutic miracle," or "miracle medicine," is not that it does not exist. The problem is that waiting for the miracle, which may or may not happen, is an all or nothing bet. And the sad reality with these bets is that the most common result is *nothing*.

When a patient or family is faced with this situation, the only thing one can do is explain that while we also want the miracle; the question is, "If the miracle does not occur, is there something we can do so that you or your family are better?" If the patient tolerates that question, it is possible that the doors are opened to do something else while we wait for the miracle to occur. This is valid both for those who place their hope in medicine as well as those who do so in a religious belief.

Let us go back to the guide's recommendation about grief.

The study of loss and past grief helps anticipate the confrontation with future loss and grief. The advice to refer our patients to appropriate psychosocial support is excellent, but we must remember that whether or not our patients and their families will follow our recommendations depends entirely on the trust they place in us.

And this very trust is closely related to the empathy they perceive in us.

We can see then that at this specific point the guide explicitly values the doctor's empathetic response. Seeing this we might ask ourselves, can empathy be taught?

That is the topic we will address below.

6.7   Can You Teach People To Be More Empathetic?

The classic way in which one learned to be empathetic was by observing their teachers, which is a method that is still alive and well in some medical schools [72].

Silently watching someone more experienced communicate can teach us many things:

How do you handle silence?
How do you let the patient know what you perceive?
How do you prepare the patient to receive bad news?
How does the communication start?
Where does the doctor sit? How far away are they from the patient? Empathy is often manifested by physical proximity to the recipient of the bad news.

From my perspective, experiencing the intimacy of the doctor's office or the care at the patient's bedside is essential in learning empathy since emotions are perceived along with their management and strategies.

The second way is to "put yourself in the patient's shoes" by acting as a patient in role-play [73].

All members of the health team should be "patients" at their own institutions at some point or another.

This is what Dr. Rosenbaum applied, after suffering from carcinoma himself and experiencing the coldness of the people in his own hospital [74, 75].

This experience is always helpful, not so much in helping health professionals to perceive the emotions that usually come with diagnosis or treatment, but rather in showing them the barriers or difficulties that the patients experience in their interaction with the health system.

These barriers or difficulties may arise from not understanding information, from the bureaucracy inherent in the health system, from the impossibility of establishing a human dialogue because they have to interact with automated systems, or even from the antipathy or lack of professionalism being shown by the health team.

All of this leads to frustration and anger.

We need to understand the emotional burden a patient deals with, which is not spurred just by fear caused by the diagnosis, but also by the lack of warmth or efficiency of the "health system."

The clinical skills exam (OSCE) is also a good way to learn this since the actor (simulated patient) can simulate situations that require the exercise of empathy by the student being examined [76, 77].

A few of the situations that can and have been examined are the emotional impact of incurability on the patient, as well as aggressive expressions during the consultation. Perhaps the most informative of these experiences was when we simulated a patient from the LGBTQ community and learned that our students were better able to treat the tumor than properly and respectfully engage with a transgender person [78]. This is a topic we will develop more fully in a later chapter.

There are different avenues aimed at improving empathy in students, which as we have discussed tends to decline as students make their way through medical school [47, 64, 66].

Improvisation has been explored, similar to excercises used in theater classes [79] by incorporating it into clinical semiotics courses [80] . There also have been projects where students visit museums and take art classes in order to improve observation skills [81], as well as using patients as storytellers to sharpen listening skills [82]; using virtual reality to stimulate empathy in students [83, 84] and even using animated graphics to promote patient-centered decision-making [85].

All of these different approaches, which have delved into the possibility of teaching empathy and the feasibility of teaching different knowledge or behaviors associated with it, have been thoroughly evaluated.

Among these works, we will highlight the one by Patel et al. [86],which emphasizes the five substantial elements that have been shown to increase the patient's perception of empathy:

1. Sitting (versus standing) during the interview.
2. Detecting patients' nonverbal cues of emotion.
3. Recognizing and responding to opportunities for compassion.
4. Nonverbal communication of caring (e.g., eye contact)
5. Verbal statements of acknowledgment, validation, and support.

These behaviors were found to improve patient perception of physician empathy and/or compassion.

As we can see, they are simple but strong strategies.

When we sit down, what does the patient perceive? That we are giving them our time.

When we detect their emotions, what does the patient perceive? That we are paying attention.

When we acknowledge these emotions and respond with compassion, what does the patient perceive? That we respect them.

When we look them in the eyes, what does a patient perceive? That we are focused on them.

Time, attention, respect, and focus. Four fundamental points to be able to listen and respond empathetically.

A map of empathy has been drawn in order to both learn and teach it [87]. This map tries to show what the person sees around them, what they say, what they want, what makes them happy, what makes them suffer, what they fear, what they hear, and what they do. It is a very useful tool to check if what we perceive is, in fact, correct.

There is no doubt that one of the most interesting instruments for the development of empathy is training in writing since it forces introspection and putting emotions into words [3, 88–92].

This double layer of "entering" oneself to discover our emotions and then "dumping" them on paper is incredibly valuable to materialize what we feel and test whether what we feel the patient is experiencing is correct or not.

But in order to be a good writer one must first be a good reader. Here, there is no doubt that the experiences narrated by great writers about their own illnesses are a huge help that can open doors to allow us to better our perception of our patients' emotions [93].

The generosity of those who master words to describe what they feel can aid us to understand our patients, who sometimes lack the subtlety to put what they feel into words. In a way, these writers can be the voices of the voiceless.

It is also very important to highlight empathy as one of the fundamental and most important characteristics of medical communication nowadays, when the rise of artificial intelligence presents new challenges in the doctor–patient relationship [94].

But this is one of the points in which our teachers function as links in a chain: what can we take from what they taught us, with some concepts that go back thousands of years, in order to incorporate into our own teachings so that our students can use them the present and better prepare themselves for an uncertain future.

Empathy is undoubtedly one of those core concepts.

6.8 Teaching Exercises

1. Individual

   (a) Do you consider yourself an empathetic person?
   (b) What do you think of the Dunning–Kruger effect?
   (c) What medicine-related work of art moves you the most? Why?
   (d) What experience during your undergraduate or graduate care practice that moved you the most?
   (e) What was the biggest mistake you made and how do you feel today compared to how you felt then?

2. Group

   (a) Form pairs and, using the work of Patrick Cairns et al. [87], make a map of each other's empathy.
   (b) Watch the movie 1991 film *The Doctor*, starring William Hurt, and discuss its content.
   (c) Which of the characters in that film do you identify with the most?
   (d) Read the book *Mortality* by Christopher Hitchens and try to identify the feelings and emotions that the author goes through.
   (e) Listen to the "Nessum Dorma" from Puccini's opera *Turandot*. Did you know that this opera was composed by Puccini while he was fighting head and neck cancer but was left unfinished because he died before finishing it? Did you know that the person who is singing it is a cancer patient who survived 20 years after a bone marrow transplant and who, on his nights in intensive care, waited anxiously for dawn to arrive? Now listen to it again with this new information.

References

1. Dr. Vidal and Benito. Empathy in the health professional's office—Articles—IntraMed. *intramed*. Published online; 2012.
2. Tan L, Le MK, Yu CC, et al. Defining clinical empathy: a grounded theory approach from the perspective of healthcare workers and patients in a multicultural setting. BMJ Open. 2021;11(9):e045224. https://doi.org/10.1136/bmjopen-2020-045224.

3. Kohut H. Introspection, empathy, and psychoanalysis: an examination of the relationship between mode of observation and theory. J Am Psychoanal Assoc. 1959;7(3):459–83.

4. Rogers CR. Empathic an unappreciated way of being. Counts Psychol. 1975;5(2):2–10.

5. Aspy DN. Empath let's get the hell on with it. Counts Psychol. 1975;5(2):10–4.

6. McGilchrist I. The matter with things: our brains, our delusions, and the unmaking of the world. London: Perspective Press; 2021.

7. Rizzo S, Melleuish G. In search of the origins of the western mind: McGilchrist and the axial age. Histories. 2021;1(1):24–41. https://doi.org/10.3390/stories1010007.

8. Wildman WJ. Engaging Iain McGilchrist: ascetical practice, brain lateralization, and philosophy of mind. Relig Brain Behav. 2019;9(4):313–8. https://doi.org/10.108 0/2153599X.2019.1604420.

9. Marias J. Person. Editorial alliance; 1997.

10. Marías J. Personal world map. Editorial alliance; 1994.

11. Mount BM. Intoxicated by my illness: and other writings on life and death. By Anatole Broyard. Hosp J. 1993;9(1):91. https://doi.org/10.1080/0742-969x.1993.11882757.

12. Frankl VE. Man's search for meaning: an introduction to logotherapy. New York: Washington Square Press; 1992.

13. Klein EA. Mrs Hattie Jones. J Clin Oncol. 2023. https://doi.org/10.1200/jco.22.02405.

14. Fernandez Ochoa LF. Intimacy and nostrity: reflection on medical secrecy. Med UPB. 2011;30(1).

15. Mamdani Z, McKenzie S, Ackermann E, et al. The cost of caring: compassion fatigue among peer overdose response workers in British Columbia. Subst Use Misuse. 2023;58(1):85–93. https://doi.org/10.1080/10826084.2022.2148481.

16. Powell SK. Compassion fatigue. Prof Case Manag. 2020;25(2):53–5. https://doi.org/10.1097/ NCM.0000000000000418.

17. Newton BW. Walking a fine line: is it possible to remain an empathic physician and have a hardened heart? Front Hum Neurosci. 2013;7:233. https://doi.org/10.3389/fnhum.2013.00233.

18. Muñoz-Miquel A. Empathy, emotions and patient-centredness: a case study on communication strategies. Hermes (Denmark). 2019;59(1):71–89. https://doi.org/10.7146/hjlcb.v59i1.116990.

19. Ioannidis JPA. Evidence-based medicine has been hijacked: a report to David Sackett. J Clin Epidemiol. 2016;73:82–6. https://doi.org/10.1016/j.jclinepi.2016.02.012.

20. Hojat M. Empathy in health professions education and patient care. New York: Springer; 2016. https://doi.org/10.1007/978-3-319-27625-0_11.

21. Hojat M, Louis DZ, Markham FW, Wender R, Rabinowitz C, Gonnella JS. Physicians' empathy and clinical outcomes for diabetic patients. Acad Med. 2011;86(3):359–64. https://doi. org/10.1097/ACM.0b013e3182086fe1.

22. Lelorain S, Gehenne L, Christophe V, Duprez C. The association of physician empathy with cancer patient outcomes: a meta-analysis. Psychooncology. 2023;32(4):506–15. https://doi. org/10.1002/pon.6108.

23. Surchat C, Carrard V, Berney A, Gaume J, Clair C. Impact of physician empathy on patient outcomes: a gender analysis. Br J Gen Pract. 2022;72(715):e99–107. https://doi.org/10.3399/ BJGP.2021.0193.

24. Lelorain S, Brédart A, Dolbeault S, Sultan S. A systematic review of the associations between empathy measures and patient outcomes in cancer care. Psychooncology. 2012;21(12):1255–64. https://doi.org/10.1002/pon.2115.

25. Marques Caetano Carreira L, Dinis S, Correia A, et al. Does the white coat influence satisfaction, trust and empathy in the doctor-patient relationship in the General and Family Medicine consultation? Interventional study. BMJ Open. 2021;11(12):e031887. https://doi.org/10.1136/ bmjopen-2019-031887.

26. Kim SS, Kaplowitz S, Johnston MV. The effects of physician empathy on patient satisfaction and compliance. Eval Health Prof. 2004;27(3):237–51. https://doi. org/10.1177/0163278704267037.

27. Adam Z, Klimeš J, Bolelouký Z, et al. Patient's benefits from physician's empathy and results of including empathy development into medical training. Klin Onkol. 2022;35(5):358–71. https://doi.org/10.48095/ccko2022358.

28. Potts LC, Bakolis I, Deb T, et al. Anti-stigma training and positive changes in mental illness stigma outcomes in medical students in ten countries: a mediation analysis on pathways via empathy development and anxiety reduction. Soc Psychiatry Psychiatr Epidemiol. 2022;57(9):1861–73. https://doi.org/10.1007/s00127-022-02284-0.

29. Steinhausen S, Ommen O, Thüm S, et al. Physician empathy and subjective evaluation of medical treatment outcome in trauma surgery patients. Patient Educ Couns. 2014;95(1):53–60. https://doi.org/10.1016/j.pec.2013.12.007.

30. Casas RS, Xuan Z, Jackson AH, Stanfield LE, Harvey NC, Chen DC. Associations of medical student empathy with clinical competence. Patient Educ Couns. 2017;100(4):742–7. https://doi.org/10.1016/j.pec.2016.11.006.

31. Frankl VE. The unconsciousness god. New York: Simon and Schuster; 1975. https://doi.org/10.2307/j.ctvt9k10d.10.

32. Kowalczyk O, Roszkowski K, Pawliszak W, et al. Religion and spirituality in oncology: an exploratory study of the communication experiences of clinicians in Poland. J Relig Health. 2022;61(2):1366–75. https://doi.org/10.1007/s10943-021-01343-1.

33. Hannan J, Sanchez G, Musser ED, et al. Role of empathy in the perception of medical errors in patient encounters: a preliminary study. BMC Res Notes. 2019;12(1):327. https://doi.org/10.1186/s13104-019-4365-2.

34. Kruger J, Dunning D. Unskilled and unaware of it: how difficulties in recognizing one's own incompetence lead to inflated self-assessments. J Pers Soc Psychol. 1999;77(6):1121–34. https://doi.org/10.1037/0022-3514.77.6.1121.

35. Pennycook G, Ross RM, Koehler DJ, Fugelsang JA. Dunning–Kruger effects in reasoning: theoretical implications of the failure to recognize incompetence. Psychon Bull Rev. 2017;24(6):1774–84. https://doi.org/10.3758/s13423-017-1242-7.

36. Coutinho MVC, Thomas J, Alsuwaidi ASM, Couchman JJ. Dunning-Kruger effect: intuitive errors predict overconfidence on the cognitive reflection test. Front Psychol. 2021;12:603225. https://doi.org/10.3389/fpsyg.2021.603225.

37. Canady BE, Larzo M. Overconfidence in managing health concerns: the Dunning–Kruger effect and health literacy. J Clin Psychol Med Settings. 2023;30(2):460–8. https://doi.org/10.1007/s10880-022-09895-4.

38. Zhou X, Jenkins R. Dunning–Kruger effects in face perception. Cognition. 2020;203:104345. https://doi.org/10.1016/j.cognition.2020.104345.

39. Dymond RF. A scale for the measurement of empathic ability. J Consult Psychol. 1949;13(2):127–33. https://doi.org/10.1037/h0061728.

40. Conklin RC, Hunt AS. An investigation of the validity of empathy measures. Couns Educ Superv. 1975;15(2):119–27. https://doi.org/10.1002/j.1556-6978.1975.tb00995.x.

41. Vodermaier A, Linden W, Siu C. Screening for emotional distress in cancer patients: a systematic review of assessment instruments. J Natl Cancer Inst. 2009;101(21):1464–88. https://doi.org/10.1093/jnci/djp336.

42. Chlopan BE, McCain ML, Carbonell JL, Hagen RL. Empathy. review of available measures. J Pers Soc Psychol. 1985;48(3):635–53. https://doi.org/10.1037/0022-3514.48.3.635.

43. DeVore C, Beck F, Clark P, Goorey N. Cognitive style as related to emotional empathy. J Dent Educ. 1989;53(9):538–41. https://doi.org/10.1002/j.0022-0337.1989.53.9.tb02345.x.

44. Hojat M, Gonnella JS, Nasca TJ, Mangione S, Vergare M, Magee M. Physician empathy: definition, components, measurement, and relationship to gender and specialty. Am J Psychiatry. 2002;159(9):1563–9. https://doi.org/10.1176/appi.ajp.159.9.1563.

45. Hojat M, Mangione S, Nasca TJ, et al. The Jefferson Scale of Physician empathy: development and preliminary psychometric data. Educ Psychol Meas. 2001;61(2):349–65. https://doi.org/10.1177/00131640121971158.

46. Glaser KM, Markham FW, Adler HM, McManus RP, Hojat M. Relationships between scores on the Jefferson Scale of physician empathy, patient perceptions of physician empathy, and humanistic approaches to patient care: a validity study. Med Sci Monit. 2007;13(7):CR291–4.

47. Chen D, Lew R, Hershman W, Orlander J. A cross-sectional measurement of medical student empathy. J Gen Intern Med. 2007;22(10):1434–8. https://doi.org/10.1007/s11606-007-0298-x.

48. Rahimi-Madiseh M, Tavakol M, Dennick R, Nasiri J. Empathy in Iranian medical students: a preliminary psychometric analysis and differences by gender and year of medical school. Med Teach. 2010;32(11):e471–8. https://doi.org/10.3109/0142159X.2010.509419.

49. Roh MS, Hahm BJ, Lee DH, Suh DH. Evaluation of empathy among Korean medical students: a cross-sectional study using the Korean version of the Jefferson scale of physician empathy. Teach Learn Med. 2010;22(3):167–71. https://doi.org/10.1080/10401334.2010.488191.

50. Hojat M, Michalec B, Veloski JJ, Tykocinski ML. Can empathy, other personality attributes, and level of positive social influence in medical school identify potential leaders in medicine? Acad Med. 2015;90(4):505–10. https://doi.org/10.1097/ACM.0000000000000652.

51. Alvaro-Gonzalez LC. The social brain: neurobiological bases of clinical interest. Rev Neurol. 2015;61(10):458–70. https://doi.org/10.33588/rn.6110.2015238.

52. Hajek A, Konig HH. Level and correlates of empathy and altruism during the Covid-19 pandemic. Evidence from a representative survey in Germany. PLoS One. 2022;17(3):e0265544. https://doi.org/10.1371/journal.pone.0265544.

53. Preston SD, deWaal FBM. Empathy: its ultimate and proximate bases. Behav Brain Sci. 2002;25(1):1–20. https://doi.org/10.1017/S0140525X02000018.

54. Eisenberg N, Fabes RA. Empathy: conceptualization, measurement, and relation to prosocial behavior. Motiv Emot. 1990;14(2):131. https://doi.org/10.1007/BF00991640.

55. Cialdini RB, Schaller M, Houlihan D, Arps K, Fultz J, Beaman AL. Empathy-based helping: is it selflessly or selfishly motivated? J Pers Soc Psychol. 1987;52(4):749–58. https://doi.org/10.1037/0022-3514.52.4.749.

56. Dutcher DD, Finley JC, Luloff AE, Johnson JB. Connectivity with nature as a measure of environmental values. Environ Behav. 2007;39(4):474–93. https://doi.org/10.1177/0013916506298794.

57. Stürmer S, Snyder M, Kropp A, Siem B. Empathy-motivated helping: the moderating role of group membership. Pers Soc Psychol Bull. 2006;32(7):943–56. https://doi.org/10.1177/0146167206287363.

58. Berenguer J. The effect of empathy in proenvironmental attitudes and behaviors. Environ Behav. 2007;39(2):15. https://doi.org/10.1177/0013916506292937.

59. Filipović AM, Bajac MB, Spaić I. Instruments of empathy-shaping in the creation of a culture of peace and non-violence. Int J Cogn Res Sci Eng Educ. 2022;10(2). https://doi.org/10.23947/2334-8496-2022-10-2-197-206.

60. Zhang L, Wang A, Xie X, et al. Workplace violence against nurses: a cross-sectional study. Int J Nurs Stud. 2017;72:8–14. https://doi.org/10.1016/j.ijnurstu.2017.04.002.

61. Hunter JA, Figueredo AJ, Becker JV, Malamuth N. Non-sexual delinquency in juvenile sexual offenders: the mediating and moderating influences of emotional empathy. J Fam Violence. 2007;22(1):43–54. https://doi.org/10.1007/s10896-006-9056-9.

62. Hartman C, Hageman T, Williams JH, Mary JS, Ascione FR. Exploring empathy and callous–unemotional traits as predictors of animal abuse perpetrated by children exposed to intimate partner violence. J Interpers Violence. 2019;34(12):2419–37. https://doi.org/10.1177/0886260516660971.

63. Fifteen TA, Parker RA, Wood DF, Benson JA. Stability of empathy among undergraduate medical students: a longitudinal study at one UK medical school. BMC Med Educ. 2011;11(1):90. https://doi.org/10.1186/1472-6920-11-90.

64. Magalhães E, Salgueira AP, Costa P, Costa MJ. Empathy in senior year and first year medical students: a cross-sectional study. BMC Med Educ. 2011;11(1):52. https://doi.org/10.1186/1472-6920-11-52.

65. Davis EL. Measurement of changes in empathy during dental school. Yearbook dentistry; 2006. https://doi.org/10.1016/s0084-3717(08)70274-5.
66. Hojat M, Mangione S, Nasca TJ, et al. An empirical study of decline in empathy in medical school. Med Educ. 2004;38(9):934–41. https://doi.org/10.1111/j.1365-2929.2004.01911.x.
67. Gilligan T, Coyle N, Frankel RM, et al. Patient-clinician communication: American Society of Clinical Oncology Consensus Guideline. J Clin Oncol. 2017;35:3618–32. https://doi.org/10.1200/JCO.
68. Nie NF, Liu ZL, Feng MX, et al. Lazarus type response to immunotherapy in three patients with poor performance status and locally advanced NSCLC: a case series and literature review. Ann Palliat Med. 2021;10(1):210–9. https://doi.org/10.21037/apm-20-2279.
69. Roesel C, Kambartel K, Kopeika U, Berzins A, Voshaar T, Krbek T. Lazarus-type tumor response to therapy with nivolumab for sarcomatoid carcinomas of the lung. Curr Oncol. 2019;26(2):e270–3. https://doi.org/10.3747/co.26.4377.
70. Ninomaru T, Okada H, Fujishima M, Irie K, Fukushima S, Hata A. Lazarus response to tepotinib for leptomeningeal metastases in a patient with MET exon 14 skipping mutation–positive lung adenocarcinoma: case report. JTO Clin Res Rep. 2021;2(3):100145. https://doi.org/10.1016/j.jtocrr.2021.100145.
71. Perumalswami CR, Jagsi R, Goold SD. Predicting a "lazarus effect" in patients with advanced cancer near the end of life: prognostic uncertainty, oncologists' emotions, and ethical questions. Am J Bioeth. 2019;19(12):57–60. https://doi.org/10.1080/15265161.2019.1675799.
72. Guilera T, Batalla I, Soler-González J. Shadowing patients: experiencing empathy in medical students. Med Educ. 2020;21(2):112–7. https://doi.org/10.1016/j.edumed.2018.06.006.
73. Rasasingam D, Kerry G, Gokani S, Zargaran A, Ash J, Mittal A. Being a patient: a medical student's perspective. Adv Med Educ Pract. 2017;8:163–5. https://doi.org/10.2147/AMEP.S121654.
74. Rosenbaum EE. A taste of my own medicine: when the doctor is the patient. New York: Random House; 1988.
75. Spiro H. Book review a taste of my own medicine: when the doctor is the patient. N Engl J Med. 1989;320(23):1525–31. https://doi.org/10.1056/nejm198906083202331.
76. Gil Deza E, De Simone G, Garcia Gerardi CF, et al. Design and validation of an Observational Standard Clinical Examination (OSCE) for clinical oncology based on ASCO/ASH curricular milestones. J Clin Oncol. 2016;34(15 Suppl):18150. https://doi.org/10.1200/jco.2016.34.15_suppl.e.
77. Gercovich D, Gil Deza E, Hirsch H, et al. Evaluation of empathy in a structured Observational Exam of Clinical Skills (OSCE) in the career of oncology at Instituto Oncológico Henry Moore-Universidad del Salvador (HM-ONCOUSAL). J Clin Oncol. 2016;34(15 Suppl):18151. https://doi.org/10.1200/jco.2016.34.15_suppl.e.
78. Gil Deza E, Abal M, Gil Deza L, et al. Caring for transgender cancer patients: shortcomings of medical education. J Clin Oncol. 2020;38(15 Suppl):11002. https://doi.org/10.1200/JCO.2020.38.15_suppl.11002.
79. Phelps M, White C, Xiang L, Swanson HI. Improvisation as a teaching tool for improving oral communication skills in premedical and pre-biomedical graduate students. J Med Educat Curri Develop. 2021;8:23821205211006411. https://doi.org/10.1177/23821205211006411.
80. Fernández-Rodríguez LJ, Bardales-Zuta VH, San-Martín M, Delgado Bolton RC, Vivanco L. Empathy enhancement based on a semiotics training program: a longitudinal study in Peruvian medical students. Front Psychol. 2020;11:567663. https://doi.org/10.3389/fpsyg.2020.567663.
81. Mukunda N, Moghbeli N, Rizzo A, Niepold S, Bassett B, DeLisser HM. Visual art instruction in medical education: a narrative review. Med Educ Online. 2019;24(1):1558657. https://doi.org/10.1080/10872981.2018.1558657.
82. Kagawa Y, Ishikawa H, Son D, et al. Using patient storytelling to improve medical students' empathy in Japan: a pre-post study. BMC Med Educ. 2023;23(1):67. https://doi.org/10.1186/s12909-023-04054-1.

83. Roswell RO, Cogburn CD, Tocco J, et al. Cultivating empathy through virtual reality: advancing conversations about racism, inequity, and climate in medicine. Acad Med. 2020;95(12):1882–6. https://doi.org/10.1097/ACM.0000000000003615.

84. Vitto C, Del Buono B, Daniel L, Rivet E, Cholyway R, Santen SA. Teaching toolbox: breaking bad news with virtual technology in the time of COVID. J Cancer Educ. 2022;37(5):1429–32. https://doi.org/10.1007/s13187-021-01975-7.

85. Sutherland T, Choi D, Yu C. "Brought to life through imagery"—animated graphic novels to promote empathic, patient-centered care in postgraduate medical learners. BMC Med Educ. 2021;21(1):66. https://doi.org/10.1186/s12909-021-02491-4.

86. Patel S, Pelletier-Bui A, Smith S, et al. Curricula for empathy and compassion training in medical education: a systematic review. PLoS One. 2019;14(8):e0221412. https://doi.org/10.1371/journal.pone.0221412.

87. Cairns P, Pinker I, Ward A, Watson E, Laidlaw A. Empathy maps in communication skills training. Clin Teach. 2021;18(2):142–6. https://doi.org/10.1111/tct.13270.

88. Torubarova I, Stebletsova A. Narrative-based medical writing: an EMP case study. J Teach Engl Specific Acad Purposes. 2021;9(1):51–9. https://doi.org/10.22190/JTESAP2101051T.

89. Ohm F, Vogel D, Sehner S, Wijnen-Meijer M, Harendza S. Details acquired from medical history and patients' experience of empathy—two sides of the same coin. BMC Med Educ. 2013;13(1):67. https://doi.org/10.1186/1472-6920-13-67.

90. Löffler-Stastka H, Datz F, Parth K, Preusche I, Bukowski X, Seidman C. Empathy in psychoanalysis and medical education—what can we learn from each other? BMC Med Educ. 2017;17(1):74. https://doi.org/10.1186/s12909-017-0907-2.

91. Liao HC, Wang YH. Storytelling in medical education: narrative medicine as a resource for interdisciplinary collaboration. Int J Environ Res Public Health. 2020;17(4):1135. https://doi.org/10.3390/ijerph17041135.

92. Savitha D, Anto T, Tv S. Introducing reflective narrative for first-year medical students to promote empathy as an integral part of physiology curriculum. Adv Physiol Educ. 2021;45(2):207–16. https://doi.org/10.1152/ADVAN.00206.2020.

93. Florijn BW, der Graaf H, Van Schoones JW, Kaptein AA. Narrative medicine: a comparison of terminal cancer patients' stories from a Dutch hospice with those of Anatole Broyard and Christopher Hitchens. Death Stud. 2019;43(9):570–81. https://doi.org/10.1080/07481187.2018.1504350.

94. Wartman SA, Combs CD. Reimagining medical education in the age of AI. AMA J Ethics. 2019;21(2):E146–52. https://doi.org/10.1001/amajethics.2019.146.

Chapter 7
Nonverbal Communication in the Consulting Room

7.1 Introduction

Words are never spoken in isolation; they are always accompanied by an environmental and gestural context.

We say what we say in a given place, at a given time of day, looking in a certain way, gesturing with our hands, covering or uncovering ourselves with our body posture, attracting or pushing others away. Even though we use the same words, in the same sequence, we never say it the same way.

Nonverbal communication was evolutionarily, contextually, and pragmatically developed prior to verbal communication. In fact, when there are discrepancies between verbal and nonverbal communication, we tend to prioritize the nonverbal message, especially in terms of the veracity of the information [1].

This is so important in medicine that Gregorio Marañón (1887–1960), probably the most important clinician in Spain and Latin America in the first half of the twentieth century, when asked about what he considered to be the most important instrument in medicine, replied without hesitation: **THE CHAIR**.

Nothing indicates to a patient that we have time, that we are focusing our attention on them, that we are putting everything aside for them, like the act of sitting down in front of the **patient**.

As you can see, it is a gesture, not a word, which says everything about the doctor's attitude. That is nonverbal communication, and it is what we will discuss in this chapter.

We have evidence that nonverbal communication was present in the animal kingdom long before the appearance of man, as well as evidence of human communication long before words could be articulated.

That implies that verbal communication helps perfect nonverbal aspects, but it is clear we continue to transmit an enormous amount of information beyond merely what we say.

© The Author(s), under exclusive license to Springer Nature Switzerland AG 2024

E. Gil Deza, *Improving Clinical Communication*, https://doi.org/10.1007/978-3-031-62446-9_7

Nonverbal communication can be nonritualized or ritualized.

Nonritual communication is related to biological phenomena: size (usually males are larger than females); sexual maturity (genital development or sexual characteristics expressed by changes in body shape, or the development of hair or feathers); availability for sexual intercourse (pheromones); identification of offspring (olfactory); aggression or stress (piloerection, changes in skin vascularization or pupillary mydriasis).

Ritualized nonverbal communication are repetitive behaviors that occur instinctively in the animal: songs or trills, dances or habitat preparation, territorial delimitation; and they can also be found in humans, though in this case they are cultural, not instinctive: clothes, attitudes, or behaviors that express our state of mind. For example, the color of mourning clothes (black in the West and white in Japan) expresses the self-absorption, isolation, and loneliness in which the person finds themselves.

7.2 Definition and History of Nonverbal Communication

Nonverbal communication is understood as the act of sending and receiving information in social relationships through the appearance, gestures, and behavior of people, as well as the environment [2].

This ability to communicate has been studied for a long time. For the purpose of this book, we will take a look at the historical summary elaborated by Knapp [3].

According to this author, the first student of nonverbal communication was Confucius, where the following dialogue between teacher and student about communicating without words is found:

1. He said: I'd like to do it without words.
2. Tze-Kung said: But, boss, if you don't say it, how can we little guys pass it on?
3. He said: How does the sky talk? The four seasons go on, everything gets born. What words does the sky use? (p. 87, Book 17, XIX).

This conviction that understanding and persuasion do not require words is one of the deepest teachings of the great teacher. Other authors highlight the same [4–6].

Simultaneously in Greece the great philosophers taught something similar: Plato, in the *Gorgias,* shows both the potential of rhetoric and its risks [7–9] and Aristotle, in his book *Rhetoric* [10], highlights the nonverbal elements of discourse: clothing, style, the sonority and the different arrangements of the voice to transmit security, sense, and conviction, to be able to persuade fellow citizens.

Let us remember that in Athens during the fifth century BC, democracy was closely related to theater, and in the theater the ability to express ideas, emotions, and show a stage reality that invited the spectator to think, reconsider, and eventually change position required great mastery of their voice and their body on the part of the actors [11–13].

Doctors should remember this relationship between theater, expressiveness, and rhetoric, and try to implement them in our courses and classes.

If the word is a cure, then rhetoric is the container, the vehicle that makes this treatment understandable and accessible.

The philosophers Cicero [14, 15] and Quintilian [16, 17] took rhetoric in the Roman Empire to its maximum expression.

These great masters of rhetoric established the relationship between the different emotions and the position of the body, the tone of voice, the direction of the gaze, the role of facial expression and gestures. Reading them is a true delight that amazes with the depth of his vision and the accuracy of his statements.

In fact, Quintilian affirms that the disharmony between what is said and the gestures or positions of the body can end up not only generating confusion in the listener but also making the whole speech hard to believe.

In the West, the influence of Christianity and the incorporation of the classics into the tradition of the Church have been notable, especially the role of Augustine of Hippo in the incorporation of Plato and the role of Thomas Aquinas in the incorporation of Aristotle into Christian philosophy.

On the topic of rhetoric, Boethius (477–524) wrote: "*An overview of the structure of rhetoric,*" and together with his *Consolations* and mathematical studies on music have constituted one of his philosophy's greatest legacies [18].

The invasion by the Ummayyad Caliphate of the Iberian Peninsula; the victory of the Franks in the Battle of Tours; the union between the King of the Franks and the Bishop of Rome; the establishment of Charlemagne as Emperor of the West; the rejection of the Muslims on the other side of the Pyrenees; and the consolidation of power in Central Europe opened a period of peace between Rome, Byzantium, and the Abbasid Caliphate, which allowed a fluid commercial and intellectual exchange between East and West.

Rhetoric was also crucial for the followers of Muhammad since the reading, exegesis, and jurisprudence of the Koranic texts were part of the cultural, religious, and political life of all communities.

During the Middle Ages, the influence of classical authors, Greeks and Romans, continued, as we can see in the universities of the time, all of which required study of the *Trivium*: grammar, logic, and rhetoric.

In the Middle Ages, a text by Thomas Wilson, *The Art of Rethorique,* in 1553 synthesizes the tips to speak in the right tone and how to correctly pronounce the English language, as highlighted by Patricia Bizzell [19–21].

Two more people deserve a special mention: Thomas Sheridan (1719–1788), actor and educator, who maintains that expressions and gestures not only serve to communicate, but they are also more primitive, natural, and universal than words.

The second is Gilbert Austin (1753–1837), who developed a sophisticated notation system to describe bodily attitude in natural conversation, with more than a hundred positions for the feet, arms, and hands [19].

This rationalist and empiricist effort to decode language was socially accompanied by the development of multiple nonverbal signals, in clothing, jewelry, or ornaments, that signaled the class, fortune, and power of those who attended an event.

One of those ornaments were fans, originating in China or Japan, which throughout the seventeenth century and until late in the twentieth century were used as a sign of distinction. There is a whole discipline called "fanology" that studies the design and use of this implement [22].

Of the many nonverbal languages that used fans, one of the most widespread was the one described by Jules Duvellroy (as we can find on the web).

At a time when there was no communication at a distance other than letters sent by post, these nonverbal signs conveyed the unmistakable signals of a lady at a safe distance.

However, the study of nonverbal language acquired a whole new dimension when the great Charles Darwin (1809–1882) incorporated photography into the study of communication and wrote: *The expression of the Emotions in man and animals*" [23].

This text studies the facial muscles of both animals and humans and their emotional response to a stimulus that is of unparalleled richness and sheds light on the evolution of nonverbal responses in different cultures.

Franz Boaz (1858–1942), considered the father of American anthropology, incorporated filming into the study of language and gestures.

Different authors, throughout the twentieth century (Traeger–Bladwhistell–Hall) extensively studied what they called paraverbal language. Body movements. Mastery of space, and speed of movement.

Jurgen Ruesh (1910–1995) is an American psychiatrist who was the first to use the expression "nonverbal communication" in a book published together with the poet, painter, literary critic, photographer, and film director Weldon Kees (1914–1955).

Paul Ekman (1934) is an American psychologist and Emeritus Professor at the University of California (San Francisco). He related facial microexpressions to emotions in communication. His hypotheses were widely disseminated through highly successful television series such as *Lie to Me* in which the protagonist uses microexpressions to detect lies.

This journey through the history of nonverbal communication from antiquity to today's TV is a preamble to the scientific study of nonverbal communication. Is it possible to assess the ability of nonverbal communication between different subjects?

7.3   Scientific Study of Nonverbal Communication

Those who wish to undertake a deeper research into nonverbal communication will find Valerie Manusov's texts very helpful [24] as she has collected the most widespread tests used in these kinds of studies.

We will select some of those tests that are used in Participant/Observer reports.

Even though we can learn a lot from the descriptions that each person makes about their own behavior and experience, these reports have severe limitations. The observation, recording, and coding of interactions by third parties are always preferable to self-examination.

Observational studies of nonverbal communication frequently employ one of the following instruments.

1. **The Social Skills Inventory**: This test was designed by Dr. Ronald E. Riggio and uses 90 items to fundamentally analyze coding ability or expressivity; decoding skill or sensitivity and the ability to regulate or control communication [25, 26].

   It is a scale that has demonstrated good reliability and internal consistency.
2. **The Emory Dyssemia Index**: This index was developed in 1994 by Elizabeth B. Love and Stephen Nowick. This test was designed to detect the presence of a deficit in the proper processing of nonverbal communication. It has been used extensively in the screening of children with communication difficulties. It analyzes seven categories: gaze and eye contact, space and touch, paralanguage, facial expression, objects/fashion, social norms, and nonverbal receptivity; ranking each in a five-point ordinal scale [27].
3. **The Touch Avoidance Measure**: This index measures a person's reaction to touching or be touched. It was designed by Andersen and Leibowitz in 1978. It is an 18-point test: 10 oriented to study the touch avoidance between people of the same sex (TAM 1) and 8 aimed at studying this construct among people of the opposite sex (TAM 2). In all cases, the observed items are classified on a five-point ordinal scale. Thus, it can be seen that married people try to avoid tactile contact with people of the opposite sex, men are more likely to avoid contact with people of the same sex than women, and older people tend to avoid tactile contact more than young people [28].
4. **The Nonverbal Perception Scale**: This instrument was designed to record nonverbal signals in a group of people and infer their moods. It has the advantage of being able to study behavior and the interpretation of behaviors in everyday life, in which interactions naturally occur, but it has the disadvantage of having great variability [29–32].
5. **The Relational Communication Scale**: This scale was created by Burgoon and Hale in 1987. It consists of 34 items and analyzes 11 topics, among which are Intimacy, Commitment, Trust, and Depth. It has shown high internal consistency and reliability [33–37].

This sample of instruments designed for the study of nonverbal communication, analyzing the interaction between two or more people, in a natural or laboratory environment, in order to assess the communication skills of children or adults, is complemented by laboratory studies in which the parameters of skin conductivity, hormone secretion, metabolite levels, and electrophysiological recordings are evaluated.

All these topics support the neurobiological reasons for nonverbal communication that we will analyze below.

7.4   Neurobiology

When we analyze the neurological component of nonverbal communication, we try to define the brain structures that are activated in the encoding and decoding of another person's bodily signals.

These studies have had an exponential development since the advent of functional magnetic resonance of the brain and have managed to demonstrate which areas of the brain are activated when subjects must interpret a certain situation.

The mirror neurons described by Giaccomo Rizzolatti [38–41] in the frontal region of primate (monkeys, apes, and humans) brains (area F5) are a set of neurons that are activated when we perform a certain action (laugh, yawn, extend our hand) and when we see another perform the same action (mirror).

The existence and role of mirror neurons is one of the foundations used to explain the theory of mind (ToM), that is, the ability to perceive the desires or emotions of another person by observing or imitating the gestures they make.

This can be studied through different tests, such as Reading the Mind in the Eyes Test (RMET) [42], in which subjects are invited to identify the emotional and mental state based on an image eyes; or the False-Belief Task, where an observer knows what another person knows, even when that knowledge is not correct, and is capable of predicting their behavior. Despite its popularity and extensive use of it, its results are subject to controversy [43, 44].

The ability to perceive desires and emotions is transferred to the interpretation of intentions and thoughts of the other, even at the risk of losing assertiveness: it is easier to imitate, and there are greater chances of getting what the other feels right than what the other thinks or wants.

This imitation system has proven to be crucial in language acquisition.

The first thing a child learns to imitate is their mother's smile, and they have a great reward when they see this imitation rewarded with greater affection from their mother.

This reward circuit, primarily focused on the release of oxytocin [45–47], is the link between the neural mirror circuit and the neurohormonal reward system that feeds back and strengthens imitative activity as a recreational activity.

Therefore, it is not just feasible to imitate but also pleasant to do it repeatedly, getting better at it with time.

Studies that delve into children's communication capacity show that after the recognition of the mother's voice that occurs from birth, the imitation of maternal gestures is crucial in the acquisition of language and in developing their communication capacity [48–51].

Understanding that the ability to emit and decode nonverbal signals in interpersonal communication is a learning and rewarding process raises the question of whether it is also something that is feasible to teach.

Is it possible to learn to communicate better in a nonverbal way?

The answer is yes. We will analyze it below.

7.5 Nonverbal Communication Teaching

A key topic for understanding the teaching of nonverbal communication is *brain plasticity.*

To summarize what we have discussed so far: there is a neural circuit (mirror neurons) that is linked to a gratification circuit (oxytocin), which is later related to language and which allows, through the theory of mind (ToM), to infer what others feel or think from their expressions and gestures. This system seems very complex. Complex enough that it makes one wonder if it could be properly developed as an adult, if one did not develop it (or developed it in an incomplete manner) during childhood.

Brain plasticity, which has mainly been studied in the rehabilitation of patients who suffered brain damage as a consequence of trauma, surgery, or a vascular accident, has been extensively demonstrated and frequently related to a dopaminergic reward circuit [52–55].

The truth is that our brain is capable of at least partially restoring loss functions by activating alternative neural circuits. While it is true that plasticity decreases with age it does not disappear.

Therefore, the first step to improve and relearn nonverbal communication skills is to see ourselves as people in need of this rehabilitation and consciously initiate a re-education process of our senses to improve our perceptive and empathetic capacity for the signals emitted by the other.

We can do this by interacting with another person, looking at photographs, or watching video recordings.

The basic exercise consists of removing sound from any recording, observing, and recording any gestures you see while trying to imagine what these gestures mean and what the speaker is feeling. Afterward, watch the whole thing again but this time with sound and see if your guesses where correct. There are numerous resources on the web that we can turn to in order to practice.

In any case, Table 7.1 summarizes the skills in which we must train.

Table 7.1 Selection of the characteristics for the teaching of nonverbal communication

Characteristic of nonverbal communication	Evidence of utility
Facial expressions	Identification of basic emotions: Joy, fear, anger, confusion, or doubt [56]
Oculesics (look at the eyes and gaze movements)	Greater empathy, satisfaction, and confidence when the gaze is held [57–60]
Gestures (movements and signals as responses of the person with whom we communicate)	Interpretation of the emotional responses of the other [61–64]
Kinesics (body language)	Relaxation, hospitality, tension, threat, and discomfort [65–67]
Proxemics (regulation of the necessary space between one and the other)	Orientation, security, comfort, privacy, olfaction, and breathing [68–72]
Haptics (somatic sensation of touching and being touched)	Trust, comfort, choice, proximity, and limit [73–76]

Once we develop these abilities by observing in silence, we can add the paralinguistic conditions: tone of voice, volume, inflection, and timber. These qualities of the voice are crucial in medicine, especially as they vividly convey emotions [77–79].

To be able to decode these conditions requires time. Taking the proper amount of time during the consultation, together with the affective tone, proximity, and the medical touch, are essential components of patient satisfaction.

There are medical situations in which all communication is nonverbal. We will analyze those below.

7.6 Nonverbal Communication in Situations Where Verbal Communication Is Not Possible

There are numerous situations or conditions that limit our ability to express or understand oral or written language: patients who have suffered trauma, people in the autism spectrum, people with dementia, young children, the elderly, and immigrants who do not speak the language, to name but a few [80–91].

Undoubtedly, the limitation of the spoken word is an important barrier in human communication, and one that should lead us to further develop the capacity for nonverbal communication.

The affectionate and serene look that reassures and shelters is one of the key elements of this communication.

The person who feels affectionately received, expected, and watched is one that more easily recovers his self-esteem and serenity.

The approach breaks the barriers of language, appearance, dirt, smell, or any other form of discrimination.

The affectionate, respectful, predictable, and friendly touch transmits affection, hope, tranquility, like the best and most powerful medicine.

One of the great Argentine pediatricians, Dr. Florencio Escardó [92], implemented kangaroo mothers for preterm infants in his service in the middle of the last century. The mother was hospitalized with the child, and she sheltered him next to her body; thus, the child was in a warm and caring environment. The mortality of these children decreased remarkably.

Gestures, paralinguistic language, and the environment communicate to the patient and their family the availability and care provided to patients.

This is increasingly important in times where there is increasing social isolation, greater violence in human relations, and greater demands on the health system. Nonverbal communication is a way for the emotional containment of the patient and their family group and helps de-escalate situations of emotional violence.

7.7 Artificial Intelligence Applied to the Study of Nonverbal Communication

A truly exciting development is the design of artificial intelligence applications to improve human communication and interactions. It is called affective computing, a field in which Rosalind Picard, an expert at the Massachusetts Institute of Technology (MIT), is a pioneer.

These technologies monitor all nonverbal communication signals, as well as electrophysiological changes in the skin or levels of neurotransmitters or hormones, to establish our mood, predict seizures in epileptic patients, determine suicidal risk, or predict our work or school performance [93–129].

The interesting thing is that they do it through the devices that we have incorporated into our daily lives: smartphones or smartwatches or other specific sensors.

Some of these techniques, especially the aid to autistic children by robots designed for verbal and nonverbal communication, have amazing results.

Therefore, it is likely that in the immediate future, in addition to training in nonverbal communication, we will have access to devices that can help us communicate better and understand the impact that words or gestures have on our and our patients' bodies.

In the meantime, we must integrate these two systems into everyday life.

7.8 Nonverbal Communication Next to Verbal Communication

In our daily life, whether family or professional, we use both verbal and nonverbal communication.

What we must be aware of is that what we communicate is essentially nonverbal. In other words, what our interlocutor fundamentally decodes is how we are, how we say what we say, where we look, what our face expresses, how far away we are, how we move our body, whether we accept or reject being touched, and what our gestures are.

We can think of verbal communication as essentially informative while nonverbal as communicative.

This explains the appearance of signal noise in any communication between what is being verbally *said* and what is being nonverbally *communicated*.

That is why we must train ourselves in this aspect of communication. The way we dress, stand, greet, and invite the patient to our consultation. How the office is arranged, the lights, the decorations, the instruments. How we sit, where we look, what we do while our patient talks, how we listen, and finally how we say what we want to say, makes all the difference in mastering this field [130–135].

We have said before that we must think of the spoken word as medicine, and we must take care of what we say as much as what we administer. We have said that verbal communication has doses, active principles, placebos, nocebos, adjuvants, and forms of administration. In this metaphor, nonverbal communication is the vehicle, the means, the way in which this remedy is administered: affectionately and warmly, distantly and icily, in proximity or at a distance, with or without commitment, with or without empathy.

While a patient may doubt the doctor's word, it is much rarer for them to doubt any nonverbal cues.

Therefore, if you are genuinely interested in caring for your patient humanely, I recommend that you pay particular attention to this aspect of communication.

One of the most important challenges is what to do with silences, which is the topic that we will see next.

7.9   Role of Silence in Human Communication

In oncology, silences are as important as words [136].

During the many meetings between doctor and patient, silence occupies an important place in oncology and in many other disciplines where patients face undesirable prognoses and must make decisions that will impact their lives.

Let us see some of them:

The silence that precedes the patient's question.
The silence that precedes the doctor's response.
The silence following the response offered.
The silence of the clinical examination.
The silence of the patient at the end of his life.
The silence of the deceased patient.

Silence is an essential part of communication in all these circumstances: it is a sign of respect, of humanity, of understanding.

Learning to handle silences can lead to not just discovering the possibility of nonverbally communicating our willingness to accompany the patient in those spaces, but also getting in touch with our own emotions [137–144].

Taking care of silences gives harmony to communication in the same way that they do as intervals between notes in a musical performance, and in fact emotions and silences have been recorded in doctor–patient communication, in the same way we write notes on music sheets [145, 146].

Communicating the diagnosis to a patient is a challenge: it usually begins with a long silence when it is bad news; but we say it immediately when it is good news.

This waiting time pre-announces that the information is not good and the patient perceives it.

If this is accompanied by preparatory words such as "what I have to tell you is not good" or "unfortunately the result is not what we wanted," it allows the patient, in some way, to receive the news more armed.

The blow is equally surprising and painful, but at least try to let the patient know what is coming.

The same happens when the established therapy fails or the disease reappears and much more when we must talk with the patient about his possible death and his wishes about the end of life.

Silence is essential for listening.

It has been said countless times that the most important tool of medical communication is the ability to listen to the patient, which means the ability to remain actively silent while the patient is speaking.

This primordial silence allows the construction of the mental image of what the patient relates, the chronology of the events from the patient's perspective; it makes it possible to distinguish the figure from the background, what the important elements of what the patient thinks have happened to and is happening to them at the moment. It helps us see how they rank their own problems.

It allows us to focus on the issues important to our patient in the *here* and *now*.

This silence has the same role as the silence of the one who draws a model, listening is seeing the portrait of the patient with our ears and seeing silently is perceiving what the patient tells us through his gaze, his gestures, his posture. This interaction of the senses of seeing and hearing is only possible through silence.

For silence to have a therapeutic effect and be integrated into a mode of communication with the patient, the doctor must first be comfortable with silence.

If the doctor does not learn to use silence, an atmosphere of tension is generated that conspires against communication.

If, on the other hand, the doctor can remain silent, attentively waiting for the patient's timing, he will have an experience similar to the contemplation described by Buddhists. A peaceful and safe atmosphere, where it is possible to get to know each other.

Anthony Back and collaborators, in their text *Compassionate Silence in the Patient-Clinician Meet. A Contemplative Approach* [147], point out three types of silences:

1. **Awkward**: This silence surprises us and sometimes reflects a distraction or is forced by a self-imposed or external interruption.

   This silence is often perceived by the patient as artificial.

   It is a nuisance, a disturbance, which destroys a climate of intimacy necessary for communication.

   Here silence makes a lot of noise: it is a sign of insensitivity, lack of preparation or opportunity.

2. **Invitational**: This is the respectful silence in which the clinician waits for the patient to "digest" the information he has received and waits for the patient's verbal and emotional response.

   At this point, silence is used as an instrument, a space, a void that can be filled by the patient's response.

   It is as if both doctor and patient allow themselves the time to let the answers flow, not impose or remove them.

3. **Compassionate**: This is the silence that arises in the conversation in which the patient has returned to himself and the doctor waits, while he feels and communicates his empathy with the sufferer.

     At this point, silence is not used as a dialogue tool but rather as an attitude on the part of the doctor, a way of being with the patient in these circumstances.

     It is a mental state that requires the clinician possess three characteristics or virtues in which they must train: attention, focus, and clear perception.
   (a) **Attention**: Refers in the first place to a moral condition, the intention of putting our whole being in the care of the patient. Being here and now, only caring for the sick; and secondly, it means to pay attention, that is to say, direct our senses to the perception of the verbal and nonverbal cues of what the patient communicates to us.
   (b) **Focus**: Refers to avoiding distractions. Our attention must be focused on different topics but our patient must always be the center of our attention.
   (c) **Clear perception**: This refers to avoiding interpretative biases. That is to say, separating what the patient says from the positive or negative impact that it has on us according to our history and experience. In other words, allowing the patient's history to guide our behavior and not the other way around.

These virtues require practice in order to be developed. For this reason, it is important that those who wish to carry them out regularly practice one of the forms of meditation that allows them to acquire that state of mind necessary to be fully alert, present in the moment, and at the same time serene and receptive to the needs of the other, without judging and without anticipating what the patient is going to say [148–150].

Silence also implies a change in the perspective of care, going from narrative care that tries to shape a discourse, filling in the gaps with the patient's or our own words and anticipating what they are going to say, to moving on to care focused on the patient.

This means having the ability to handle silence from the behavioral point of view as an invitational instrument and from the contemplative point of view as an instrument of perception.

It is an incredibly enriching experience to be able to carry out a silent and deeply intimate encounter with the patient in any situation, but particularly with those patients who find themselves at the end of their lives.

Learning to be silent is therapeutic for both the patient and the doctor since it makes communication between the two healthier and more tolerable [151].

There are programs that have been specifically designed to monitor the dying and there is clear evidence of their usefulness for medical humanization. They remove the professional from thinking of himself as an exclusively rational being whose task is oriented to solving problems and repositions him as a person whose vocation is the care of the suffering [152].

If human evolution is closely linked to this ability to decode words and silences, the technological revolution has incorporated this economy of nonverbal communication into robotics and communication on social networks.

7.10   Nonmedical Applications of Nonverbal Communication: Robotics, Emojis, and Emoticons

Many times when referring to hyperrational and emotionless humans, we say that they are robotic, and in fact that is the image that many members of the community have of scientists and researchers [153].

The truth is that the robots that began simply with the aim of carrying out mechanical and routine tasks in the manufacture of objects have had a notable evolution and today they are part of our daily life and we usually communicate with them, such as when we request products or services through Chatbots.

The narrative regarding robot–human interaction both in literature and in the cinema shows a gradual humanization in the faces, gestures, and decisions of robots [154–158].

At the same time, prosthetic replacement technology means that more and more humans walk with prosthetic legs, listen with hearing aids, see with implanted lenses, feed ourselves with infusion pumps, and clean our blood with dialysis machines. Therefore, we can see that the human–machine interaction is notably more intimate than we think and the border between a humanized robot and a "roboticized" human is getting closer and closer.

In fact, in order to avoid unnecessary ethical conflicts, robots should be considered objects since it would be a mistake to see them as people [159].

The neatness of the design and the materials used for the construction of physical robots and the realism of the human avatars in virtual reality achieve amazing effects when it comes to interacting with people.

Not only have they been endowed with human voices but they have incorporated nonverbal language with remarkable efficiency.

The second field where nonverbal language has generated a revolution is in the use of emojis or emoticons [160].

Emoticons add emotional context to written communication, and the study of their design has shown a high correlation between the different designs and the emotional context they provide, which can be positive (joy, happiness, success), neutral (understanding, agreement), or negative (grief, anger, depression) [161].

In the previously cited article by Novak et al., we can see a map of the emojis and their relationship with positive or negative feelings.

Refining the design of emojis by incorporating nonverbal facial cues reduces the ambiguity of their interpretation [162].

This is regardless of the language of the text [163]. And also its interpretation is easy and fast, which is key for the younger generations, given the evidence that the duration of the focus of human attention has been reduced to 8 s due to the use of digital technology [164].

Certainly the possibility of studying the nonverbal expression of emotions through emojis has made it possible to detect moods in patients and students [165–167]; in public health, it has allowed the issuance of clearer messages about the risks and preventive measures [168–170]; they facilitate the understanding of the evolutions reported by patients [171, 172] . The emotional impact of the recent Covid-19 pandemic was studied in the emoticons used by the population and hospitalized patients [173–175]; and lastly, it has also been used in medical teaching by teachers and students to understand and memorize concepts [169, 170, 176, 177].

Therefore, the knowledge of nonverbal expressions in communication has led us to capture them in representative figures that are used as a complement or in replacement of texts in digital communications and are increasingly used for the transmission of emotions whose interpretation is usually unequivocal. They have also proven to be universal, easily understood by many different languages. Finally, they are used to monitor patients or the emotional state of the population and to clarify the language of public health messages.

The use of emojis not only gives an emotional tone to a short message (which would otherwise be noticeably longer), but also clarifies the emotional impact of the recipient and improves communication.

Nonverbal language proficiency in face-to-face interaction is now also nonverbal language proficiency in textual exchange on social media.

7.11 Teaching Exercises

1. Personal

   (a) Do you consider that you pay attention to the nonverbal signals that your patient expresses?

   (b) Have you seen with the eyes of a patient the environment in which you receive them? Do you feel that it is a cosy, intimate, warm environment?

   (c) What part of your body language most clearly expresses your affection for your patients: your body attitude, your look, your proximity, your serenity, your ritual, your touch, your hug?

   (d) Experience the silence. During one of the meetings with your colleagues or patients, be quiet, focus on your breathing and the sensations in your body. Experience the sensations you have: are you relaxed, tense, anxious, fearful? Observe the face, the hands, the body of your interlocutor. Focus on the moment. What do you observe new, different? What detail did you miss? Use those feelings to continue the dialogue.

   (e) Do you have command of the language of emoticons? Try to consciously use them in your next text messages and observe their effect.

   (f) Have you used emoticons in your classes? If not, use them and see the impact on your students.

2. In a group

   (a) Get together as a group and randomly distribute cards with an emotion (Anger, Joy, Disappointment, Love, Frustration, etc.) and each person who receives the card must express that emotion in a nonverbal way. Observe what happens with the body, the face, the position of the hands, the movements, the breathing, the way of walking, in each emotion and record what allowed you to intuit the emotion of your colleague.

(b) Separate the participants into senders and receivers, place both groups at a distance of 3 or 4 m. Give senders a card with a message; it can be positive ("You must tell him that he won the lottery") or negative ("You must tell him that his son died in an accident"). Observe the body language of the person who must transmit the message and stop them before they reach their recipient. Ask the recipient if they are going to receive a positive or negative message and why they think so. Once they receive the message, observe the impact it had on the receiver. Then switch roles in each group. This will allow you to study kinetics and proxemics in human communication.

(c) Choose a video interview publicly available from which you can analyze nonverbal communication. Extract frames to show the group and analyze the body positions, hands, faces, and ask them to try to deduce the emotional state of the speaker. Then play the video for them to confirm or refute their claims.

(d) Gather the group in a circle and train them to notice their breath. With your eyes closed, regulate your breathing by inhaling for a count of 1–4 and exhaling for a count of 4–1 for 2 min. Then ask them to perceive the air entering through their nostrils, passing through the choanae and the pharynx, how the air enters through the larynx and the trachea and inflates the lung. Ask them to try to perceive the instant that separates inspiration from expiration. At the moment that you perceive the sounds that surround you, that is the ideal state to open your eyes and perceive reality moment by moment, for a few minutes.

References

1. Editorial. Non-verbal communication in general practice. J R Coll Gen Pract. 1980;30:323–4.
2. Manusov V, Patterson ML. The SAGE handbook of nonverbal communication. New York: SAGE Publications; 2006.
3. Knapp ML. An historical overview of nonverbal research. In: The SAGE handbook of nonverbal communication. New York: SAGE Publications; 2006. https://doi.org/10.4135/9781412976152.n1.
4. Rosemont H. A reader's companion to the Confucian analects. New York: Springer; 2013. https://doi.org/10.1057/9781137303394.
5. Chang HC. Language and words: communication in the analects of Confucius. J Lang Soc Psychol. 1997;16(2):107. https://doi.org/10.1177/0261927X970162001.
6. Yi SH. Persuasion without words: Confucian persuasion and the supernatural. Humanities (Switzerland). 2019;8(4):182. https://doi.org/10.3390/h8040182.
7. Doyle J. Socrates and Gorgias. Phronesis. 2010;55(1):1–25. https://doi.org/10.1163/003188610X12589452898769.
8. Wilburn J. Gorgias on knowledge and the powerlessness of logos. Humanities (Switzerland). 2023;12(1):9. https://doi.org/10.3390/h12010009.

9. Tusi J. Between rhetoric and sophistry: the puzzling case of Plato's Gorgias. Apeiron. 2020;53(1):59. https://doi.org/10.1515/apeiron-2018-0099.
10. Aristotle. In: Kennedy GA, editor. On rethoric. Oxford: Oxford University Press; 1991.
11. Major WE. The court of comedy: Aristophanes, rhetoric, and democracy in fifth-century Athens; 2013. https://doi.org/10.1080/00335630.2015.1057936.
12. Csapo E, Goette HR, Green JR, et al. Theatre and autocracy in the ancient world. Berlin: De Gruyter; 2022. https://doi.org/10.1515/9783110980356.
13. Robson M. Performing democracy. Anglia. 2018;136(1):154–70. https://doi.org/10.1515/ang-2018-0014.
14. Cicero MT. De Oratore: books I-II; 1942.
15. Mankin D. Cicero: of Oratores book III; 2011. https://doi.org/10.1017/9780511778292.
16. Quintilian Q, Marcus F. Institution oratory. In: Oxford classical texts: M. Fabi Quintilian: Institution Oratories: twelve books, vol. 1. Oxford: Oxford University Press; 2017. p. 1–6. https://doi.org/10.1093/oseo/instance.00170757.
17. Gerbrandy P. Quintilian's Institute oratory as a literary work. Hermes (Germany). 2020;148(1):86. https://doi.org/10.25162/HERMES-2020-0006.
18. Beechy T. The legacy of Boethius in medieval England: the consolation and its afterlives. J Engl Ger Philol. 2020;119(3):417. https://doi.org/10.5406/jenglgermphil.119.3.0417.
19. Enos T, Bizzell P, Herzberg B. The rhetorical tradition: readings from classical times to the present. Coll Compos Commun. 1991;42(1):99. https://doi.org/10.2307/357551.
20. Bizzell P. Rhetoric in the European tradition. Rhetor Soc Q. 1992;22(3):59. https://doi.org/10.1080/02773949209390961.
21. Bizzell P. Persuasion and argument: coterminous? Pedagogy. 2005;5(2):317. https://doi.org/10.1215/15314200-5-2-317.
22. Davies H. Fanology: hand-fans in the prehistory of mobile devices. Mob Media Commun. 2019;7(3):303–21. https://doi.org/10.1177/2050157919846181.
23. Darwin C. The expression of the emotions in man and animals. Oxford: Oxford University Press; 2013. https://doi.org/10.1017/cbo9781139833813.
24. Manusov VL. The sourcebook of nonverbal measures: going beyond words. London: Routledge; 2014. https://doi.org/10.4324/9781410611703.
25. Riggio RE, Watring KP, Throckmorton B. Social skills, social support, and psychosocial adjustment. Pers Individ Dif. 1993;15(3):275. https://doi.org/10.1016/0191-8869(93)90217-Q.
26. Riggio RE. Assessment of basic social skills. J Pers Soc Psychol. 1986;51(3):649. https://doi.org/10.1037/0022-3514.51.3.649.
27. Love EB, Nowicki S, Duke MP. The Emory dyssemia index: a brief screening instrument for the identification of nonverbal language deficits in elementary school children. J Psychol Interdiscip Appl. 1994;128(6):703. https://doi.org/10.1080/00223980.1994.9921302.
28. Andersen PA, Leibowitz K. The development and nature of the construct touch avoidance. Environ Psychol Nonverb Behav. 1978;3(2):89. https://doi.org/10.1007/BF01135607.
29. Burgoon JK, Buller DB, Hale JL, de Turck MA. Relational messages associated with nonverbal behaviors. Hum Commun Res. 1984;10(3):351. https://doi.org/10.1111/j.1468-2958.1984.tb00023.x.
30. Burgoon JK, Birk T, Pfau M. Nonverbal behaviors, persuasion, and credibility. Hum Commun Res. 1990;17(1):140–69. https://doi.org/10.1111/j.1468-2958.1990.tb00229.x.
31. Denault V, Plusquellec P, Jupe LM, et al. The analysis of nonverbal communication: the dangers of pseudoscience in security and justice contexts. Anuario de Psicologia Juridica. 2020;30(1):1. https://doi.org/10.5093/apj2019a9.
32. Burgoon JK, Wang X, Chen X, Pentland SJ, Dunbar NE. Nonverbal behaviors "speak" relational messages of dominance, trust, and composure. Front Psychol. 2021;12:624177. https://doi.org/10.3389/fpsyg.2021.624177.
33. Hartmark-Hill J. Critical synthesis package: relational communication scale (RCS). MedEdPORTAL. Published online 2013. https://doi.org/10.15766/mep_2374-8265.9454.

34. Rubin RB, Palmgreen P, Sypher HE. Relational communication scale. In: Communication research measures. London: Routledge; 2020. https://doi.org/10.4324/9781003064343-52.
35. Hale JL, Burgoon JK, Householder B. The relational communication scale. In: The sourcebook of nonverbal measures: going beyond words. London: Routledge; 2014.
36. Gallagher TJ, Hartung PJ, Gerzina H, Gregory SW, Merolla D. Further analysis of a doctor-patient nonverbal communication instrument. Patient Educ Couns. 2005;57(3):262. https://doi.org/10.1016/j.pec.2004.06.008.
37. Gallagher TJ, Hartung PJ, Gregory SW. Assessment of a measure of relational communication for doctor-patient interactions. Patient Educ Couns. 2001;45(3):211. https://doi.org/10.1016/S0738-3991(01)00126-4.
38. Fadiga L, Fogassi L, Pavesi G, Rizzolatti G. Motor facilitation during action observation: a magnetic stimulation study. J Neurophysiol. 1995;73(6):2608. https://doi.org/10.1152/jn.1995.73.6.2608.
39. Rizzolatti G, Fogassi L, Gallese V. Neurophysiological mechanisms underlying the understanding and imitation of action. Nat Rev Neurosci. 2001;2(9):661. https://doi.org/10.1038/35090060.
40. Rizzolatti G, Fadiga L, Gallese V, Fogassi L. Premotor cortex and the recognition of motor actions. Cogn Brain Res. 1996;3(2):131. https://doi.org/10.1016/0926-6410(95)00038-0.
41. Rizzolatti G, Craighero L. The mirror-neuron system. Annu Rev Neurosci. 2004;27:169–92. https://doi.org/10.1146/annurev.neuro.27.070203.144230.
42. Kittel AFD, Olderbak S, Wilhelm O. Sty in the mind's eye: a meta-analytic investigation of the nomological network and internal consistency of the "reading the mind in the eyes" test. Assessment. 2022;29(5):872. https://doi.org/10.1177/1073191121996469.
43. Bloom P, German TP. Two reasons to abandon the false belief task as a test of theory of mind. Cognition. 2000;77(1):B25. https://doi.org/10.1016/S0010-0277(00)00096-2.
44. Wellman HM, Cross D, Watson J. Meta-analysis of theory-of-mind development: the truth about false belief. Child Dev. 2001;72(3):655. https://doi.org/10.1111/1467-8624.00304.
45. Harvey AR. Links between the neurobiology of oxytocin and human musicality. Front Hum Neurosci. 2020;14:350. https://doi.org/10.3389/fnhum.2020.00350.
46. Ho SS, MacDonald A, Swain JE. Associative and sensorimotor learning for parenting involves mirror neurons under the influence of oxytocin. Behav Brain Sci. 2014;37(2):203. https://doi.org/10.1017/S0140525X1300232X.
47. Stewart AL, Field TA, Echterling LG. Neuroscience and the magic of play therapy. Int J Play Ther. 2016;25(1):4. https://doi.org/10.1037/pla0000016.
48. Bakker M, Kaduk K, Elsner C, Juvrud J, Gredebäck G. The neural basis of non-verbal communication-enhanced processing of perceived give-me gestures in 9-month-old girls. Front Psychol. 2015;6:59. https://doi.org/10.3389/fpsyg.2015.00059.
49. Kawai E, Takagai S, Takei N, Itoh H, Kanayama N, Tsuchiya KJ. Maternal postpartum depressive symptoms predict delay in non-verbal communication in 14-month-old infants. Infant Behav Dev. 2017;46:33–45. https://doi.org/10.1016/j.infbeh.2016.11.006.
50. Smith J, Eadie T, Levickis P, Bretherton L, Goldfeld S. Predictive validity of verbal and non-verbal communication and mother–child turn-taking at 12 months on language outcomes at 24 and 36 months in a cohort of infants experiencing adversity: a preliminary study. Int J Lang Commun Disord. 2018;53(5):969–80. https://doi.org/10.1111/1460-6984.12408.
51. Balconi M, Fronda G. The use of hyperscanning to investigate the role of social, affective, and informative gestures in non-verbal communication. Electrophysiological (EEG) and inter-brain connectivity evidence. Brain Sci. 2020;10(1):29. https://doi.org/10.3390/brainsci10010029.
52. Rosenzweig MR, Bennett EL. Psychobiology of plasticity: effects of training and experience on brain and behavior. Behav Brain Res. 1996;78(1):57. https://doi.org/10.1016/0166-4328(95)00216-2.

53. Weiller C, Chollet F, Friston KJ, Wise RJS, Frackowiak RSJ. Functional reorganization of the brain in recovery from striatocapsular infarction in man. Ann Neurol. 1992;31(5):463. https://doi.org/10.1002/ana.410310502.

54. Deroide N, Nih LR, Tran Dinh RY, Lévy B, Kubis N. Cerebral plasticity: from bench to bedside in stroke treatment. Rev Med Interne. 2010;31(7):486. https://doi.org/10.1016/j.revmed.2009.08.014.

55. Templar-Eynon S. Neuropsychological rehabilitation: effects of auditory training on cortical plasticity, attention, and working memory in receptive aphasia. In: Dissertation abstracts international: section B: the sciences and engineering, vol. 68(1-B). Ann Arbor: University Microfilms; 2007.

56. Mandal MK, Awasthi A. Understanding facial expressions in communication: cross-cultural and multidisciplinary perspectives. New York: Springer; 2015. https://doi.org/10.1007/978-81-322-1934-7.

57. Bowman JM, Compton BL. Interpersonal oculesics: eye-related signals of attraction, interest, and connection. In: Nonverbal communication in close relationships. London: Routledge; 2022. https://doi.org/10.1007/978-3-030-94492-6_1.

58. Eltuzerova G. Elements of oculesics in literary text and their semantics. Bull Sci Pract. 2021;7(5):580. https://doi.org/10.33619/2414-2948/66/65.

59. Fesharaki F. Nonverbal communication of pharmacists during counseling leading to patient satisfaction: evidence from Iranian retail market. Atl J Commun. 2019;27(1):62. https://doi.org/10.1080/15456870.2019.1540241.

60. Gabbott M, Hogg G. An empirical investigation of the impact of non-verbal communication on service evaluation. Eur J Mark. 2000;34(3–4):384. https://doi.org/10.1108/03090560010311911.

61. Michela B, Giulia F. Gesture in hyperscanning during observation. Inter-brain connectivity. Neuropsychol Trends. 2020;28:59. https://doi.org/10.7358/neur-2020-028-bal2.

62. Ramos-Cabo S, Vulchanov V, Vulchanova M. Gesture and language trajectories in early development: an overview from the autism spectrum disorder perspective. Front Psychol. 2019;10:1211. https://doi.org/10.3389/fpsyg.2019.01211.

63. Belío-Apaolaza HS, Hernández Muñoz N. Emblematic gestures learning in Spanish as L2/FL: interactions between types of gestures and tasks. Lang Teach Res. 2021;7:1–33. https://doi.org/10.1177/13621688211006880.

64. Rochmah SN, Swandhina M, Maulana RA. Child gesture as a form of non-verbal communication; 2020. https://doi.org/10.2991/assehr.k.200303.071.

65. Jolly S. Understanding body language: Birdwhistell's theory of kinesics. Corp Commun Int J. 2000;5(3):133. https://doi.org/10.1108/13563280010377518.

66. Affini LN. A study of kinesics category and the manifestation towards a toddler attitudes. Eternal. 2018;8(2) https://doi.org/10.26877/eternal.v8i2.3048.

67. Hans A, Hans E. Kinesics, haptics and proxemics: aspects of non-verbal communication. IOSR J Hum Soc Sci Ver IV. 2015;20(2).

68. Burgoon JK, Jones SB. Toward a theory of personal space expectations and their violations. Hum Commun Res. 1976;2(2):131. https://doi.org/10.1111/j.1468-2958.1976.tb00706.x.

69. Rios-Martinez J, Spalanzani A, Laugier C. From proxemics theory to socially-aware navigation: a survey. Int J Soc Robot. 2015;7(2):137. https://doi.org/10.1007/s12369-014-0251-1.

70. Ballendat T, Marquardt N, Greenberg S. Proxemic interaction: designing for a proximity and orientation-aware environment. In: ACM international conference on interactive tabletops and surfaces, ITS 2010; 2010. https://doi.org/10.1145/1936652.1936676.

71. Kim J, de Dear R. Workspace satisfaction: the privacy-communication trade-off in open-plan offices. J Environ Psychol. 2013;36:18–26. https://doi.org/10.1016/j.jenvp.2013.06.007.

72. Bailenson JN, Blascovich J, Beall AC, Loomis JM. Interpersonal distance in immersive virtual environments. Pers Soc Psychol Bull. 2003;29(7):819. https://doi.org/10.1177/0146167203029007002.

73. Feygin D, Keehner M, Tendick F. Haptic guidance: experimental evaluation of a haptic training method for a perceptual motor skill. In: Proceedings—10th symposium on haptic interfaces for virtual environment and teleoperator systems, HAPTICS 2002; 2002. https://doi.org/10.1109/HAPTIC.2002.998939.
74. Coles TR, Meglan D, John NW. The role of haptics in medical training simulators: a survey of the state of the art. IEEE Trans Haptics. 2011;4(1):51. https://doi.org/10.1109/TOH.2010.19.
75. Ernst MO, Banks MS. Humans integrate visual and haptic information in a statistically optimal fashion. Nature. 2002;415(6870):429. https://doi.org/10.1038/415429a.
76. Lederman SJ, Klatzky RL. Haptic perception: a tutorial. Atten Percept Psychophys. 2009;71(7):1439. https://doi.org/10.3758/APP.71.7.1439.
77. Ray EB, Ray GB. The relationship of paralinguistic cues to impression formation and the recall of medical messages. Health Commun. 1990;2(1):47. https://doi.org/10.1207/s15327027hc0201_4.
78. Kee JWY, Khoo HS, Lim I, Koh MYH. Communication skills in patient-doctor interactions: learning from patient complaints. Health Prof Educ. 2018;4(2):97. https://doi.org/10.1016/j.hpe.2017.03.006.
79. Devillers L, Vidrascu L. Real-life emotions detection with lexical and paralinguistic cues on human-human call center dialogs. In: Proceedings of the annual conference of the international speech communication association, INTERSPEECH, vol. 2; 2006. https://doi.org/10.21437/interspeech.2006-275.
80. Voetmann SS, Hvidt NC, Viftrup DT. Verbalizing spiritual needs in palliative care: a qualitative interview study on verbal and non-verbal communication in two Danish hospices. BMC Palliat Care. 2022;21(1):3. https://doi.org/10.1186/s12904-021-00886-0.
81. Hogrefe K, Ziegler W, Weidinger N, Goldenberg G. Non-verbal communication in severe aphasia: influence of aphasia, apraxia, or semantic processing? Cortex. 2012;48(8):952–62. https://doi.org/10.1016/j.cortex.2011.02.022.
82. Hillen MA, de Haes HCJM, Verdam MGE, Smets EMA. Trust and perceptions of physicians' nonverbal behavior among women with immigrant backgrounds. J Immigr Minor Health. 2018;20(4):963–71. https://doi.org/10.1007/s10903-017-0580-x.
83. Rexach L. Palliative care in dementia. Eur Geriatr Med. 2012;3:131–40. https://doi.org/10.1016/j.eurger.2012.01.015.
84. Härgestam M, Hultin M, Brulin C, Jacobsson M. Trauma team leaders' non-verbal communication: video registration during trauma team training. Scand J Trauma Resusc Emerg Med. 2016;24(1):37. https://doi.org/10.1186/s13049-016-0230-7.
85. Ronald Mac Keith P, Abercrombie MLJ. Section of paediatrics parent-staff communication in a children's unit, vol. 65; 1972. p. 335.
86. Stepanikova I, Zhang Q, Wieland D, Eleazer GP, Stewart T. Non-verbal communication between primary care physicians and older patients: how does race matter? J Gen Intern Med. 2012;27(5):576–81. https://doi.org/10.1007/s11606-011-1934-z.
87. Nimbalkar SM, Raval H, Bansal SC, Pandya U, Pathak A. Non-verbal communication in a neonatal intensive care unit: a video audit using non-verbal immediacy scale (NIS-O). Indian J Pediatr. 2018;85(11):1025–7. https://doi.org/10.1007/s12098-018-2680-6.
88. Harrison A. Experimental investigation of non-verbal communication in eating disorders. Psychiatry Res. 2021;297:113732. https://doi.org/10.1016/j.psychres.2021.113732.
89. Alcântara PL, Wogel AZ, Rossi MIL, Neves IR, Sabates AL, Puggina AC. Effect of interaction with clowns on vital signs and non-verbal communication of hospitalized children. Rev Paul Pediatr. 2016;34(4):432–8. https://doi.org/10.1016/j.rppede.2016.02.011.
90. Yamaguchi M, Takeda K, Onishi M, Deguchi M, Higashi AT. Non-verbal communication method based on a biochemical marker for people with severe motor and intellectual disabilities. J Int Med Res. 2006;34:30.
91. My non verbal communication skills made a big difference.
92. Wikipedia. Florencio Escardó. https://es.wikipedia.org/wiki/Florencio_Escard%C3%B3.

93. Rudovic O, Lee J, Dai M, Schuller B, Picard RW. Personalized machine learning for robot perception of affect and engagement in autism therapy. Sci Robot. 2018;3:eaao6760. http://robotics.sciencemag.org/.

94. Picard RW, Boyer EW. Smartwatch biomarkers and the path to clinical use. Med. 2021;2(7):797–9. https://doi.org/10.1016/j.medj.2021.06.005.

95. Bickmore T, Giorgino T, Green N, Picard R. Special issue on dialog systems for health communication. J Biomed Inform. 2006;39(5):465–7. https://doi.org/10.1016/j.jbi.2006.02.002.

96. Picard R, Wolf G. Guest Editorial sensor informatics and quantified self. IEEE J Biomed Health Inform. 2015;19(5):1531. https://doi.org/10.1109/JBHI.2015.2462372.

97. McHill AW, Sano A, Hilditch CJ, et al. Robust stability of melatonin circadian phase, sleep metrics, and chronotype across months in young adults living in real-world settings. J Pineal Res. 2021;70(3):e12720. https://doi.org/10.1111/jpi.12720.

98. McDuff D, Gontarek S, Picard RW. Remote detection of photoplethysmographic systolic and diastolic peaks using a digital camera. IEEE Trans Biomed Eng. 2014;61(12):2948–54. https://doi.org/10.1109/TBME.2014.2340991.

99. Sano A, Phillips AJ, Yu AZ, et al. Recognizing academic performance, sleep quality, stress level, and mental health using personality traits, wearable sensors and mobile phones. Int Conf Wearable Implant Body Sens Netw. 2015;2015:10.1109/BSN.2015.7299420.

100. Coppersmith DDL, Wang SB, Kleiman EM, et al. Real-time digital monitoring of a suicide attempt by a hospital patient. Gen Hosp Psychiatry. 2023;80:35–9. https://doi.org/10.1016/j.genhosppsych.2022.12.005.

101. Onorati F, Regalia G, Caborni C, et al. Prospective study of a multimodal convulsive seizure detection wearable system on pediatric and adult patients in the epilepsy monitoring unit. Front Neurol. 2021;12:724904. https://doi.org/10.3389/fneur.2021.724904.

102. Sano A, Yu AZ, McHill AW, et al. Prediction of happy-sad mood from daily behaviors and previous sleep history. In: Proceedings of the annual international conference of the IEEE Engineering in Medicine and Biology Society, EMBS, vol. 2015-November. Institute of Electrical and Electronics Engineers Inc.; 2015. p. 6796–6799. https://doi.org/10.1109/EMBC.2015.7319954.

103. Jaques N, Taylor S, Azaria A, Ghandeharioun A, Sano A, Picard R. Predicting students' happiness from physiology, phone, mobility, and behavioral data. Int Conf Affect Comput Intell Interact Workshops. 2015;2015:222–8. https://doi.org/10.1109/ACII.2015.7344575.

104. Taylor S, Sano A, Ferguson C, Mohan A, Picard RW. Quantifyme: an open-source automated single-case experimental design platform. Sensors (Switzerland). 2018;18(4):1097. https://doi.org/10.3390/s18041097.

105. Ghandeharioun A, Azaria A, Taylor S, Picard RW. "Kind and grateful": a context-sensitive smartphone app utilizing inspirational content to promote gratitude. Psychol Well Being. 2016;6(1):9. https://doi.org/10.1186/s13612-016-0046-2.

106. Fletcher RR, Dobson K, Goodwin MS, et al. ICalm: wearable sensor and network architecture for wirelessly communicating and logging autonomic activity. IEEE Trans Inf Technol Biomed. 2010;14(2):215–23. https://doi.org/10.1109/TITB.2009.2038692.

107. Phillips AJK, Clerx WM, O'Brien CS, et al. Irregular sleep/wake patterns are associated with poorer academic performance and delayed circadian and sleep/wake timing. Sci Rep. 2017;7(1):3216. https://doi.org/10.1038/s41598-017-03171-4.

108. Fischer D, McHill AW, Sano A, et al. Irregular sleep and event schedules are associated with poorer self-reported well-being in US college students. Sleep. 2020;43(6):1–12. https://doi.org/10.1093/sleep/zsz300.

109. Sano A, Chen W, Lopez-Martinez D, Taylor S, Picard RW. Multimodal ambulatory sleep detection using LSTM recurrent neural networks. IEEE J Biomed Health Inform. 2019;23(4):1607–17. https://doi.org/10.1109/JBHI.2018.2867619.

110. Pedrelli P, Fedor S, Ghandeharioun A, et al. Monitoring changes in depression severity using wearable and mobile sensors. Front Psychiatry. 2020;11:584711. https://doi.org/10.3389/fpsyt.2020.584711.

111. Kim ES, Moskowitz JT, Kubzansky LD. Introduction to special issue: interventions to modify psychological well-being and population health. Affect Sci. 2023;4(1):1–9. https://doi.org/10.1007/s42761-023-00184-3.
112. Kubzansky LD, Kim ES, Boehm JK, et al. Interventions to modify psychological well-being: progress, promises, and an agenda for future research. Affect Sci. 2023;4:174. https://doi.org/10.1007/s42761-022-00167-w.
113. Sano A, Taylor S, McHill AW, et al. Identifying objective physiological markers and modifiable behaviors for self-reported stress and mental health status using wearable sensors and mobile phones: observational study. J Med Internet Res. 2018;20(6):e210. https://doi.org/10.2196/jmir.9410.
114. Doré BP, Morris RR, Burr DA, Picard RW, Ochsner KN. Helping others regulate emotion predicts increased regulation of one's own emotions and decreased symptoms of depression. Pers Soc Psychol Bull. 2017;43(5):729–39. https://doi.org/10.1177/0146167217695558.
115. McDuff D, Gontarek S, Picard RW. Improvements in remote cardiopulmonary measurement using a five band digital camera. IEEE Trans Biomed Eng. 2014;61(10):2593–601. https://doi.org/10.1109/TBME.2014.2323695.
116. Picard RW. Future affective technology for autism and emotion communication. Philos Trans R Soc B Biol Sci. 2009;364(1535):3575–84. https://doi.org/10.1098/rstb.2009.0143.
117. Reynolds C, Picard R. Ethical evaluation of displays that adapt to affect. Cyberpsychol Behav. 2004;7:662.
118. Chen W, Hernandez J, Picard RW. Estimating carotid pulse and breathing rate from near-infrared video of the neck. Physiol Meas. 2018;39(10):10NT01. https://doi.org/10.1088/1361-6579/aae625.
119. Kleiman EM, Turner BJ, Fedor S, et al. Digital phenotyping of suicidal thoughts. Depress Anxiety. 2018;35(7):601–8. https://doi.org/10.1002/da.22730.
120. Bickmore T, Gruber A, Picard R. Establishing the computer-patient working alliance in automated health behavior change interventions. Patient Educ Couns. 2005;59(1):21–30. https://doi.org/10.1016/j.pec.2004.09.008.
121. Poh MZ, Loddenkemper T, Reinsberger C, et al. Convulsive seizure detection using a wrist-worn electrodermal activity and accelerometry biosensor. Epilepsia. 2012;53(5):e93. https://doi.org/10.1111/j.1528-1167.2012.03444.x.
122. Lopez-Martinez D, Picard R. Continuous pain intensity estimation from autonomic signals with recurrent neural networks. Annu Int Conf IEEE Eng Med Biol Soc. 2018;2018:5624–7. https://doi.org/10.1109/EMBC.2018.8513575.
123. Nock MK, Kleiman EM, Abraham M, et al. Consensus statement on ethical & safety practices for conducting digital monitoring studies with people at risk of suicide and related behaviors. Psychiatr Res Clin Pract. 2021;3:57–66. https://doi.org/10.1176/appi.
124. Goldenholz DM, Moss R, Jost DA, et al. Common data elements for epilepsy mobile health systems. Epilepsia. 2018;59(5):1020–6. https://doi.org/10.1111/epi.14066.
125. Bhatkar V, Picard R, Staahl C. Combining electrodermal activity with the peak-pain time to quantify three temporal regions of pain experience. Front Pain Res. 2022;3:764128. https://doi.org/10.3389/fpain.2022.764128.
126. El Kaliouby R, Picard R, Baron-Cohen S. Affective computing and autism. Ann N Y Acad Sci. 2006;1093:228–48. https://doi.org/10.1196/annals.1382.016.
127. Johnson KT, Picard RW. Advancing neuroscience through wearable devices. Neuron. 2020;108(1):8–12. https://doi.org/10.1016/j.neuron.2020.09.030.
128. Picard RW. Affective medicine: technology with emotional intelligence. Amsterdam: IOS Press; 2001. http://www.media.mit.edu/affect
129. Poh MZ, McDuff DJ, Picard RW. Advancements in noncontact, multiparameter physiological measurements using a webcam. IEEE Trans Biomed Eng. 2011;58(1):7–11. https://doi.org/10.1109/TBME.2010.2086456.

130. Kelly M, Svrcek C, King N, Scherpbier A, Dornan T. Embodying empathy: a phenomenological study of physician touch. Med Educ. 2020;54(5):400–7. https://doi.org/10.1111/medu.14040.

131. Davies P. Non-verbal communication with patients. Br J Nurs. 1994;3(5):220–3.

132. Kacperek L. Non-verbal communication: the importance of listening. Br J Nurs. 1994;6(5):275–9.

133. Abney DH, Dale R, Louwerse MM, Kello CT. The bursts and lulls of multimodal interaction: temporal distributions of behavior reveal differences between verbal and non-verbal communication. Cogn Sci. 2018;42(4):1297–316. https://doi.org/10.1111/cogs.12612.

134. Mast MS. On the importance of nonverbal communication in the physician-patient interaction. Patient Educ Couns. 2007;67(3 special issue):315–8. https://doi.org/10.1016/j.pec.2007.03.005.

135. Kemper KJ, Shaltout HA. Non-verbal communication of compassion: measuring psychophysiologic effects. BMC Complement Altern Med. 2011;11:132. https://doi.org/10.1186/1472-6882-11-132.

136. Bartels J, Rodenbach R, Ciesinski K, Gramling R, Fiscella K, Epstein R. Eloquent silences: a musical and lexical analysis of conversation between oncologists and their patients. Patient Educ Couns. 2016;99(10):1584. https://doi.org/10.1016/j.pec.2016.04.009.

137. McHenry M, Parker PA, Baile WF, Lenzi R. Voice analysis during bad news discussion in oncology: reduced pitch, decreased speaking rate, and nonverbal communication of empathy. Support Care Cancer. 2012;20(5):1073–8. https://doi.org/10.1007/s00520-011-1187-8.

138. Hoerger M, Epstein RM, Winters PC, et al. Values and options in cancer care (VOICE): study design and rationale for a patient-centered communication and decision-making intervention for physicians, patients with advanced cancer, and their caregivers. BMC Cancer. 2013;13:188. http://www.biomedcentral.com/1471-2407/13/188

139. Gibbings-isaac D, Iqbal M, Tahir MA, Kumarapeli P, De lusignan S. The pattern of silent time in the clinical consultation: an observational multichannel video study. Fam Pract. 2012;29(5):616–21. https://doi.org/10.1093/fampra/cms001.

140. Bruneau TJ. Communicative silences: forms and functions. J Commun. 1973;23:17.

141. Ephratt M. The functions of silence. J Pragmat. 2008;40(11):1909–38. https://doi.org/10.1016/j.pragma.2008.03.009.

142. Rockwell SL, Woods CL, Lemmon ME, et al. Silence in conversations about advancing pediatric cancer. Front Oncol. 2022;12:894586. https://doi.org/10.3389/fonc.2022.894586.

143. Sabbadini A. Listening to silence. Br J Psychother. 1991;7(4):406–15.

144. Visser LNC, Tollenaar MS, van Doornen LJP, de Haes HCJM, Smets EMA. Does silence speak louder than words? The impact of oncologists' emotion-oriented communication on analogue patients' information recall and emotional stress. Patient Educ Couns. 2019;102(1):43–52. https://doi.org/10.1016/j.pec.2018.08.032.

145. Margulis EH. Moved by nothing: listening to musical silence. J Music Theory. 2007;51(2):245–76. https://doi.org/10.1215/00222909-2009-003.

146. Alexander SC, Garner DK, Somoroff M, Gramling DJ, Norton SA, Gramling R. Using music[al] knowledge to represent expressions of emotions. Patient Educ Couns. 2015;98(11):1339–45. https://doi.org/10.1016/j.pec.2015.04.019.

147. Back AL, Bauer-Wu SM, Rushton CH, Halifax J. Original articles: Compassionate silence in the patient-clinician encounter: a contemplative approach. J Palliat Med. 2009;12(12):1113.

148. Verhaeghen P. Mindfulness as attention training: meta-analyses on the links between attention performance and mindfulness interventions, long-term meditation practice, and trait mindfulness. Mindfulness (N Y). 2021;12(3):564–81. https://doi.org/10.1007/s12671-020-01532-1.

149. Verhaeghen P. Mindfulness and meditation training. In: Cognitive training: an overview of features and applications. Basel: Springer Nature Switzerland AG; 2021. https://doi.org/10.1007/978-3-030-39292-5_17.

150. Jha AP, Krompinger J, Baime MJ. Mindfulness training modifies subsystems of attention. Cogn Affect Behav Neurosci. 2007;7(2):109. https://doi.org/10.3758/CABN.7.2.109.

151. Suchman AL, Matthews DA. What makes the patient-doctor relationship therapeutic? Exploring the connexional dimension of medical care. Ann Intern Med. 1988;108(1):125–30.

152. Rushton CH, Sellers DE, Heller KS, Spring B, Dossey BM, Halifax J. Impact of a contemplative end-of-life training program: being with dying. Palliat Support Care. 2009;7(4):405–14. https://doi.org/10.1017/S1478951509990411.

153. Sosa N, Rios K. The utilitarian scientist: the humanization of scientists in moral dilemmas. J Exp Soc Psychol. 2019;84:103818. https://doi.org/10.1016/j.jesp.2019.103818.

154. Hanson D. Humanizing interfaces: an integrative analysis of the aesthetics of humanlike robots; 2007.

155. Cypess R, Kemper S. The anthropomorphic analogy: humanising musical machines in the early modern and contemporary eras. Organ Sound. 2018;23(2):167. https://doi.org/10.1017/S1355771818000043.

156. Madani K. Robots' vision humanization through machine-learning based artificial visual attention. In: Communications in computer and information science, vol. 1055 CCIS; 2019. https://doi.org/10.1007/978-3-030-35430-5_2.

157. Payr S. In search of a narrative for human–robot relationships. Cybern Syst. 2019;50(3):281–99. https://doi.org/10.1080/01969722.2018.1550913.

158. Bowles T, Pauletto S. Emotions in the voice: humanising a robotic voice. In: Proceedings of the 7th sound and music computing conference, SMC 2010; 2010.

159. Bryson JJ. Robots should be slaves; 2010. https://doi.org/10.1075/nlp.8.11bry.

160. Dirgayasa IW. EMOJI, a breakthrough in contemporary communication (a literature review). J Lang Lit Teach. 2022;4(2):63. https://doi.org/10.35529/jllte.v4i2.63-76.

161. Novak PK, Smailović J, Sluban B, Mozetič I. Sentiment of emojis. PLoS One. 2015;10(12):e0144296. https://doi.org/10.1371/journal.pone.0144296.

162. Boutet I, Guay J, Chamberland J, Cousineau D, Collin C. Emojis that work! Incorporating visual cues from facial expressions in emojis can reduce ambiguous interpretations. Comput Hum Behav Rep. 2023;9:100251. https://doi.org/10.1016/j.chbr.2022.100251.

163. Dürscheid C, Siever UCM. Beyond the alphabet—communication with emojis. Zeitschrift fur Germanistische Linguistik. 2017;45(2):256.

164. Borreli L. Human attention span shortens to 8 seconds due to digital technology: 3 ways to stay focused. Medical Daily.

165. Herring AMR, Craven MP, Mughal F, et al. Potential of using visual imagery to revolutionise measurement of emotional health. Arch Dis Child. 2020;105(7):690. https://doi.org/10.1136/archdischild-2019-317758.

166. Donovan D. Mood, emotions and emojis: conversations about health with young people. Ment Health Pract. 2016;20(2):23. https://doi.org/10.7748/mhp.2016.e1143.

167. Danesi M. Emotional wellbeing and the semiotic translation of emojis. In: Exploring the translatability of emotions. Cham: Palgrave Macmillan; 2022. https://doi.org/10.1007/978-3-030-91748-7_12.

168. Sinha S, Shrivastava A, Paradis C. A survey of the mobile phone-based interventions for violence prevention among women. Adv Soc Work. 2020;19(2):493. https://doi.org/10.18060/22526.

169. Willoughby JF, Liu S. Do pictures help tell the story? An experimental test of narrative and emojis in a health text message intervention. Comput Human Behav. 2018;79:75. https://doi.org/10.1016/j.chb.2017.10.031.

170. Lotfinejad N, Assadi R, Aelami MH, Pittet D. Emojis in public health and how they might be used for hand hygiene and infection prevention and control. Antimicrob Resist Infect Control. 2020;9(1):27. https://doi.org/10.1186/s13756-020-0692-2.

171. Morelle AM, de Lima GE, D'Agustini N, Venero FC, Barrios CH. Real-time detection of patient-reported outcomes (PRO) through an app: a Brazilian experience. J Clin Oncol. 2019;37(15 Suppl):e23059. https://doi.org/10.1200/jco.2019.37.15_suppl.e23059.

172. Corrêa RE, Velho PE, Fornazzaro MF, Tolocka RE. Perceived levels of stress, emotions and physical activity in outpatients with diffuse connective tissue diseases. Ital J Dermatol Venerol. 2022;157(4):348–54. https://doi.org/10.23736/S2784-8671.22.07280-2.
173. Stoikos S, Izbicki M. Multilingual emoticon prediction of tweets about COVID-19. In: Proceedings of the third workshop on computational modeling of people's opinions, personality, and emotion's in social media; 2020.
174. Al-Rawi A, Siddiqi M, Morgan R, Vandan N, Smith J, Wenham C. COVID-19 and the gendered use of emojis on twitter: infodemiology study. J Med Internet Res. 2020;22(11):e21646. https://doi.org/10.2196/21646.
175. Fadhil A, Schiavo G, Wang Y, Yilma BA. The effect of emojis when interacting with conversational interface assisted health coaching system. In: ACM international conference proceeding series; 2018. https://doi.org/10.1145/3240925.3240965.
176. Mahaffey AL. "N.A.M.E." FUN! Emojis may illustrate structure-function relationships of neurotransmitters to health professions students. Adv Physiol Educ. 2021;45(4):895–901. https://doi.org/10.1152/ADVAN.00123.2021.
177. Marzouk S, He S, Lee J. Emoji education: how students can help increase health awareness by making emojis. JMIR Med Educ. 2022;8(4):e39059. https://doi.org/10.2196/39059.

Chapter 8
Patient Needs: A Communication Map

8.1 Introduction

The mental map of communication with our patients, at least in oncology, involves understanding the needs of the patient at each stage of the disease.

We will analyze this technique in the specialty that I practice, clinical oncology, and which I develop at greater length in my book "On Cancer and Its Demons," [1] but it is easily adaptable to other specialties. The important thing to keep in mind is that the first step in communicating with the patient is to have an overview of their situation in order to be more open and attentive to what they might need.

Throughout our practical experience, the following points seem to be priorities when accompanying someone from diagnosis to death.

Each of these points will be developed throughout this chapter and we have also added a subheading in order to try to put our patient's emotional perspective into words.

1. The moment of diagnosis is: "The unexpected truth."
2. The patient's staging is: "The transitory truth."
3. The prognosis is: "The uncertain truth."
4. The treatment is: "The understandable truth."
5. The follow-up is: "The truth sought."
6. Recurrence is: "The feared truth."
7. Research is: "The neutral truth."
8. Error is: "The irritating truth."
9. Alternative treatments are: "The paradoxical truth."
10. Death is: "The ultimate truth."
11. Mourning is: "The remembered truth."

We will now begin to explore this map.

E. Gil Deza, *Improving Clinical Communication*,
https://doi.org/10.1007/978-3-031-62446-9_8

8.2   Node 1: The Moment of Diagnosis Is: "The Unexpected Truth"

A cancer diagnosis, whether made in white on black or pronounced by a doctor, confronts us with an unexpected truth.

The concept of unexpected is very similar to that of unwanted: this is not an impossible truth, it is not a truth that we have not thought about, it is simply one we hoped would not touch us, that someone else would win this lottery, at least this time.

Denial is the most common reaction to the possibility of cancer.

It is an expression of denial in the face of death.

The word cancer has connotations of pain, suffering, and death, which is why it is one of the most feared diseases of the twentieth and twenty-first centuries, as explained by Susan Sontag who suffered from not one but three cancers (breast, uterus, and leukemia secondary to myelodysplasia) and lived 29 years after her first diagnosis and 14 after her second one [2–7].

Therefore, the patient who sees this word written in a diagnosis or receives the information for the first time from their doctor is often shocked.

Diagnosis communication strategies have been outlined in multiple guidelines, but in our practice we continue to use the rule called "SPIKES," which is an acronym created by Buckman et al. [8, 9], and which masterfully summarizes care in communicating the truth. In medicine, it is used for all communication nodes, but fundamentally for diagnostic truth.

"SPIKES" is a six stage bad news communication protocol which means:

- Setting and starting: There is a big difference between improvisation and spontaneity. Improvising happens when one is not mentally clear about what they're going to say or what they're going to do: this is extremely dangerous. Spontaneity happens when someone has mentally and physically planned the conversation they are going to have with the patient or their family, but is nonetheless open to reacting with empathy to what the patient feels or needs.
- Perception: "Before you speak, ask". Assess what the patient's thoughts, emotions, and fears are. Have they been informed of what they have or what is wrong with them? What do you think they know and understand of what you have told them?
- Invitation: Invite the patient to express what they want to know about what's happening to them, about treatment alternatives, and about the possible evolution of the disease.
- Knowledge: Provide, in a slow and empathetic way, the knowledge that the patient needs. Prepare the patient for what you are going to say, say it and then wait for their reaction.
- Emotions: Evaluate the emotions the patient is feeling with empathetic responses.
- Strategy and summary: this must be planned before starting the conversation: what are the diagnostic or therapeutic proposals that I'm going to present to the patient so they can think about pursuing them or not.

The simplicity of these recommendations and their proven usefulness in different fields of medicine have made them extremely popular [10–15], and we highly recommend them.

8.3   Node 2: The Staging of the Patient Is: "The Transitory Truth"

The second communicative node consists of the staging of the cancer patient [16–21].

The classification of diseases, from the taxonomic point of view, is a nineteenth- and twentieth-century effort.

In the nineteenth century, Rudolf Virchow systematized the cytopathological and histopathological diagnosis of human diseases.

In the twentieth century, from the actuaries' lists, the IDC (International Disease Classification) arose, which is now in its 11th edition and is a coded list of ailments [22–25].

The systematic evaluation of the volume of oncological diseases is relatively recent in medicine and its birth can be placed in the middle of the twentieth century. Especially in regards to systematic classification using the TNM system (Tumor-Nodes-Metastases), which is now in its eighth edition [26–28].

The index of general state of activity of the patient, the performance status, was introduced by David Karnofsky, of the fathers of oncology. It is a ten-point ordinal scale, where 100 is a patient with no activity limitations, asymptomatic with no signs of disease and 0 is deceased [29–32].

These three axes—what disease you have, how widespread it is, and how much it affects your performance status—continue to be the classic prognostic tripod in oncology. Today the molecular and genetic profile of the ailments is added as predictors of response to treatments.

In order to determine how widespread the disease is, we use clinical examination [33–35] (about a third of all patients who arrive at the first consultation do so with a clinically detectable disseminated tumor) for evidence of metastasis in:

– Skin: palpable or visible cutaneous or subcutaneous nodules.
– Nodes: especially supraclavicular, axillary, or inguinal.
– Clinically detectable pleural effusion.
– Visceral involvement: disturbances of gait, speech, or consciousness due to brain metastases; jaundice or hepatomegaly due to liver metastases; ascites due to peritoneal compromise.
– Bone involvement: pain on percussion.

However, many times, the patient does not have clinical evidence of disseminated disease, and it is detected through images: ultrasound, scintigraphy, computed tomography, magnetic resonance imaging or PET scan.

In some tumors, metastases is detected by elevated values in some chemical elements found in blood: biological markers such as PSA (Prostate); Beta human chorionic gonadotropin (Tumors of the placenta or germ cell tumors); Alpha fetoprotein (hepatocarcinoma or germ cell tumors); LDH (rapid growing tumors); CEA or CA19-9 (Digestive tumors); CA 125 (ovarian tumors).

What is important to understand from the point of view of communication is that staging is a transitory truth: "Today we have this stage." However, it's also at the same time a static concept: since the stage of the patient's disease always refers to the first consultation in which an oncologist sees a patient.

But it also has a dynamic component: a patient can be diagnosed in the initial stages of the disease and then progress to more advanced stages, or they may be diagnosed in advanced stages and improve, in some cases managing to make the disease disappear.

What are the advantages of the **static** concept of staging: the comparison of populations. Since all patients are staged in the first consultation, this makes the study of the evolution of diseases in homogeneous groups comparable.

However, from the patient's point of view, every time we study the disease, they feel that they're taking an exam, where they'll get a passing grade if we find nothing and they'll fail if we find anything.

This dynamic of staging and follow-up tests for some patients is exhausting, as it is very similar to studies to reassure a condition.

8.4   Node 3: The Prognosis Is: "The Uncertain Truth"

The most recognized ability of Hippocratic doctors 25 centuries ago was not so much their diagnostic or therapeutic ability, but their ability to issue accurate forecasts about the evolution of a patient's disease [36–42].

We must clarify that this was of great practical importance. For Greek doctors, medicine should focus on potentially curable diseases and should not fall into the arrogance of treating incurable diseases. That could lead them to fall into the sin of "Hubris," the excessive pride that leads them to go against the design of the gods.

Therefore, respect for the figure of the doctor trained at the Cos school was based on the seriousness with which he established the future evolution of an ailment.

Thus we can see in the Hippocratic Corpus numerous references to the signs that indicate high mortality: drowsiness, breathing, emaciation, decreased urine, the characteristics of fevers, types of cranial injuries, etc.

It must be pointed out that such successes are based on observation and experience. Due to the therapeutic limitations of the time, many patients, when they were seen, were very close to death.

Therefore, many of these prognoses were of near or imminent death.

Today, on the other hand, the prognosis involves months at least, and several years at most, which makes it even more uncertain.

Therefore the prognostic communication must, above all, make this fact relevant: all statements about the future are conditional and uncertain [43–46].

But what is conditionality?

Today many ailments are diagnosed subclinically, that is, before they give rise to symptoms such as changes in laboratory values or in images.

In many patients, at least in oncology, the greatest source of information for decision-making is the primary tumor, and less frequently the metastases, and we know that there are subtle but consistent differences between the two.

Most patients have comorbidities (this is the name given to the coexistence of different diseases in one person) such as hypertension, diabetes, or liver or kidney disorders. Each of these conditions has in itself a specific prognosis.

In addition to all of the above, we are seeing more and more elderly patients, which, in medicine, is relatively new. We have thousands of years of experience with pediatric patients, but barely 50 years with geriatric patients. Age alone already determines a certain life expectancy.

Finally, everything we know about the prognosis comes from series of patients seen in the past. Therefore, even when the patient's condition is similar to a patient seen 10 years ago, we are trying to predict how the path moves forward by looking in the rearview mirror.

It's vital that our patient understand these epistemic conditions about what we are going to communicate.

What is uncertainty?

Uncertainty simply means that the future is unknowable. We are not seeing it, we are merely imagining it and the image we form of it is significantly influenced by the past.

This explains the fallibility of our claims. We **believe** that tomorrow will be the same as today, but we **know** that it will be slightly different.

Furthermore, while it is possible that tomorrow will be the same as today, it is highly unlikely that in 1 year the situation will be the same as today and it is absolutely probable that in 5 years it will be very different from today.

However, it is very difficult for us to imagine what we will be like in 5 years. Our own self-image 5 years from now is completely foreign to our current selves.

Just because probabilities are more accurate the closer the event is does not mean that our margin of error isn't high. A study carried out in seriously ill patients hospitalized in intensive care units reveals that the error rate goes from 10% in the 48-h survival prognosis to 50% in the 1-month survival prognosis.

Imagine what happens when what we are forecasting is 5 or 10 years away.

We have to keep one thing in mind though: it is more likely to hit the magnitude than the date. It is one thing to say "he has a few days left to live" (which can vary between 1 and 30 days) and another is to say he dies in 4 days.

The same is true for a forecast in months or years.

The two things that are important in communicating the forecast are: outlook and motive.

What do we understand by outlook?

When we propose the prognosis to a patient, it is good to do it in at least three scenarios: pessimistic, realistic, and optimistic.

The pessimistic (worst) and optimistic (best) scenarios are unlikely scenarios. They are not impossible but they are infrequent, and therefore surprising.

The realistic scenario is the most likely.

One of the communication problems is that social networks highlight and amplify improbable scenarios, especially optimistic ones. People are exposed to testimonials of patients who have evolved very well with different treatments.

Quantitatively, these examples are few, but the dissemination of their cases makes these situations available to everyone and generates anguish and hope at the same time.

It's useful to visualize the prognostic outlook as those three possible evolutions and highlight the magnitude more than the number: weeks, months, years; few or many; It is more accurate than raising a certain number; a number that is both usually wrong and is unforgettable, both for the patient and his family.

"Few months" is more accurate than "3 months" although the number that most arises when we say few is 3.

The second point is more important: motive.

Why is knowing the patient's prognosis important?

The question isn't trying to ascertain our right to know this information or not, but rather it seeks to understand the reasons for looking for this information, and also trying to see if it is possible to optimize the endeavor.

Hardly anyone asks for a forecast simply out of curiosity, most have a reason: many times relates to something concrete such as a certain event (anniversaries, completion of tasks or studies, delegation of tasks or responsibilities, trips or goals) other times it relates to a condition (not I want to die in the Hospital or I prefer to go home), while others have different reasons for why they want to know the expectations of cure or survival of a disease.

Whatever the reasons might be, they are not simply why the patient wants to know their prognosis, they are also frequently why the patient wants to live and we must always bear in mind Nietzsche's phrase: "He who has a why to live for can bear almost any how."

Therefore, we can use the moment of communicating the prognosis as an opportunity to learn how the patient handles uncertainty, to expose our limitations and conditioning factors, to train ourselves in communicating with ambiguity and to learn the reasons why a patient wants to live.

Patients who don't tolerate uncertainty and doctors who are inflexible in their statements tend to be an explosive combination; on the contrary, patients who are tolerant of uncertainty and humble and flexible doctors can have a more peaceful coexistence.

8.5   Node 4: The Treatment Is: "The Understandable Truth"

Every time a patient agrees to undergo a treatment, they place their trust first in their doctor and secondly in the understanding of their disease, prognosis, and therapeutic alternatives.

All medical treatment essentially has two objectives: to prolong life and improve quality of life, ideally both.

All other targets are non-medical.

Extending life is relatively simple to understand and difficult to achieve. It simply means adding one more day of life to a treated population relative to an untreated population. Difficult to demonstrate because prospective, randomized studies are needed, with prolonged follow-ups to confirm that this happens and even then, it's impossible to know if this addition has been achieved in a patient because we have no one to compare it with.

This results in a very solid parameter, but one that is nonetheless restricted to populations rather than individual patients.

Quality of life is another matter. In the first place, it is usually difficult to understand what exactly is good quality of life? How do we compare the quality of life between different people? How do we compare our own quality of life at different ages? How do we integrate the gray areas in which something improved while something else worsened in relation to the quality of our life?

All of this means that it's quite frequent for patient and doctor to make a sort of "negotiation" between longevity and quality of life.

This is an ongoing negotiation, because at each meeting when the treatments that the patient is receiving are re-evaluated, their tolerability is compared and the treatment objectives are re-evaluated. It is very reasonable that as we approach the end we demedicalize the patient.

De-prescription in geriatrics should be the rule, and polypharmacy the exception, which is exactly the opposite of what happens today.

In oncology, there are many therapeutic alternatives [47–51] and we have tried to summarize them in Fig. 8.1 [1].

All these alternatives are valid:

1. **"Wait and see"** (WS): is an option when the tumors are of low aggressiveness (Gleason 6 prostate cancer, luminal A breast tumors, superficial melanomas) and the treatments do not offer the possibility of prolonging survival. It is also an option when incurable situations are asymptomatic and the results of the treatments are similar whether the patient has symptoms or not.
2. **"Surgery":** is the most widely used option for localized tumors and in some circumstances, for disseminated tumors, with one or very few metastasis sites.
3. **"Radiotherapy":** is frequently used after conservative surgeries (for example, on the breast, head and neck, esophagus, larynx, anus), for the treatment of painful bone metastases or for the treatment of bleeding tumors.
4. **"Hormonotherapy":** is the term used for the use of hormonal treatments in tumors sensitive to these drugs: breast, prostate, and endometrial cancer, among

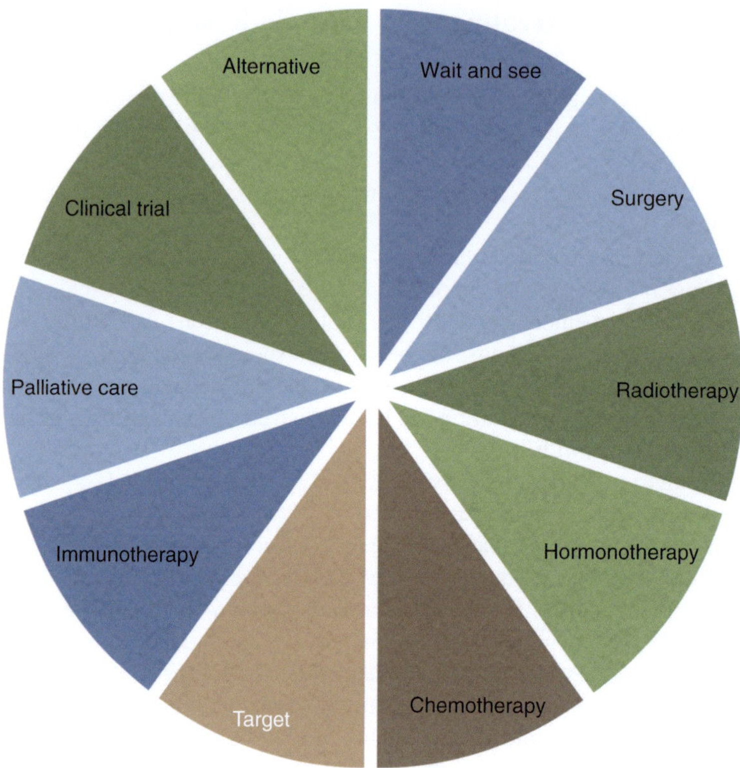

Fig. 8.1 Therapeutic approach for a cancer patient

others. In general, they are tumors that grow slowly and express receptors that can be blocked or modulated by hormones.

5. **"Chemotherapy":** is the term reserved for the use of drugs capable of killing abnormal cells. They were discovered after the Second World War and act mostly at the DNA level, which is a molecule located in the nucleus of the cell and in charge of transmitting genetic information. Their toxicity mainly affects normal cells that divide rapidly: white blood cells, platelets, germ cells, hair follicles, and cells of the intestinal mucosa.

6. **"Target":** refers to molecular targets that can be modified by the administration of specific drugs that block a certain growth pathway, the most widely used are those that block epidermal growth receptors (EGFR, HER2neu), but also block cytoplasmic enzymes such as Kinases that phosphorylate proteins and activate certain processes and in other cases block vessel formation, as is the case with Bevacizumab and other antiangiogenic drugs. They are usually more tolerable than chemotherapy drugs and have fewer adverse effects.

7. **"Immunotherapy":** refers to the use of substances that modify the immune system. In the case of organ transplants or autoimmune diseases, immunosup-

pressive substances are used, designed to reduce the activity of the immune system. The adverse effect of the suppression of immunity is the appearance of infections and tumors. In the case of cancer, substances are used to activate the immune system in order to eradicate the abnormal cells that have appeared. The adverse effect of immunostimulation is the appearance of autoimmune diseases and inflammatory reactions in different parts of the body.

8. **"Palliative care":** refers to the use of treatments aimed at calming the physical or psychological symptoms caused by the disease or the treatments, including the patient and their family. Palliative treatments should be implemented from the first consultation, because even though they are the scientifically recommended treatments for when the patient is incurable and especially at the end of their life, they are useful enough to be implemented from day 1. This way they not only make the treatments more tolerable and increase treatment adherence, they also have an impact on survival.

9. **"Clinical trial":** is an option that is always present. The difference with the previous eight points is that in this case, the treatment is depersonalized (the patient is never more an object of study than in a clinical trial) and the objective of the treatment is not to benefit the patient in the first place but to obtain a useful response for science. If the patient freely and generously wishes to participate in obtaining knowledge, they may benefit, but that is not the objective of a study. The fundamental ethics of a clinical trial is ignorance of an answer that we need to obtain. If someone knows the answer, it is unethical for them to investigate.

10. **"Alternative treatments":** refers to treatments that are not based on evidence but on belief. These treatments have not been tested according to scientific methodology, they are often based on testimonial successes and when they are scientifically studied, unfortunately most of them are not useful.

When we are going to communicate to a patient the therapeutic alternatives for their ailment, it is good to have this wheel of topics in mind, at least in the case of cancer patients, because if we go through them one by one, explaining the reasons why they are or aren't useful alternatives, the patient understands (a) that we have made the effort to analyze all of them and (b) they will select, together with the doctor, the treatment that they consider the most tolerable and the best for them.

8.6   Node 5: The Follow-Up Is: "The Truth Sought"

After establishing a treatment, the patient is followed up on. Clinical follow-up has, in the first place, the objective of evaluating tolerance to the established treatment [52–58].

Adherence to treatment depends on whether it is well tolerated, easy to administer, and the personality of the patient.

Follow-up builds loyalty and helps to achieve goals: weight loss, physical activity, glycemic control, taking antibiotics and, in the case of cancer patients, assessing the toxicities of treatments.

The second objective of clinical follow-up is to assess the effectiveness of what we are doing: Did the blood pressure go down? Has the pulse regularized? Was blood glucose controlled? Did the tumor shrink?

In other words, we seek to know if we are on the right track or not and for that we look for signs that the treatment is failing.

Therefore, the concept of the clinical examination in the follow-up can confirm whether what we are doing is correct, whether it is well tolerated and is effective or, on the contrary, demonstrate that it is not working.

This is the truth we are looking for: for our patient, here and now, does this work?

Many times, the success of our chosen treatment is confirmed, but other times, we're faced with the fact that our chosen treatment isn't working and this generates anguish in the patient.

It is very important that the patient understands, from the very first moment, the objective of the follow-up plan we establish.

In the particular case of cancer patients, it is very important that the patient understands that the objective of follow-up **isn't to detect small or asymptomatic metastases.**

One of the errors that we must correct from the beginning is the concept of "early detection of metastases".

Why?

Because it just doesn't exist.

Just as it has been shown that detecting relatively small primary tumors is a good thing because it manages to cure more patients (at least as a more or less proven hypothesis), it's also true that up till now, there is no evidence that in most tumors (there may be some exception with lymphomas, germ cell tumors, colon, and some others), the detection of a subclinical metastasis allows curing more patients or significantly prolonging life when compared to clinically detected metastases.

Clearly those patients in whom asymptomatic small-volume disease is detected live longer than those in whom symptomatic large-volume disease is detected, but it is possible that the time they gain is not due to treatments but to the time it takes for small-volume metastatic diseases to become large-volume ones.

We can see then how the follow-up is seen by the patient as a moment that generates a lot of anxiety. If it confirms that everything is fine, this will be a momentary relief until the next control, but if it shows that something is wrong, treatment should be adjusted or changed.

In the case of cancer, we are also faced with the possible detection of a recurrence, which is one of the most feared truths.

8.7 Node 6: The Recurrence Is: "The Feared Truth"

The recurrence of oncological disease is a devastating moment for the patient and a moment of breakdown of trust in the doctor–patient relationship [59–64].

Usually, the initial diagnosis of cancer is a surprise in the patient's life, which frequently leads them to change habits and lifestyles and to undergo treatments which are often toxic or affect his quality of life.

Somehow, the patient establishes a series of implicit pacts with life and with the treating physician so that the disease does not reappear.

The detection of recurrent disease confronts the patient with the same fears that they believed were averted, they feel betrayed and question all the sacrifices or suffering to which they were subjected because they feel that everything has been useless.

It is a moment in which the doctor's understanding and their support are needed more than ever to get out of the state of shock and analyze the reasonable therapeutic alternatives that exist.

The doctor should not feel that questioning the patient is a personal attack, they must understand that it's a necessary step to rebuild trust.

There is a particularly difficult point which occurs when the patient complains of a certain ailment without studies having shown any lesions. This is often seen as a mistake rather than a limitation.

Let me explain: a negative study does not certify the absence of disease. A negative study simply means that if there is disease, it's below the study's detection limit (1 cm in Ultrasound, 0.7 cm in CAT scan, and 0.5 cm in PET scan).

These values seem very small but a 1 cm tumor has billions of cells and a 0.5 cm tumor has hundreds of millions of cells. Therefore from the point of view of the images, they are small, but biologically speaking, they are a huge population of cells.

So it is very important that when the studies do not show disease we should happily share this finding but with some caveats, and if the patient continues to feel the discomfort we reaffirm our trust in their experience and re-examine the area in question more frequently.

There are special situations in which recurrence is still curable (single lesions, especially in the Central Nervous System or in regional nodes after a sentinel node in breast cancer).

In most tumors, however, recurrence in multiple sites isn't curable.

It is very common for all tumors to have second or third lines of treatment for advanced cancer. It should be noted that second lines in oncology rarely manage to make the disease disappear and the duration of the benefit of these treatments is usually short-lived.

That is why many patients in these conditions ask for...

8.8 Node 7: Research Is: "The Neutral Truth"

In all circumstances in which doctors use what we call "Evidence-Based Medicine," we carry out an extrapolation exercise.

We extrapolate general knowledge from clinical trials or treatment guidelines (which synthesize clinical trials) to a particular case, that of our patient.

If our patient's characteristics are similar to the inclusion criteria of those who participated in the study and they lack the exclusion criteria of those who couldn't participate, then it is possible that the results we obtain are similar.

At this point, we must recognize that it is highly unlikely that we will obtain the same result as those reported in the studies.

There are multiple explanations. Patient selection, researcher's experience, publication bias, scientific fraud, the excellence of the centers in which the studies have been carried out, or simply random chance. All of these and more mean that most of the time, the efficacy of treatments is maximum and toxicity is minimal in research studies.

Therefore one must expect the benefit to our patient to be less and the harm to be greater.

The second extrapolation is from personal experience. We must be very alert to the bias that our accumulated experience introduces into our judgment. Good results lead us to "trust" a treatment and bad results lead us to "distrust" them.

Therefore one pours that influence into decision-making during the consultation.

The third extrapolation one makes is between the expected results and the patient's values. One tries that the decision made is one that respects what the patient wants for their life.

Many times we succeed, but other times, unfortunately, we do not.

As we see in medical practice, what we do through extrapolation is to apply knowledge: knowledge we learned from clinical trials, from the experience with our patients, and from dialogue with our patient.

A clinical trial is exactly the opposite.

The ethical foundation of clinical research is ignorance of the result.

We investigate what we do not know.

We investigate to find out.

Participation in the search for knowledge is one of the most generous acts that a patient can do, since they put their life in service of obtaining knowledge. Knowledge which will be of great use to the community as a whole, but is never guaranteed to be of use to the individual patient.

If, in medical practice, the ideal is to personalize treatment, in a clinical trial, the patient must adapt to the requirements of the study.

Today clinical trials are regulated at both the national and international levels.

You cannot research anything you want, nor can you do so with whatever methods you want [65–75].

International regulations are formally expressed in the World Medical Association's Helsinki Declaration.

This is a document that embodied what was expressed by the Nuremberg Code, which was promulgated after the trial of 23 doctors who experimented on human beings in the Nazi death camps [76–78].

That was the first Never Again in the History of Medicine.

From then on, we made a commitment that the human being would never again be treated as a means, but would always be respected as an end in itself.

Obtaining knowledge had to have the express and free authorization of the person to be involved (informed consent) and was to be preceded by experimentation on animals to study its toxicity.

The result is that nowadays, drug experiments in humans are designed in four phases (I–IV) and are preceded by phase 0, which is animal experimentation, as can be seen in Table 8.1.

Until the 1990s, clinical evidence in oncology was divided into three sources: (a) studies sponsored by the pharmaceutical industry (which had the best results and least toxicity); (b) academic studies not sponsored by the industry that obtained intermediate results and increased toxicity; (c) observational studies in the real world not sponsored by the industry that obtained the worst results and the highest toxicity.

Table 8.1 Phases of pharmacological experimentation with human beings

Phase 0	This phase precedes human experimentation. The drug is studied in at least three species to determine its metabolism and toxicity. From this perspective, all human pharmacology since the second half of the twentieth century is preceded by veterinary pharmacology
Phase I	This phase seeks to determine the pharmacodynamics and pharmacokinetics of a drug in humans. It establishes the maximum tolerable doses (MTD: What is the maximum dose that we can administer) and the limiting dose toxicity (TDL: What is the toxicity that prevents increasing the dose). This phase can be carried out in healthy volunteers
Phase II	This phase seeks to determine the efficacy of a drug in a certain pathology. It evaluates the rate of responses, the duration of the response, and the frequency and severity of toxicities in a population affected by a certain disease. It is usually carried out in a population that oscillates between 20 and 50 patients. Therefore, they are highly selected patients
Phase III	These are studies that are carried out comparing two or more populations treated with the drug being researched (frequently associated with conventional treatment) and compares it with another population treated with the standard treatment. If treatment assignment is random, the study is called randomized. They are trials that incorporate hundreds or thousands of patients who are selected according to strict inclusion and exclusion criteria. In general, they are carried out in more than one center (multicenters) and evaluate overall survival (time from diagnosis to death), quality of life, response rate, progression-free time (time until the disease worsens), or disease-free time (time until the disease returns). They are extremely expensive and the logistics of carrying them out are complex
Phase IV	They are pharmacovigilance studies that are carried out after the drug is marketed and is being applied or consumed by the general population. It seeks to see the efficacy and tolerance of the drug in the real world

Today practically all academic studies and most of the "real world" studies are sponsored by the pharmaceutical industry and their results are similar in efficacy and toxicity, which is hardly credible. Then we have the office experience, which is anecdotal and sometimes reflects what has been published and sometimes does not.

From this perspective, while information has been gained, knowledge free of bias has been lost. At least when it comes to oncology.

The certain thing is that research is essential to obtain and to develop knowledge and in spite of all its defects, it continues being the only way to know the truth.

When a patient has an incurable disease, and especially when therapeutic resources based on evidence or experience have been exhausted, many patients seek clinical trials.

The first precaution that we must take is that, if possible, the physician carrying out the trial shouldn't be the one treating the patient. This is to prevent the patient from mistaking the intent of the trial.

The clinical trial does not seek to benefit a patient, it seeks to obtain knowledge.

When the doctor who treats a patient is the one who suggests a study, this can be confusing for the patient.

Communication between researcher and research subject is totally different from that between doctor and patient.

The researcher must communicate in a neutral way so that the patient chooses freely.

They must rigorously inform what is known and what is unknown, they must highlight the objective of the study and help everyone involved understand the informed consent that patients and witnesses must sign.

The researcher must refrain from giving an opinion in favor of the study and at all times they must emphasize the free participation of the patient and the opportunity to leave the study without this impairing the patient's relationship with their doctor.

Researchers must emphasize the need for commitment to carry out clinical visits, laboratory studies, and images.

They should also highlight the free nature of the trial. It is unethical to charge a patient to obtain knowledge from them.

They must have emergency care protocols and precautions for the provision of medication free of charge in the event that the product is approved for marketing.

In developed countries, trials must be registered with the national or regional authority, which implies that the study has been reviewed and approved by the authorities.

It is important to note that the Helsinki Declaration is mandatory for all doctors in the world and establishes that if the legislation in the respective countries is more restrictive, the national legislation must be applied. If a nation's legislation is less restrictive, however, one must still apply the rules outlined in the Declaration [79–81].

Studies that have not been reviewed by an independent ethics committee or are not supervised by authorities should be distrusted.

The best advice I can give to a patient who is about to participate in a clinical trial is to be accompanied by someone they trust, so that there are two people who listen and ask the researcher questions. The patient should also take the consent form home so that they can read it carefully and write down any questions that arise from reading.

In the United States, only 3% of patients agree to participate in a clinical study.

Therefore, patients seek research studies, but most of them refrain from participating.

8.9   Node 8: Error: "The Irritating Truth"

Many believe that the worst news a doctor could deliver is cancer diagnosis or a prognosis of incurability or death, and that may be true from the patient's perspective, but from the doctor's perspective, the worst news to deliver is that you have made a mistake [82–91].

For a long time, errors in medicine were handled wrongly, in at least two different ways.

The first way was by hiding the error, and in the few cases when it wasn't hidden, it was instead both blurred and hidden.

Today we know that hiding and disguising an error only leads to worse results than being honest and open about it.

The second way in which error handling was wrong was attributing the error to personal failure.

More time was wasted in finding a culprit than in studying what caused the error in the first place and how to prevent it from happening again.

Today we know that many medical errors are the consequence of poorly designed or poorly controlled processes.

In the particular case of oncology, we know that approximately between 1% and 3% of biopsies are wrong.

Before, we would have blamed the pathologist for that responsibility, his lack of training, lack of care in sample processing, etc. Today we know that the safest way to prevent this error from reaching the patient consists not only in implementing a sample traceability system from the biopsy to the histological preparation, but also that all preparations with a malignant diagnosis are seen at least by two independent pathologists.

Review of the histological preparation lowers the error rate from 1% to 0.0001%. Not acknowledging and hiding the error perpetuates it. Recognizing it and establishing a detection system avoids it.

Prescriptive error rate is also in the order of 1% when done manually. Electronic prescription with alerts for maximum and minimum doses, as well as drug interactions, significantly improves patient safety.

Something similar occurs with the traceability of laboratory studies or the image analysis.

It is very likely that artificial intelligence will allow us to develop systems to increase patient safety in all these fields.

However, even when the error rate can be minimized, error is unfortunately unavoidable.

Fewer will be produced, perhaps a lot fewer, but some will always be produced.

Therefore training and protocolization in the discussion of medical error is essential.

First inform the insurance company that an error has been made.

Second, summon the patient or family to a meeting to discuss the issue.

Thirdly, make sure to have someone with you (especially your boss or director).

Prepare all the information and choose a suitable setting for the discussion of the error.

Consider that when communicating bad news, the vulnerable person is the patient. In this particular case, when discussing an error, the vulnerable party is the doctor.

Fourthly, act with honesty and humility.

Slowly and calmly explain why you have summoned the patient and family.

Describe the error as it happened.

Show how you discovered it and what you did to minimize the consequences of the error.

Have all the material ordered and available to hand out, in case the family wants to review it or make a copy.

Listen carefully to family members' questions or reactions and respond humbly to both.

Offer to solve the problems caused by you (or the institution).

Offer to refer the patient to another colleague for continued care.

This open, honest, and transparent way of discussing the error is the one that obtains the best results for both patient and professional.

It is true that there may be very complex situations, especially if the patient or family members are intolerant of errors, but most people are understanding of human errors if they are approached with humility and respect.

The worst that can happen is that they not only find out the mistake before you expose it, but they find out that you tried to hide it, because then the problem is that the patient and family feel cheated.

Repentance before being found out leads to open and honest discussion of the mistake; repentance after being found out is a hypocritical excuse. We do not regret the mistake we made, we are ashamed of having been discovered.

The error breaks the childish confidence in the infallibility of the doctor or the system, but if it is properly discussed and its consequences resolved or avoided, it generates a new, more adult trust, no longer built on a false sense of infallibility but rather in transparency and honesty.

Table 8.2 shows you the sequence that we established at the Henry Moore Institute for handling medical errors.

Table 8.2 Recommendations for managing medical error in oncology. (Henry Moore Institute)

1. Order all the material you reviewed and notify the insurance company
2. Call the patient and his family for an interview
3. Prepare the site properly
4. Be accompanied by your boss or director
5. Explain the mistake humbly and slowly
6. Apologize honestly and take responsibility
7. Shut up and wait to see what the patient and family understand
8. Do not react to aggression
9. If there is a solution, propose it and assume the costs
10. If there is no solution, ask if they want to change the professional

8.10   Node 9: Alternative Treatments Are: "The Paradoxical Truth"

Alternative treatments are frequently used by patients with chronic diseases in general and are very frequent in those diagnosed with cancer [92–98].

These are treatments that patients do not tell doctors about unless specifically asked.

In general, they are grouped into three areas: alternative medicines, alternative drugs, and alternative techniques or technologies.

Alternative medicines are usually presented as esoteric medicines (Chinese, Hindu, Aztec, Prehistoric, Shamanic, Alien, etc.); in some cases, they have their own classification of diseases, while in others they apply modern diagnostic standards.

Alternative medicines are presented as treatments discovered in an accidental or unexpected way (for example, Bach Flowers were indicated by a talking lily to Dr. Bach in Scotland).

Alternative techniques or technologies use creative names: Magnetic Resonance; Quantum Activator; Alpha waves, etc.

The truth is that all of these claim to have an efficacy that has not been scientifically studied or which has not been demonstrated (as is the case with homeopathy).

Its enormous dissemination through the media and social networks is often due to the testimonials of patients, some of them famous, who say they have benefited from these treatments.

The point of diffusion and acceptance is not so much its effectiveness as its safety. The hypothesis that leads many patients to undergo these treatments is that, apart from the financial toxicity (some are certainly not cheap), they do not produce any other adverse effect.

This means that many patients ask themselves: why not try it if it can't harm me?

This is the most important point to discuss with the patient: treatments that have not been adequately studied for their efficacy have also not been adequately studied for their safety, nor for the safety of their preparation, storage, or distribution.

In other words, most of them pass under the radar of health controls.

Let us remember that one of the cases that led to the founding of what would later become the Food and Drug Administration in the USA was the contamination of a cough syrup with methyl alcohol in the 1920s. In my own country of Argentina, there was a notorious case of propolis candies, used to treat flu symptoms, also contaminated with methyl alcohol in the 1990s.

The patients who were affected by this contaminant thought that what they consumed was safe, because it was natural.

This idea of safety, security, and natural origin is one of the most widespread ideas among those who practice and consume alternative medicines.

Other similar ideas are diets (some of them highly restrictive); use of gases such as ozone (ozone therapy); infusions such as teas made from different leaves or flowers; pseudopsychological therapies (stories of past lives) or visualization methods (Simonton) to increase the effectiveness of drugs or radiation.

Also included in these self-administered treatments are dietary or multivitamin supplements, which are available over the counter and are promoted as repairing or restorative agents for health.

Some of these treatments can generate states of anxiety or anguish, others may have limitations because they modify one or more intracellular processes, even at low doses.

The key to communication is for the patient to have the confidence to tell their doctor what they are doing, because if they have any limitations they should discontinue it (remember that in the case of oral cancer drugs, grapefruit juice may be prohibited, because it modifies the absorption of oncological drugs).

For the patient to have that confidence, it is useful for the doctor to avoid judging the reasons that leads the patient to seek these treatments or their relatives to recommend them.

Keep in mind that most patients place a trust in a treatment that they think is safe, while knowing that they are may be being deceived.

Somehow a false hope is more tolerable than a lack of hope.

Many times, what the patient needs is our commitment to accompany them in what they decide to do.

Frequently, after trying 1 or 2 months, patients abandon these treatments and have the peace of mind of "having tried everything."

8.11   Node 10: Death Is: "The Ultimate Truth"

In his book "Night Colloquia in Jerusalem" Cardinal Carlo Maria Martini maintains that death is the last and most important challenge of the Faith [99, 100].

Nobody knows how they will behave until then.

Death represents the insurmountable existential limit.

"Nobody who has a brain stops thinking when faced with death. No one who has a heart stops feeling in the face of death" said Gregorio Marañón, one of the greatest Spanish doctors of the last century.

Death is what makes us all equal. It is, according to Fernando Savater, what humanizes us.

Whatever our birth, whatever our fortune, with good or bad luck, we will all find ourselves having to depart when the end comes.

It is not often that death is discussed with patients and yet it is probably the most enriching of conversations.

It is not a conversation that can be faced as soon as we know someone, but after a period of time, and especially after several lines of treatment, it is reasonable to raise the subject [101–108].

It is very reasonable that someone does not want to think or talk about it, and therefore we should not go beyond the statement and make it clear that if they wish, when they wish, we can talk about this topic.

What advantage does it have?

We did a study at the Institute in which we retrospectively evaluated the clinical histories of a hundred patients assisted from the diagnosis of cancer until their death.

There we found that 70 of them had talked about death and 30 had not. We paired them by diagnosis and verified that all had received similar treatments according to the pathology; that they all had similar lifespans after being diagnosed with metastases; but that those with whom death was discussed were chemotherapy-free for three and a half months before dying and nine out of ten had died at home with palliative care; while those who were not spoken to received chemotherapy up to 1 days before dying and died in sanatoriums or hospitals.

In other words, talking did not change their longevity, but it did change the type of treatment they received and the place in which they died.

I can't say for certain whether talking about the subject was the right choice or not, since the patient or the doctor may not have given themselves that opportunity; Nor could I affirm that the quality of life was different, since it is possible that for some patients receiving treatment and dying in sanatoriums is what they consider most appropriate for their lives.

What I can affirm is that in our experience, being able to talk about death allows the patient who wishes to die at home with palliative care and without chemotherapy to be able to do so.

This is a conversation that requires intimacy and mutual knowledge. It takes time and trust.

Some ways to start talking about them is to ask the patient, in view of the fact that the treatments are not managing to control the disease, what they want us to do and, in the event that there are no therapeutic options, what do they think would be the most appropriate course of action.

Another way is to talk about palliative care.

One can also ask if, in the event that the patient loses consciousness, what are the limits of care they want: intensive therapy, intubation, resuscitation, etc.

Most patients appreciate this opportunity to talk about it and feel calmer doing so, it is as if they have a pending matter that they can now resolve.

A more challenging conversation that usually happens is with relatives, especially if the patient did not express their wishes.

Worse still is when the patient is unconscious and a family member interprets that the patient's wishes were for life support measures and another interprets that they were not.

In these cases, the role of the doctor is many times that of a mediator between extreme positions, trying to reconcile emotions to try to provide the most reasonable care without injuring any of the parties.

This is of enormous importance for the last node.

Caring for survivors.

8.12   Node 11: Mourning Is: "The Remembered Truth"

Grief is one of the worst studied stages of life [109–118].

It is one of the most important debts in the history of medicine.

Historically, most family members received support from their peers and relief from religion.

But in a society that tends more and more to individualism, with families scattered in different regions of the world and an increasingly secularized society, the problems of mourning are more and more evident.

What do we know?

That the more unexpected and violent a death is, the more shocking it is.

That the younger the deceased was, the more difficult the mourning is (in fact, for most families the death of a child is a devastating event and many cause pathological mourning).

That in the event that the death can't be confirmed (wars, catastrophes, or kidnappings), it is more difficult to grieve. Without confirmation, the mind turns to hopes of their survival rather than grief.

We will focus below on the most frequent deaths, which are deaths caused by chronic diseases: cancer, Alzheimer's, cardiopulmonary diseases, or simply old age.

The first thing to note is that our death experience has changed in the twenty-first century compared to previous centuries.

Today there is a great virtual presence of death. In the media, social networks, and virtual games, where almost anything is killed, and many times one dies in a horrifying but playful and remote way.

At the same time as this omnipresent presence of death and violence, there is a great inexperience of the dying and death. Philippe Ariès, the great historian of death in the West, has shown it with absolute clarity.

We live in a great dichotomy: presence of virtual death and concealment of real death.

In the West, most patients die in hospitals.

The difficulty of implementing palliative care, hospices, and death at home is largely due to changes in family structures (fewer children, multiple partners, dispersal of the family for work reasons, independence of the wife and smaller housing units) but also, and not to a small extent, in the desire not to see the patient die at home.

One of the reasons that is most frequently outlined is the lack of elements for the treatment of the patient's decompensation (serums, oxygen, sedatives, nursing), forgetting that when a patient is in home palliative care, when death occurs, it is necessary to alleviate the anguish and allow him to die in peace, not prolong the agony with support measures that most of the time cause an unnecessary prolongation of suffering.

Another of the difficulties in the implementation of palliative care is the pro-euthanasia movement (or its variant, which is assisted suicide), which consists of killing or making it easier for the patient to kill themselves to alleviate suffering.

One of the reasons why many patients choose this path is to relieve their relatives of the suffering of caring for them. This arises many times in the care of the bereavement of relatives who commit suicide.

This feeling generates great ambivalence: on the one hand, they seek consolation in the fact that the patient's will was finally done and, on the other, they feel partly responsible for the irreversible decision they made.

What are the keys to communication in grief?

It is advisable to have a closing meeting of the clinical case with the patients whenever possible and if they require it, since this allows us to review the history of the patient's disease, the treatments carried out, and the reasons and objectives with which they were implemented.

This meeting allows the free expression of emotions and clarifies the doubts that many relatives had and did not previously express: the most frequent is how much the deceased knew and wanted.

Although there is increasing insistence that, as far as possible, a written record of the patient's wishes be left (living will or will of therapeutic limitation), there are still many patients who do not fill out these documents.

Undoubtedly, when these documents exist, they are irrefutable proof of the expression of the patient's will and usually provide a great relief to the bereaved.

Another important point to highlight in communication with family members during grief are some common experiences that have been collected.

The feeling of disbelief is common in the first days or weeks. Many seem to be living an experience similar to that moment before waking up, half-awake, yet still half asleep, where there is a vague idea of reality and it is not easy to distinguish between a dream and reality.

That unreality between what is lived, what is felt, and what is known is a frequent component.

This is often accompanied by the perception or vivid memory of the voice, the aromas, or the presence of the deceased person, many times with an intimate sensation of seeing them again in places the patient frequented: the kitchen, the dining room, the desk.

The sadness due to the loss, the feeling of injustice, the pain for the absence, which become deeper as the days pass after the death.

It is important to highlight that the moment of greatest emptiness and pain occurs approximately after 3 months, where the feeling of absence is accompanied by the conviction that the deceased will not return.

Until then, there may be fantasies of a miraculous return, but at that moment, a physical sensation of irreversibility is present.

Then, little by little, the pain of loss becomes an intimate presence. The memory returns in the form of words, anecdotes, or advice, which often appear unexpectedly but opportunely for decision making.

If after 3 months the depression deepens, it is advisable to consult for the evaluation of prolonged grief.

An important point is that, if possible, the bereaved should avoid making irreversible decisions in the first year of mourning (moving, selling, or bequeathing items), since these decisions can later bring a lot of regret.

Finally, we must know that in the face of certain losses, such as the death of a child, there is a wound that divides our life in two, one part that was stopped at the tragic moment of the loss, and another that is built from there, as if it were the course of two different beings.

What should we keep in mind?

That mourning crystallizes certain moments of the patient's life and illness, that the family member can remember with extreme precision and is capable of repeating word for word what we said.

That ability to vividly remember where we were, what we were doing, how our relative was doing, and what the doctor said is remarkable and persists many years after the relative's death.

Therefore we must be careful with our words and our gestures in these extreme moments of our patients and their families.

In summary: these 11 nodes that go from diagnosis to mourning have specific challenges and elements in common. This map of communication with our patient helps us to empathetically prepare ourselves to dialogue and deliberate with our patient to choose the treatment alternatives that best suit their needs.

8.13 Teaching Exercises

1. Personal

    (a) When you're preparing to communicate something to your patient, do you have a mental map of the communication nodes?
    (b) What is easier for you to communicate: the diagnosis, the prognosis, or the therapeutic alternatives? Why?
    (c) Have you had to report a medical error? What precautions did you take?
    (d) Have you accompanied relatives in mourning? What did they remember with greater precision from the experiences lived by the patient?

2. Group

   (a) Get together as a group and discuss the communication nodes that you find
       in the clinical course of a certain ailment.
   (b) In pairs, practice delivering news of diagnostic, prognostic, therapeutic error
       and end of life. Observe the difficulties in starting the different conversa-
       tions that the participants have.
   (c) As a group, design a damage minimization strategy for the communication
       of a medical error in which the right (healthy) kidney was removed from a
       patient instead of the left kidney (affected by a 6 cm renal tumor) because
       the wrong side was recorded in the admission history. (Try to fulfill the fol-
       lowing roles: administrator, legal adviser, surgeon, anesthetist, staff doctor
       who made the mistake.)

References

1. Gil Deza E. Of cancer and its demons. 1st ed. Authorship; 2019.
2. Sunday S. Illness as more than metaphor. New York. Published online.
3. Sunday S. Illness as a metaphor. In: AIDS and its metaphors; 1991.
4. Sontag S. Illness as metaphor and AIDS. Soc Sci Med. 1989;29(11):1235–42.
5. Fernandez MB. Illness as metaphor: an approach from the hermeneutics of Paul Ricoeur. In-keys of Thought. 2023;3. https://doi.org/10.46530/ecdp.v0i33.602.
6. Chan S. The pain of Susan Sontag. Glob Soc. 2010;24(3):369. https://doi.org/10.1080/13600826.2010.485559.
7. Jurecic A. Illness as narrative; 2012. https://doi.org/10.1136/medhum-2012-010322.
8. Buckman RAR. Breaking bad news: the SPIKES strategy. Commun Oncol. 2005;2(2):138.
9. Baile WF, Buckman R, Lenzi R, Glober G, Beale EA, Kudelka AP. SPIKES—a six-step protocol for delivering bad news: application to the patient with cancer. Oncologist. 2000;5(4):302. https://doi.org/10.1634/theoncologist.5-4-302.
10. Dubé C. Practical plans for difficult conversations in medicine: strategies that work in breaking bad news by Robert Buckman, MD, PhD. Am J Lifestyle Med. 2011;5(3):293. https://doi.org/10.1177/1559827611398192.
11. Farrell TW, Reed J, Roffers M. Beyond SPIKES: key principles to enhance communication in difficult conversations. J Clin Oncol. 2014;32(31 Suppl):138. https://doi.org/10.1200/jco.2014.32.31_suppl.138.
12. F. C. Communication of bad news: how is the students' perspective concerning a lecture? Psychooncology. 2014;23.
13. Kraushaar H, Garber N, Ross D. Implementing a pediatric resident curriculum to improve confidence with breaking bad news to patients and their families. Pediatrics. 2021;147(3_MeetingAbstract):534. https://doi.org/10.1542/peds.147.3ma6.534.
14. Bosch Bayard RI, Blanco Aspiazu MA, Rodríguez Blanco AL. Cómo debemos comunicar malas noticias en tiempos de pandemia. Rev habanera cienc méd. 2021;20(4).
15. Prabavathy S. Breaking bad news—a psychological approach. Pondicherry J Nurs. 2017;10(3):27. https://doi.org/10.5005/pjn-10-3-27.
16. Carr DT. Is staging of cancer of value? Cancer. 1983;51(12 Suppl):2503–5. https://doi.org/10.1002/1097-0142(19830615)51:12+<2503::AID-CNCR2820511320>3.0.CO;2-2.
17. Fielding R. Communicating risk: doctor's recommendation is decision making in uncertain conditions. BMJ. 2003;327(7428):1404. https://doi.org/10.1136/bmj.327.7428.1404-a.

18. Thompson JF, Scolyer RA. Cooperation between surgical oncologists and pathologists: a key element of multidisciplinary care for patients with cancer. Pathology. 2004;36(5):496. https://doi.org/10.1080/00313020412331283897.

19. Cohen SM, Maciejewski R, Nelson JE, et al. The messenger matters: relative influence of oncologists versus other care team members on advanced cancer patients' illness understanding. J Clin Oncol. 2016;34(15 Suppl):6545. https://doi.org/10.1200/jco.2016.34.15_suppl.6545.

20. Russell BJ, Ward AM. Deciding what information is necessary: do patients with advanced cancer want to know all the details? Cancer Manag Res. 2011;3(1):191. https://doi.org/10.2147/CMR.S12998.

21. Barba D, León-Sosa A, Lugo P, et al. Breast cancer, screening and diagnostic tools: all you need to know. Crit Rev Oncol Hematol. 2021;157:103174. https://doi.org/10.1016/j.critrevonc.2020.103174.

22. Hirsch JA, Nicola G, McGinty G, et al. ICD-10: history and context. Am J Neuroradiol. 2016;37(4):596. https://doi.org/10.3174/ajnr.A4696.

23. van der Linden R, Bolt T, Veen M. 'If it can't be coded, it doesn't exist'. A historical-philosophical analysis of the new ICD-11 classification of chronic pain. Stud Hist Philos Sci. 2022;94:121–32. https://doi.org/10.1016/j.shpsa.2022.06.003.

24. Almeida MSC, de Sousa Filho LF, Rabello PM, Santiago BM. International classification of diseases—11th revision: from design to implementation. Rev Saude Publica. 2020;54:104. https://doi.org/10.11606/s1518-8787.2020054002120.

25. Harrison JE, Weber S, Jakob R, Chute CG. ICD-11: an international classification of diseases for the twenty-first century. BMC Med Inform Decis Mak. 2021;21:206. https://doi.org/10.1186/s12911-021-01534-6.

26. Gospodarowicz MK, Miller D, Groome PA, Greene FL, Logan PA, Sobin LH. The process for continuous improvement of the TNM classification. Cancer. 2004;100(1):1. https://doi.org/10.1002/cncr.11898.

27. Tnm T, Denoix P, Uicc T, et al. TNM history, evolution and milestones. Published online; 1987.

28. Bertero L, Massa F, Metovic J, et al. Eighth edition of the UICC classification of malignant tumours: an overview of the changes in the pathological TNM classification criteria—what has changed and why? Virchows Arch. 2018;472(4):519. https://doi.org/10.1007/s00428-017-2276-y.

29. Armstrong TS, Mendoza T, Gning I, et al. Validation of the M. D. Anderson symptom inventory (MDASI-BT). J Clin Oncol. 2006;24(18 Suppl). https://doi.org/10.1200/jco.2006.24.18_suppl.1546.

30. Pochettino F, Visconti G, Godoy D, et al. Association between Karnofsky performance status and outcomes in cancer patients on home parenteral nutrition. Clin Nutr ESPEN. 2023;54:211. https://doi.org/10.1016/j.clnesp.2023.01.020.

31. Krikorian JG, Daniels JR, Brown BW, Hu MSJ. Variables for predicting serious toxicity (vinblastine dose, performance status, and prior therapeutic experience): chemotherapy for metastatic testicular cancer with cis-dichlorodiammineplatinum(II), vinblastine, and bleomycin. Cancer Treat Rep. 1978;62(10):1455.

32. Yates JW, Chalmer B, McKegney FP. Evaluation of patients with advanced cancer using the karnofsky performance status. Cancer. 1980;45(8):2220. https://doi.org/10.1002/1097-0142(19800415)45:8<2220::AID-CNCR2820450835>3.0.CO;2-Q.

33. Ludvik NR, Mizrahi M. S1588 the value of inspection: physical exam reveals pancreatic malignancy. Am J Gastroenterol. 2020;115(1):S808. https://doi.org/10.14309/01.ajg.0000708400.16818.48.

34. Paydar I, Oermann EK, Knoll M, et al. The value of the history and physical for patients with newly diagnosed brain metastases considering radiosurgery. Front Oncol. 2016;6:40. https://doi.org/10.3389/fonc.2016.00040.

35. Miles KA, Voo SA, Groves AM. Additional clinical value for PET/MRI in oncology: moving beyond simple diagnosis. J Nucl Med. 2018;59(7):1028. https://doi.org/10.2967/jnumed.117.203612.

36. Demaitre L. The art and science of prognostication in early university medicine. Bull Hist Med. 2003;77(4):765. https://doi.org/10.1353/bhm.2003.0164.

37. Askitopoulou H, Nyktari V, Papaioannou A, Stefanakis G, Konsolaki E. The origins of oral medicine in the Hippocratic collected works. J Oral Pathol Med. 2017;46(9):689. https://doi.org/10.1111/jop.12615.

38. van der Eijk PJ. Divination, prognosis and prophylaxis: the Hippocratic work "on dreams" (De victu 4) and its near eastern background. Stud Anc Med. 2004;27:187. https://doi.org/10.1163/9789047414315_011.

39. Karagiannis TC. The timeless influence of Hippocratic ideas on diet, salicylates and personalized medicine. Hell J Nucl Med. 2014;17(1):2.

40. Brigić A, Hasanović M, Pajević I, Aljukić N, Hamidović J, Jakovljević M. Principles of Hippocratic medicine from the perspective of modern medicine. Psychiatr Danub. 2021;33:1340.

41. Papavramidou N, Fee E, Christopoulou-Aletra H. Jaundice in the hippocratic corpus. J Gastrointest Surg. 2007;11(12):1728. https://doi.org/10.1007/s11605-007-0281-1.

42. Thomas JM, Cooney LM, Fried TR. Prognosis reconsidered in light of ancient insights—from Hippocrates to modern medicine. JAMA Intern Med. 2019;179(6):820. https://doi.org/10.1001/jamainternmed.2019.0302.

43. Razavi D. Uncertainty and hope in cancer patients. Psychother Psychosom. 2013;82:1–134.

44. Olver IN. Evolving definitions of hope in oncology. Curr Opin Support Palliat Care. 2012;6(2):236. https://doi.org/10.1097/SPC.0b013e3283528d0c.

45. Brown R, Bylund CL, Eddington J, Gueguen JA, Kissane DW. Discussing prognosis in an oncology setting: initial evaluation of a communication skills training module. Psychooncology. 2010;19(4):408. https://doi.org/10.1002/pon.1580.

46. Boeriu E, Borda A, Miclea E, et al. Prognosis communication in pediatric oncology: a systematic review. Children. 2023;10(6):972. https://doi.org/10.3390/children10060972.

47. Li Z, Zou J, Chen X. In response to precision medicine: current subcellular targeting strategies for cancer therapy. Adv Mater. 2023;35(21):e2209529. https://doi.org/10.1002/adma.202209529.

48. Benjamín Walbaum G, Francisco Acevedo C, Diego Carrillo B, et al. Her2 positive breast cancer: current systemic therapy and local experience. Rev Cir (Mex). 2023;75(1). https://doi.org/10.35687/s2452-454920230011653.

49. Ohishi T, Kaneko MK, Yoshida Y, Takashima A, Kato Y, Kawada M. Current targeted therapy for metastatic colorectal cancer. Int J Mol Sci. 2023;24(2):1702. https://doi.org/10.3390/ijms24021702.

50. Huitink JM, Teoh WHL. Current cancer therapies—a guide for perioperative physicians. Best Pract Res Clin Anaesthesiol. 2013;27(4):481. https://doi.org/10.1016/j.bpa.2013.09.003.

51. Waks AG, Winer EP. Breast cancer treatment: a review. JAMA J Am Med Assoc. 2019;321(3):288. https://doi.org/10.1001/jama.2018.19323.

52. Dent J, Topping A, Ferguson C, et al. To follow up or not? A new model of supportive care for early breast cancer. J Clin Oncol. 2011;29(15 Suppl):9098. https://doi.org/10.1200/jco.2011.29.15_suppl.9098.

53. Ohlsson B, Breland U, Ekberg H, Graffner H, Tranberg KG. Follow-up after curative surgery for colorectal carcinoma—randomized comparison with no follow-up. Dis Colon Rectum. 1995;38(6):619. https://doi.org/10.1007/BF02054122.

54. Scherman P, Hansdotter P, Holmberg E, et al. High resection rates of colorectal liver metastases after standardized follow-up and multimodal management: an outcome study within the COLOFOL trial. HPB. 2023;25(7):766. https://doi.org/10.1016/j.hpb.2023.03.003.

55. van Ommen-Nijhof A, Steenbruggen TG, Capel L, et al. Survival and prognostic factors in oligometastatic breast cancer. Breast. 2023;67:14. https://doi.org/10.1016/j.breast.2022.12.007.

56. Zhukovsky DS, Soliman P, Liu D, et al. Patient engagement with early stage advance care planning at a Comprehensive Cancer Center. Oncologist. 2023;28(6):542. https://doi.org/10.1093/oncolo/oyad015.

57. Brands MT, Swinkels IJ, Aarts AMWM, et al. Value of routine follow-up in oropharyngeal squamous cell cancer patients treated with curative intent. Head Neck. 2023;45(3):586. https://doi.org/10.1002/hed.27269.

58. Misplon S, Marneffe W, Himpe U, Hellings J, Demedts I. Evaluation of the implementation of value-based healthcare with a weekly digital follow-up of lung cancer patients in clinical practice. Eur J Cancer Care (Engl). 2022;31(6):e13653. https://doi.org/10.1111/ecc.13653.

59. Tralongo P, Dal Maso L, Surbone A, et al. Use of the word "cured" for cancer patients—implications for patients and physicians: the Siracusa charter. Curr Oncol. 2015;22(1):38. https://doi.org/10.3747/co.22.2287.

60. Schapira MM, Fletcher K, Ganschow PS, et al. Use and complexity of numeric concepts and terms in breast cancer treatment consultations. J Gen Intern Med. 2016;31(2):S452.

61. Rosenberg CA, Flanagan C, Brockstein B, et al. Promotion of self-management for post treatment cancer survivors: evaluation of a risk-adapted visit. J Cancer Surviv. 2016;10(1):206. https://doi.org/10.1007/s11764-015-0467-6.

62. Winner M, Wilson A, Ronnekleiv-Kelly S, Smith TJ, Pawlik TM. A singular hope: how the discussion around cancer surgery sometimes fails. Ann Surg Oncol. 2017;24(1):31. https://doi.org/10.1245/s10434-016-5564-x.

63. Saxena RK. Communicating bad news in oncology practice. Indian J Health Stud. 2019;1(1):115. https://doi.org/10.56490/ijhs.2019.1106.

64. Thota V, Paravathaneni M, Konduru S, Baralo B, Mulla S, Thirumaran R. Breaking bad news in the oncologic population: residents' perspective. J Clin Oncol. 2021;39(15 Suppl):e24113. https://doi.org/10.1200/jco.2021.39.15_suppl.e24113.

65. Golombek SG, Van Den Anker J, Rose K. Clinical trials in children: ethical and practical issues. Int J Pharm Med. 2007;21(2):121. https://doi.org/10.2165/00124363-200721020-00002.

66. Cahan E. Ethical or exploitative—should prisoners participate in COVID-19 vaccine trials? Science (1979). Published online 2020. https://doi.org/10.1126/science.abe7861.

67. Raymond J, Long H. Science and ethics, therapeutic misconception and mirage. J Neuroradiol. 2008;35(5):268. https://doi.org/10.1016/j.neurad.2008.04.004.

68. Martins IRM. The digital patient—the research behind collaborative care and analytics. Orphanet J Rare Dis. 2018;13.

69. Budin-Ljøsne I, Teare HJA, Kaye J, et al. Dynamic consent: a potential solution to some of the challenges of modern biomedical research. BMC Med Ethics. 2017;18(1):4. https://doi.org/10.1186/s12910-016-0162-9.

70. Holm M, Alvariza A, Fürst C-J, et al. Recruitment of participants to research with a RCT design in palliative homecare settings-health care professionals experiences. Palliat Med. 2016;30(6).

71. Bicudo E. Pharmaceutical research, democracy and conspiracy. International Clinical Trials in Local Medical Institutions. London: Routledge; 2016. https://doi.org/10.4324/9781315600321.

72. Bell JA, Balneaves LG. Cancer patient decision making related to clinical trial participation: an integrative review with implications for patients' relational autonomy. Support Care Cancer. 2015;23(4):1169–96.

73. Campbell B. Informed consent in developing countries: myth or reality. Hanover: Darmouth University; 2008.

74. Triantafillidis JK, Peros G. Ethical issues related to chemotherapy in patients with gastric cancer. Ann Gastroenterol. 2007;20(3).

75. Saesen R, Van Hemelrijck M, Bogaerts J, et al. Defining the role of real-world data in cancer clinical research: the position of the European Organisation for Research and Treatment of Cancer. Eur J Cancer. 2023;186:52. https://doi.org/10.1016/j.ejca.2023.03.013.

76. The Nuremberg code. Trials of war criminals before the Nuremberg military tribunals under control council law. US government Printing Office; 1949;vol. 2(10).

77. Alderman SS, Taylor T. Trials of war criminals before the Nuernberg Military Tribunals. Columbia Law Rev. 1951;51(3):407. https://doi.org/10.2307/1119299.

78. Schütz M, Braswell H, Ethicizing history. Bioethical representations of Nazi medicine. Bioethics. 2023;37(6):581. https://doi.org/10.1111/bioe.13168.

79. Carlson RV, Boyd KM, Webb DJ. The revision of the declaration of Helsinki: past, present and future. Br J Clin Pharmacol. 2004;57(6):695. https://doi.org/10.1111/j.1365-2125.2004.02103.x.

80. Molina JL, Tubaro P, Casilli A, Santos-Ortega A. Research ethics in the age of digital platforms. Sci Eng Ethics. 2023;29(3):17. https://doi.org/10.1007/s11948-023-00437-1.

81. Davis S. Declaration of Helsinki: can it still serve as a north star for ethics in regulatory trials? Perspect Clin Res. 2023;14(1):1. https://doi.org/10.4103/picr.picr_247_22.

82. Palanki B. Errors of the intellect: a neglected aspect in teaching. J Eng Educ Transform. 2021;34(3):109. https://doi.org/10.16920/jeet/2021/v34i3/152121.

83. Cooper AB, Chidwick P, Cybulski P, Sibbald R. Checklist to meet ethical and legal obligations in the consent pathway for critically ill patients (ChELO): a quality improvement project and case studies. Can J Crit Care Nurs. 2015;26(3):16.

84. Swinfen D, Labuschagne M, Joubert G. Disclosing medical errors: how do we prepare our students? BMC Med Educ. 2023;23(1):191. https://doi.org/10.1186/s12909-023-04125-3.

85. Hobgood C, Hevia A, Hinchey P. Profiles in patient safety: when an error occurs. Acad Emerg Med. 2004;11(7):766. https://doi.org/10.1197/j.aem.2003.11.023.

86. McLennan S. The law as a barrier to error disclosure: a misguided focus? Trends Anaesth Crit Care. 2018;19:1. https://doi.org/10.1016/j.tacc.2018.02.002.

87. Gibelli F, Turrina S, De Leo D. Medical error disclosure in the Italian healthcare context: a delicate balance between ethical obligations and the principle of non-self-incrimination. Patient Educ Couns. 2022;105(7):1976. https://doi.org/10.1016/j.pec.2022.03.003.

88. Pathak Y. Medication errors: an ethical analysis. Biomed J Sci Tech Res. 2022;45(2). https://doi.org/10.26717/bjstr.2022.45.007162.

89. Alharbi W, Cleland J, Morrison Z. Addressing medication errors in an adult oncology department in Saudi Arabia: a qualitative study. Saudi Pharm J. 2019;27(5):650. https://doi.org/10.1016/j.jsps.2019.03.007.

90. Hannawa A. Principles of medical ethics: implications for the disclosure of medical errors. Medicoleg Bioeth. Published online 2012. https://doi.org/10.2147/mb.s25040.

91. Martin-Fumadó C, Morlans M, Torralba F, Arimany-Manso J. Medical errors communication. Ethical and medicolegal issues. Med Clin (Barc). 2019;152(5):195. https://doi.org/10.1016/j.medcli.2018.07.013.

92. Stöcker A, Mehnert-Theuerkauf A, Hinz A, Ernst J. Utilization of complementary and alternative medicine (CAM) by women with breast cancer or gynecological cancer. PLoS One. 2023;18(5):e0285718. https://doi.org/10.1371/journal.pone.0285718.

93. Akeeb AA, King SM, Olaku O, White JD. Communication between cancer patients and physicians about complementary and alternative medicine: a systematic review. J Integr Complement Med. 2023;29(2):80. https://doi.org/10.1089/jicm.2022.0516.

94. Ng JY, Bhatt HA, Raja M. Complementary and alternative medicine mention and recommendations in pancreatic cancer clinical practice guidelines: a systematic review and quality assessment. Integr Med Res. 2023;12(1):100921. https://doi.org/10.1016/j.imr.2023.100921.

95. Standish LJ, Malani SM, Lynch K, et al. Integrative Oncology's 30-year anniversary: what have we achieved? A North American naturopathic oncology perspective. Integr Cancer Ther. 2023;22:15347354231178911. https://doi.org/10.1177/15347354231178911.

96. Nejat N, Rahbarian A, Mehrabi F, Rafiei F. Complementary and alternative medicine application in cancer patients in Iran. J Cancer Res Clin Oncol. 2023;149(6):2271. https://doi.org/10.1007/s00432-022-04317-2.

97. Lee JW, Lee DY, Kim D. Knowledge and attitude about alternative treatment in cancer patient. Keimyung Med J. 2023;42(1):38. https://doi.org/10.46308/kmj.2022.00248.

98. Rivera Núñez LA, Borja Cabrera AR, Argotti Zumbana MS, Valarezo Cabrera VX, Vilca Ruiz AS. Alternative therapies applied to oncological patients for pain management. Sapienza Int J Interdiscip Stud. 2023;4(1). https://doi.org/10.51798/sijis.v4i1.609.

99. Faccini AC. Teacher, pastor and prophet. Carlo Maria Martini; 2021. https://doi.org/10.2307/j.ctv2175hvm.

100. Martini CM. Last interview with card. Carlos Maria Martini. Brazilian Ecclesiastical Magazine. 2019;72(288). https://doi.org/10.29386/reb.v72i288.827.

101. Gonella S, Basso I, Clari M, Dimonte V, Di Giulio P. A qualitative study of nurses' perspective about the impact of end-of-life communication on the goal of end-of-life care in nursing home. Scand J Caring Sci. 2021;35(2):502. https://doi.org/10.1111/scs.12862.

102. von Blanckenburg P, Riera Knorrenschild J, Hofmann M, et al. Expectations, end-of-life fears and end-of-life communication among palliative patients with cancer and caregivers: a cross-sectional study. BMJ Open. 2022;12(5):e058531. https://doi.org/10.1136/bmjopen-2021-058531.

103. Evenblij K, Ten Koppel M, Smets T, Widdershoven GAM, Onwuteaka-Philipsen BD, Pasman HRW. Are care staff equipped for end-of-life communication? A cross-sectional study in long-term care facilities to identify determinants of self-efficacy. BMC Palliat Care. 2019;18(1):1. https://doi.org/10.1186/s12904-018-0388-z.

104. Omilion-Hodges LM, Swords NM. Communication matters: exploring the intersection of family and practitioner end of life communication. Behav Sci. 2017;7(1):15. https://doi.org/10.3390/bs7010015.

105. Im J, Mak S, Upshur R, Steinberg L, Kuluski K. "Whatever happens, happens" challenges of end-of-life communication from the perspective of older adults and family caregivers: a qualitative study. BMC Palliat Care. 2019;18(1):113. https://doi.org/10.1186/s12904-019-0493-7.

106. Kopp ML, Mayberry ALM. An end-of-life communication performance rubric: reliability assessment. J Hosp Palliat Nurs. 2021;23(5):429. https://doi.org/10.1097/NJH.0000000000000772.

107. Olsson MM, Windsor C, Chambers S, Green TL. A scoping review of end-of-life communication in international palliative care guidelines for acute care settings. J Pain Symptom Manag. 2021;62(2):425. https://doi.org/10.1016/j.jpainsymman.2020.11.032.

108. Payongayong JV, Thomas-Hawkins C, Jarrín OF, Barberio J, Hain DJ. Effects of end-of-life communication knowledge, attitudes, and perceived behavioral control on end-of-life communication behaviors among nephrology nurse practitioners. Nephrol Nurs J. 2022;49(3):213. https://doi.org/10.37526/1526-744x.2022.49.3.213.

109. McLean E, Singer J, Laurita E, Kahler J, Levin C, Papa A. Perception of grief responses: are maladaptive grief responses and the stages of grief considered normal? Death Stud. 2022;46(6):1414. https://doi.org/10.1080/07481187.2021.1983890.

110. Maciejewski PK, Zhang B, Block SD, Prigerson HG. An empirical examination of the stage theory of grief. JAMA. 2007;297(7):716. https://doi.org/10.1001/jama.297.7.716.

111. Avis KA, Stroebe M, Schut H. Stages of grief portrayed on the internet: a systematic analysis and critical appraisal. Front Psychol. 2021;12:12. https://doi.org/10.3389/fpsyg.2021.772696.

112. Gregory C. The five stages of grief an examination of the Kubler-Ross model. Psycom. 2019;4(Maret):1–13.

113. Brooks MP. Listening to layers of loss. J Autoethnography. 2023;4(2):174. https://doi.org/10.1525/joae.2023.4.2.174.

114. Tullis JA. Death of an ex-spouse: lessons in family communication about disenfranchised grief. Behav Sci. 2017;7(2):16. https://doi.org/10.3390/bs7020016.

115. Liew CH. Family grief communication, self-construal, and the functioning of grieving college students. West Lafayette: Purdue University; 2020.
116. Kamm S, Vandenberg B. Grief communication, grief reactions and marital satisfaction in bereaved parents. Death Stud. 2001;25(7):569–82. https://doi.org/10.1080/074811801753184291.
117. Weber M, Alvariza A, Kreicbergs U, Sveen J. Adaptation of a grief and communication family support intervention for parentally bereaved families in Sweden. Death Stud. 2021;45(7):528. https://doi.org/10.1080/07481187.2019.1661883.
118. Li Y, Chan WCH, Marrable T. "I never told my family I was grieving for my mom": the not-disclosing-grief experiences of parentally bereaved adolescents and young adults in Chinese families. Fam Process. 2023;63:379. https://doi.org/10.1111/famp.12865.

Chapter 9
Special Communication Needs: LGBTQ Patient Care

9.1 Introduction

If we were to distill the experience most members of the LGBTQ community associate with healthcare into one word, it would be traumatic.

If we delved a little deeper into that experience, we would see that it is mainly composed of fear, contempt, helplessness, and prejudice [1–4].

They feel judged, or worse, condemned, by people who do not understand what is happening to them and who furthermore consider that how they choose to live their lives is both wrong and disorderly.

These same people believe that those in the community live in an environment of moral perdition and that they are responsible for the illnesses they suffer, either because they are a consequence of their choices or punishment for their perversions.

In order to understand what the other person is experiencing, we must at least be able to imagine what an LGBTQ+ person feels throughout their life.

First of all, we must understand that the decision to change gender or sexuality is usually a surprise for the patient.

It is not something sought after, but rather something that emerges as a situation of discomfort with one's own body and one's own sex; initially experiencing it as strange and wrong [5–7].

It is possible that this is only a temporary situation; a time of self-reflection and exploration, but it is also quite possible that this is a permanent change.

This self-perceived situation generates insecurity and, especially when seen as wrong, is frequently denied and silenced so as not to scandalize the person's own family and friends for fear of rejection [8–11].

This usually leads to a double life: one is the representation of the person as imagined and desired by social or moral canons and the other is the hidden life of the person who expresses their desires and real experiences: to themselves, and

E. Gil Deza, *Improving Clinical Communication*,
https://doi.org/10.1007/978-3-031-62446-9_9

sometimes to others in a community where they can feel like an honest person and free to be who they are without being judged or excluded [12–15].

This double life is often exhausting, since these people must behave like consummate actors who repeat their lines perfectly under penalty of being discovered as impostors, fakes, a shame to those closest to them.

Hence, at some point, the "coming out" occurs, with reactions ranging from acceptance to rejection; the latter, in some cases, homicidal in certain communities.

Therefore, when we are in front of a patient from the LGBTQ community, it is good to ask about this aspect of their life, because there we will find how many times these people have been deceived, defrauded, stigmatized, subjected to ridicule or violence; by their parents, police or judicial authorities, teachers, and even religious representatives.

And we will soon discover that the health system and many doctors have been hostile to them as well.

Therefore, before thinking that they are distrustful or "paranoid," it would be good to know their life stories.

It is always easier to judge than to know, but many times, it is enough to know a little about the misfortunes that the other has experienced to stop judging.

It is by no means our intention to make a detailed and exhaustive list of the violence that many patients suffer, but some of the most frequent topics that patients refer are: domestic violence; expulsion from home in adolescence; domestic, school, police, or church abuse; bullying and school expulsion; incitement to consume alcohol, tobacco, and drugs; prostitution and human trafficking; criminal and police violence; judicial indifference; incarceration; rejection in emergency rooms or hospitals.

Listening to some of the stories of patients who are barely over 20 years old is both touching and terrifying.

It is touching because one perceives the effort and desire to survive along with the extreme fragility and vulnerability that explains the high rate of suicides in the LGBTQ community [16] and it's terrifying because it shows the kind of things people are capable of doing to others when they see them alone, vulnerable, and in need: when your next-door neighbor can be a monster, the world is no longer a safe place.

Many of their stories remind survivors of extermination camps, civil wars, or great catastrophes.

Similarities between expressions of racism and homophobia are not unusual, as are the painful experiences in health care of people discriminated against for reasons of race, religion, gender, or sexual orientation [17, 18].

A significant number of members of the LGBTQ community must travel long distances to be treated in places where they do not feel ashamed [19], and others have had to forcibly emigrate from their homeland to avoid being persecuted [20].

Therefore, understand that many of our patients' attitudes of distrust can be fully justified by the life stories they have had to live.

Secondly, if you are genuinely interested in communicating properly with them, respect them.

The word respect is frequently used to establish distance, but the truth is that it is made up of two Latin terms: re (to return to) and spectare (to observe). That is to say, respect is the attitude by which we stop our walk and retrace our steps to carefully observe something or someone whom we had seen superficially.

Respect is the antipode of indifference.

In order to show respect, we must know more precisely what certain terms that are used to refer to conditions of the LGBTQ+ community mean. To do so, we have transcribed in full the glossary proposed by the eighth version of Standards of Care for the Health of Transgender and Gender Diverse People [21]:

CISGENDER refers to people whose current gender identity corresponds to the sex they were assigned at birth.

DETRANSITION is a term sometimes used to describe an individual's retransition to the gender stereotypically associated with their sex assigned at birth.

EUNUCH refers to an individual assigned male at birth whose testicles have been surgically removed or rendered non-functional and who identifies as a eunuch. This differs from the standard medical definition by excluding those who do not identify as eunuch.

EUNUCH-IDENTIFIED: An individual who feels their true self is best expressed by the term eunuch. Eunuch-identified individuals generally desire to have their reproductive organs surgically removed or rendered non-functional.

GENDER: Depending on the context, gender may reference gender identity, gender expression, and/or social gender role, including understandings and expectations culturally tied to people who were assigned male or female at birth. Gender identities other than those of men and women (who can be either cisgender or transgender) include transgender, nonbinary, genderqueer, gender neutral, agender, gender fluid, and "third" gender, among others; many other genres are recognized around the world.

GENDER-AFFIRMATION refers to being recognized or affirmed in a person's gender identity. It is usually conceptualized as having social, psychological, medical, and legal dimensions. Gender affirmation is used as a term in lieu of transition (as in medical gender-affirmation) or can be used as an adjective (as in gender-affirming care).

GENDER-AFFIRMATION SURGERY (GAS) is used to describe surgery to change primary and/or secondary sex characteristics to affirm a person's gender identity.

GENDER BINARY refers to the idea there are two and only two genders, men and women; the expectation that everyone must be one or the other; and that all men are male, and all women are female.

GENDER DIVERSE is a term used to describe people with gender identities and/or expressions that are different from social and cultural expectations attributed to their sex assigned at birth. This may include, among many other culturally diverse identities, people who identify as nonbinary, gender expansive, gender nonconforming, and others who do not identify as cisgender .

GENDER DYSPHORIA describes a state of distress or discomfort that may be experienced because a person's gender identity differs from that which is physically and/or socially attributed to their sex assigned at birth. Gender Dysphoria is also a diagnostic term in the DSM-5 denoting an incongruence between the sex assigned at birth and experienced gender accompanied by distress. Not all transgender and gender-diverse people experience gender dysphoria.

GENDER EXPANSIVE is an adjective often used to describe people who identify or express themselves in ways that broaden the socially and culturally defined behaviors or beliefs associated with a particular sex. Gender creative is also sometimes used. The term gender variant was used in the past and is disappearing from professional usage because of negative connotations now associated with it.

GENDER EXPRESSION refers to how a person enacts or expresses their gender in everyday life and within the context of their culture and society. Expression of gender through physical appearance may include dress, hairstyle, accessories, cosmetics, hormonal and surgical interventions as well as mannerisms, speech, behavioral patterns, and names. A person's gender expression may or may not conform to a person's gender identity.

GENDER IDENTITY refers to a person's deeply felt, internal, intrinsic sense of their own gender.

GENDER INCONGRUENCE is a diagnostic term used in the ICD-11 that describes a person's marked and persistent experience of an incompatibility between that person's gender identity and the gender expected of them based on their birth-assigned sex.

INTERSEX refers to people born with sex or reproductive characteristics that do not fit binary definitions of female or male.

MISGENDER/MISGENDERING refers to when language is used that does not correctly reflect the gender with which a person identifies. This may be a pronoun (he/him/his, she/her/hers, they/them/theirs) or a form of address (sir, Mr.).

NONBINARY refers to those with gender identities outside the gender binary. People with nonbinary gender identities may identify as partially a man and partially a woman or identify as sometimes a man and sometimes a woman, or identify as a gender other than a man or a woman, or as not having a gender at all. Nonbinary people may use the pronouns they/them/theirs instead of he/him/his or she/her/hers. Some nonbinary people consider themselves to be transgender or trans; some do not because they consider transgender to be part of the gender binary. The shorthand NB or "enby" is sometimes used as a descriptor for non-binary. Examples of nonbinary gender identities are genderqueer, gender diverse, genderfluid, demigender, bigender, and agender.

RETRANSITION refers to second or subsequent gender transition whether by social, medical, or legal means. A retransition may be from one binary or nonbinary gender to another binary or nonbinary gender. People may retransit more than once. Retransition may occur for many reasons, including evolving gender identities, health concerns, family/societal concerns, and financial issues.

SEX ASSIGNED AT BIRTH refers to a person's status as male, female, or intersex based on physical characteristics. Sex is usually assigned at birth based on appearance of the external genitalia. AFAB is an abbreviation for "assigned female at birth." AMAB is an abbreviation for "assigned male at birth."

SEXUAL ORIENTATION refers to a person's sexual identity, attractions, and behaviors in relation to people on the basis of their gender(s) and or sex characteristics and those of their partners . Sexual orientation and gender identity are distinct terms.

TRANSGENDER or trans are umbrella terms used to describe people whose gender identities and/or gender expressions are not what is typically expected for the sex to which they were assigned at birth. These words should always be used as adjectives (as in "trans people") and never as nouns (as in "transgenders") and never as verbs (as in "transgendered").

TRANSGENDER MEN or **TRANS MEN** or **MEN OF TRANS EXPERIENCE** are people who have gender identities as men and who were assigned female at birth. They may or may not have undergone any transition. FTM or Female-to-Male are older terms that are falling out of use. **TRANSGENDER WOMEN** or **TRANS WOMEN** or **WOMEN OF TRANS EXPERIENCE** are people who have gender identities as women and who were assigned male at birth. They may or may not have undergone any transition . MTF or Male-to-Female are older terms that are falling out of use.

TRANSITION refers to the process whereby people usually change from the gender expression associated with their assigned sex at birth to another gender expression that better matches their gender identity. People may transition socially by using methods such as changing their name, pronoun, clothing, hair styles, and/or the ways that they move and speak. Transitioning may or may not involve hormones and/or surgeries to alter the physical body. Transition can be used to describe the process of changing one's gender expression from any gender to a different gender. People may transition more than once in their lifetimes.

TRANSPHOBIA refers to negative attitudes, beliefs, and actions concerning transgender and gender-diverse people as a group. Transphobia may be enacted in discriminatory policies and practices on a structural level or in very specific and personal ways. Transphobia can also be internalized, when transgender and gender-diverse people accept and reflect such prejudice about themselves or other transgender and gender diverse people. While trans-phobia sometimes may be a result of unintentional ignorance rather than direct hostility, its effects are never benign. Some people use the term anti-transgender bias instead of transphobia.

This is not an exhaustive glossary, but we found it to be a laudable effort to provide technical clarity to expressions that are used in a polysemic way in everyday life and especially in the media.

The clearest gesture of respect to the non-binary or transgender person is "How do you want us to refer to you?" which is the same as, "What is your preferred pronoun or name?"

As the Jesuit priest James Martin says in his book "*Building Bridges*" [22], the name is much more than an accident: God changes Abran's name to Abraham to reveal a new reality, Christ changes Simon's name to Peter to make him head of the Church and Paul changes his name Saul to go from persecutor to disciple. Even Catholic Popes choose a name that represents them and shows what actions they will carry out during their pontificate.

Therefore, changing your name means starting a new stage in life and hence the need to respect this decision.

It is more than courtesy, it is the first sign of affection for the other, and affection is a formidable medicine.

Many transgender people refer to their previous name of choice as a "dead name" and perceive it as aggression or at least insensitivity when they are called by the name they have left behind.

Of the efforts that have been made to build bridges between the healthcare system and the LGBTQ community, three of them are crucial: (a) to stop considering the choice of gender or sexuality a mental illness; (b) to recognize and register patients from the LGBTQ community in order to evaluate the incidence and evolution of the conditions that afflict them specifically: and (c) to highlight the lack of specific knowledge for the care of members of this community.

We will analyze all three topics.

Clear evidence of the evolution of medicine with respect to the problem of gender and sexuality is the change in terms that we have made over time, as highlighted by Mumford, Fraser, and Knudson: in the mid-1960s, the term transvestism was incorporated for the first time as a category of sexual deviation; in 1975, the term transsexualism was incorporated as a category of sexual disorder and deviation; in 1979, the term "gender disphoria" was used for the first time; in 1980, the third edition of DSM and the tenth edition of ICD in 1990 use the term "gender identity disorder"; in 2019, the 11th edition of the DSM moved the diagnoses related to gender identity and sexual orientation from the chapter "Mental and behavioral disorders" to the chapter "Conditions related to sexual health" and introduced the term "gender incongruence" in order to depathologize this condition [23].

Today numerous scientific societies, including the American Society of Clinical Oncology (ASCO) of the United States, call members of the LGBTQ community as "Sexual and Gender Minorities" (SGMs) and recommend that gender identity and sexual orientation be recorded in the Medical Records [24, 25].

As an example of the difficulty to find historical records on the care of transgender patients, Dr. Cathcart-Rake and his collaborators showed that in the Mayo Clinic Tumor Registry's registry of 385,820 patients from 1972 to 2017, they only found one case [26]. Perceiving and recording our patients' gender and sexual orientation is the first step to dismantling the barriers to their access to the health system and respectful treatment.

Some of the situations that we must resolve include: the lack of knowledge about the effectiveness of treatments due to low participation in clinical trials [27]; the lack of medical information for health education for members of the LGBTQ community [28]; The fact that LGBTQ community has a higher incidence of smokers [29], among other reasons because tobacco promotion campaigns were designed specifically for them [30]; the fact they are affected by comorbidities that are related to cancer (HPV) [31] and require specific antiviral treatments such as HIV [32].

All of these situations require that doctors and all members of the health team find humility, especially what Albert and collaborators call "cultural humility" [33]. In their article, these authors highlight: "A minority (20–40%) of oncology clinicians (physicians, nurses, and advanced practitioners) feel knowledgeable to address Sexual Gender Minority-specific health disparities, but a majority (70–80%) want education regarding the unique health needs of SGM patients with cancer."

This lack of knowledge in medical training was what we highlighted in our own experience, which we will analyze below.

9.2 An Educational Void

In 2018, we had the first experience of caring for a transgender patient with cancer at our institution.

This was a person whose biological sex at birth was male and then underwent gender reaffirmation treatment to become a woman. This transwoman patient still had an ID with her previous deadname and suffered from localized prostate cancer that had to be treated with surgery or radiotherapy.

After analyzing her case and evaluating the therapeutic alternatives, the patient respectfully, but with great firmness, told us that she appreciated our advice but that she had not felt respected as a woman when they called her by her deadname in the waiting room.

We apologized and assured her that this would not happen again, but we became aware of our ignorance on this subject and asked for help in informing us on this point.

She was the one who provided us with the first guide in this regard.

When we discussed it with the team, we interpreted that we were facing a generational problem: we had grown up in a binary world and did not understand the reality of a more complex world; the consensus was that if we studied the same phenomenon in our graduate students, we would not find any difficulty regarding this topic.

That motivated us to design the experiment that we implemented in an Objective structured Clinical Examination [34] (OSCE) in 2019.

The OSCE [35–52] is an exam of clinical skills in which the student goes through different clinical stations in a given period of time. In each station, there is an actor playing a patient suffering from a certain ailment or symptom; or the student may have to interpret a report or establish a differential diagnosis using images of a patient or a genetic report.

The Instituto Henry Moore-Universidad del Salvador (USAL) OSCE is an exam for first- and second-year students, carried out once a year since 2015. It lasts 4 h and is done on the second Saturday of November at Instituto Oncológico Henry Moore. The institute is an outpatient care facility, and is used exclusively during that day for this examination.

It consists of eight stations distributed as follows: two stations with simulated patients (one incurable, one curable), two stations to evaluate team work (the ethics committee, and the tumor board) and four stations for individual work (paper reading comprehension, differential diagnosis with patient images, genetic report interpretation, and scans interpretation) [53, 54].

In 2020, [55] the work we carried out in 2019 at Station 2 was selected for oral presentation at the American Society of Clinical Oncology (ASCO) congress (Fig. 9.1).

The inspiration for our station was Robert Eads (Fig. 9.2), a transman patient with ovarian cancer who was refused treatment by a dozen doctors in the 1990s. His final year of life was the focus of the 2001 documentary *Southern Comfort*.

All our actors were trained with this documentary and it's a highly recommended watch for anyone interested in this subject.

The most important facts for our station case were:

- The fact that he was born female, had been married and had two children.
     We added a family history of breast cancer.
- Ten years before the consultation, he'd had a bilateral mastectomy and had started testosterone therapy.
- Three weeks before the consultation he'd had a complete resection of a Stage IIIC ovarian cancer.

What did we wish to evaluate in each student?

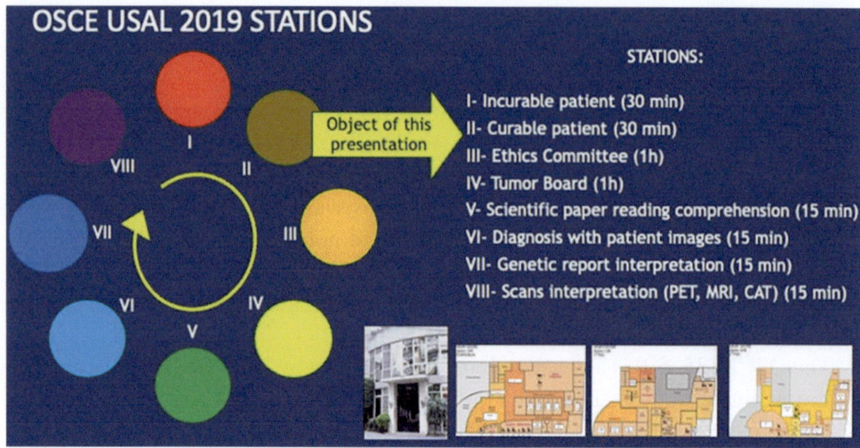

Fig. 9.1 OSCE 2019 design to evaluate care of transgender patients

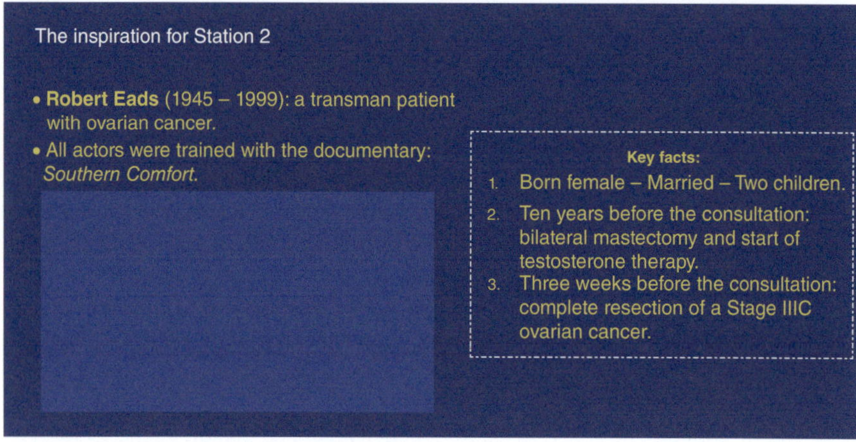

Fig. 9.2 Inspirational life story for training actors

(a) Their knowledge of the transman condition.
(b) The use of the patient's preferred pronouns.
(c) Whether they discontinued testosterone therapy or not.
(d) If they recommended a genetic study.
(e) If they treated the ovarian cancer according to NCCN guidelines.
(f) And if they had any Moral discomfort with transgender patient care.

How did we evaluate these points? With three different instruments:

– An observer evaluation in the form of a checklist, completed in real time
– An electronic health record that the student filled out during the evaluation.
– A recording of each student to verify and analyze after the session.

The results were:

(a) Five students (20%) were unaware of the transman condition.
(b) Three students (12%) did not use the patient's preferred gender pronoun.
(c) Seventeen students (68%) discontinued testosterone therapy.
(d) Most students (92%) recommended a genetic study.
(e) Everyone treated ovarian cancer according to NCCN guidelines.
(f) None expressed moral discomfort with patient care.

In other words, **we found that our students were better prepared to treat the cancer than the patient,** and specifically lacked knowledge and skills to properly care for a transgender patient.

In other words, we were not facing a generational problem when it came to the care of patients from the LGBTQ community, but rather a problem of medical ignorance that went beyond the material available to educate us.

Before presenting our work, we reviewed all the study plans of oncology courses taught in our country and found that the topic of cancer in LGBTQ patients was only discussed in relation to AIDS and there was no communication module oriented to specific care regarding LGBTQ patients [32].

This leads to the question: What kind of doctors do we want our students to be? What kind of doctors do we want to be?

In a pluralistic, diverse, and democratic society, caring for our patient's values and outlook on life are just as important as technical or oncological knowledge when it comes to establishing a trusting and healthy doctor–patient relationship.

This conclusion led to an immediate learning on our part as teachers of future oncologists: this reality must be addressed in their medical training.

And with this in mind, we added a new module to the curriculum so as to address the specific needs of LGBTQ cancer patients as of 2020.

As a side note, it is interesting to highlight that the students themselves reflected on their lack of education for caring for LGBTQ patients during their final exams. And we were more than eager to participate in more discussions and continue learning on this topic.

Therefore, the essential problem is whether we want to see and care for our fellow citizens of the LGBTQ community or, on the contrary, we want them to continue to be invisible, a topic that we will address below.

9.3   The Problem of Invisible Patients

There is a well-known saying in Spanish: "There is no worse blind man than he who does not want to see."

Medicine, many times in its history, did not want to see and made serious mistakes: it did not want to see that getting sick was natural until Hippocrates separated human illness from sin or the capricious will of the gods; it did not want to see that it was possible to operate without pain until the birth of anesthesia; it did not want to see that pus was not necessary for the healing of wounds until Lister demonstrated that antisepsis saved lives; it did not want to operate in a regulated manner until Halstead demonstrated that radical surgery cured some patients; it did not want to see the risk of radiation until it was unfortunately too late; it did not want to see the warning signs with which the Covid 19 pandemic might have been avoided [56].

Not seeing is the greatest oversight we can make in the practice of our art [57].

The invisible patient, the invisible illness, the invisible symptom are causes of abandonment, suffering, and death.

LGBTQ patients have treated doctors with more care and affection than they received in return most of the time [18].

The visibility of the patient from the LGBTQ community doesn't just depend on the doctor and the health team.

Without a doubt society and politics have a lot to do with it. Considering homosexuality or transgenderism a social stigma is one of the reasons for invisibility [58]. In developed societies, a genuine effort is being made to develop awareness of the value of respect for the human person and avoiding all types of discrimination [59].

Understanding what is happening and learning from our mistakes and limitations can be the way to improve access to health and care for all patients [60].

All members of the health team must be trained in developing care and communication skills with patients from the LGBTQ community [61, 62].

Such training must cover the entire spectrum of health care: from prevention [63] and treatments to palliative care [64] such as grief [65], in both adults [66] and young people [67].

When we stop to observe what happens to patients from the LGBTQ community, we are amazed [68, 69].

The word amazement is made up of two terms "a," which means without, and "shadow."

We can now see clearly where before there was darkness, and the first thing we see is our insensitivity to the suffering of a fellow human being.

A society that expels, a community that excludes and marginalizes, a system that places barriers to access, are all manifestations of insensitivity and inhumanity.

An inhuman medicine does not cure, it does not relieve, it does not console and it does not protect, that is to say, it is not real medicine [70].

Instead, recovering sensitivity and humanity is a great cure for a medicine sick with indifference and distancing [71].

Value others and their differences. Accepting others as they are and assisting them with warmth and respect makes us better doctors and better doctors are always a blessing.

9.4   A Vulnerable Population

A marginalized, excluded population with barriers to access the healthcare system is a vulnerable population.

From a family point of view, they frequently leave home at an early age and that puts them in a precarious situation [72].

Youth in the LGBTQ community have higher rates of alcoholism and smoking [73].

They suffer higher rates of bulimia and anorexia during their adolescence and youth.

From a social point of view, they have more school dropouts, greater obstacles in getting a job, and greater difficulties in keeping it [74].

This often leads to prostitution being one of the only job options that many of them have [31].

It is a group with a low birth rate, a higher abortion rate, a low breastfeeding rate, and a low sexual protection rate [75, 76].

These situations of abandonment, social isolation, unemployment, and poverty are conditions of illness. The person who has best studied the social determinants of health or illness is Sir Michael Marmot and he observed that segregated members of the LGBTQ community or any other excluded minority experience also affects their health [77–82].

The impact of alcoholism on disadvantaged groups and its devastating effects on health is well documented [83].

Preventable premature deaths make poverty and marginalization more devastating diseases than any other [84, 85].

The impact of stress and anxiety due to malnutrition and social conditions of poverty and unhealthiness are not exclusive to the West, it has also been demonstrated in Eastern societies, so we could say that it is universal [86].

Finally, we must not forget that the most important epidemic to come in the developed world is the loneliness epidemic. Isolation, especially in the elderly, generates depression due to lack of social ties [87].

The awareness of this vulnerability generated by social rejection should motivate us to generate feelings of inclusion, dialogue, and protection of people from the LGBTQ community.

All differences in a multiethnic and multicultural society are reasonable as long as they do not affect the life and health of others.

That should be an insurmountable limit: the life of others and respect for their person are values higher than the belief that their life choice is wrong, unnatural, immoral, deviant, or sinful. All terms with which we try to avoid our responsibility.

Probably the philosopher who has studied this topic the most is Emmanuel Levinas and his sense of infinite responsibility toward the other [88–91].

Thinking that the other person may be making a wrong choice should not be a reason to ignore their care; on the contrary, we must be even more understanding and respectful.

In order to have fluid and truthful medical communication with a patient from the LGBTQ community, we must create an inclusive health system.

9.5   A Safe Environment: A Respectful Look—A Kind Word

To generate an inclusive place of care, we must start by changing ourselves and recovering the sense of openness and proximity that gave rise to our profession.

In the West, the maximum representative of proximity is reflected in the parable of the Good Samaritan (Lk X, 29–37) from the Gospel of Saint Luke (who was a doctor):

The Parable of the Good Samaritan

[25] On one occasion, an expert in the law stood up to test Jesus. "Teacher," he asked, "what must I do to inherit eternal life?"

[26] "What is written in the Law?" I have replied. "How do you read it?"

[27] He answered, "'Love the Lord your God with all your heart and with all your soul and with all your strength and with all your mind'[a]; and, 'Love your neighbor as yourself'. [b]"

[28] "You have answered correctly," Jesus replied. "Do this and you will live."

[29] But he wanted to justify himself, so he asked Jesus, "And who is my neighbor?"

[30] In reply Jesus said: "A man was going down from Jerusalem to Jericho, when he was attacked by robbers. They stripped him of his clothes, beat him and went away, leaving him half dead. [31] A priest happened to be going down the same road, and when he saw the man, he passed by on the other side. [32] So too, a Levite, when he came to the place and saw him, passed by on the other side. [33] But a Samaritan, as he traveled, came where the man was; and when he saw him, he took pity on him. [34] He went to him and bandaged his wounds, pouring on oil and wine. Then he put the man on his own donkey, brought him to an inn and took care of him. [35] The next day he took out two denarii [c] and gave them to the innkeeper. 'Look after him', he said, 'and when I return, I will reimburse you for any extra expense you may have'.

[36] "Which of these three do you think was a neighbor to the man who fell into the hands of robbers?"

[37] The expert in the law replied, "The one who had mercy on him."

Jesus told him, "Go and do likewise."

It is interesting to think that this evangelical parable has lost its force because we have nothing against the Samaritans, but at the time Jesus pronounced it, it was scandalous.

The Samaritans for the Jews were heretics and reprobates, therefore a good Samaritan was impossible, it was literally an oxymoron.

To have an idea of its strength, we should make the effort to imagine what behavior or ideology generates such repulsion in us that it is impossible to imagine that it can be saved.

Returning to the figure of the Samaritan, nothing prevents him from being close: his religion, his culture, his health, his business... nothing, he gets off the horse, medically assists the badly injured, puts him on his horse, takes him to the inn, takes care of him during the night and when he leaves he leaves money so that the injured person can be left in the care of the innkeeper and assures that he will pay off the debt upon his return.

This contrasts with the attitudes of the three remaining characters: the robbers, the priest and the Levite, the first are the cause of the damage, while rest are ignorant of the suffering. Pope Francis in his encyclical Fratelli tutti, does not hesitate to classify the latter accomplices.

Therefore, the first gesture is to become aware of the damage we can cause to another with our rejection or our indifference.

This must be accompanied by technical training to competently assist the needs of members of the LGBTQ community, in this sense, a text to start with is the Standards of Care version 8 [21] and all guidelines that address the prevention, diagnosis, and treatment of health conditions in this group of patients.

What does a safe environment consist of?

When Dr. Juno Obedin-Maliver discussed our work at ASCO 2020, she presented the following slide [7] (Fig. 9.3).

Their observations were excellent, but this slide in particular left me thinking for a long time because of the simplicity and depth of what it says:

Building a safer and more inclusive system requires knowing:
What happens to the patient when they approach that door?
How do you find it if it's not visible?
How do you access it?
How easy is it to open?

Only knowing the experiences of our patients can help us in this aspect.

Building a safer system requires knowing what happens behind the door, in the office, in the intimacy of the doctor–patient relationship.

If a patient is attacked in word or deed by a doctor at our institution, we are all responsible.

For too long in medicine, victims have had to give all kinds of explanations while members of the health team looked the other way.

That is why we must establish a system of zero tolerance for the mistreatment of a patient, similar to that established against any sexual assault: not in my office, not in my emergency room, not in my apartment, not in my institution.

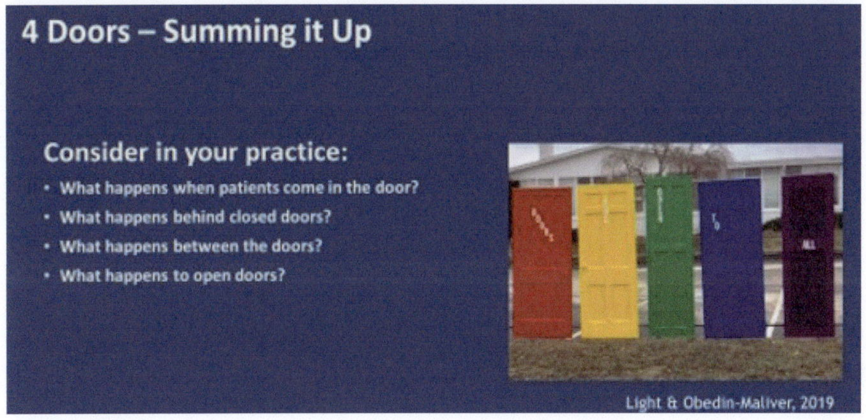

Fig. 9.3 Doors to be opened

What happens between the doors? Building a more secure system requires communication between professionals. We live in a world that is increasingly interconnected but unfortunately also more isolated. We must leave our own isolation with the computer and cell phone and not be afraid to share the problems or dilemmas of healthcare practice with all members of the health team.

Everyone's looks help us see more clearly.

And finally, what happens if we open the doors? What do we fear? What prejudices lead us to want them to remain closed?

A more inclusive system includes us all.

A safer system protects us all.

A more accessible system serves us all.

What are the minimum requirements that a safe system for the LGBTQ community must have?

We can think of the answer to this question from the "top" or from the "bottom," that is, from society or from the intimacy of the encounter with a patient.

In any case, both paths are necessary.

I prefer to think about it from the minimum to the maximum, from the act to the policy, and not the other way around, but it is simply a preference.

The first step to a safe system is that the doctor and the health team are convinced of the person's right to respectful and dignified treatment, under any condition and circumstance.

Sometimes you only have power over the nine square meters of your office and not much else. Well, let those nine square meters be a place in which any patient from the LGBTQ community feels respected, listened to, treated with kindness and appropriateness.

Have you trained to assist them?

Do you understand the value of their choice and their name?

Are you interested in what your patient feels and suffers?

Do you defend their rights?

Do you make sure your medication is appropriate?

Do you monitor their health the same way you do other patients?

Do we understand that when our practice is hostile, the patient will be exposed to unsafe medications and treatments that no one will control?

That is the first change and the most important of all.

The next step is to join with other members of the health team interested in caring for these people and form a multidisciplinary care service in which quality medical care can be provided that respects the most modern standards [21].

The following hierarchy is an open, respectful, and inclusive institution.

This has an effect on the entire medical community, to prevent patients from having to travel to receive the care to which they are entitled, allowing them to do so in any area close to the place where they live [92].

This should end up forming a society that is respectful of the human rights of all its members and, above all, promotes unrestricted respect for the rights of the minorities that make it up.

From the level of the polis to the intimacy of the office, commitment to caring for others and promoting their rights improves us all.

In the specific field of oncology, this is crucial [32, 72, 93–97].

Proper assistance does not only involve applying what is already known but also investigating how we can improve what we already know.

9.6   New Knowledge in a Different Society

Probably the sociologist who most clearly saw the structure and dynamics of modern society is Zygmunt Bauman [98–104].

In his different texts, Bauman reflects the changes that have occurred in modern societies with respect to identity, belonging, and links between their members.

The concept of "liquid societies" is the one that best describes the dynamics of modern relationships and structures.

Before, duty defined identity and human relationships, obedience was a highly appreciated virtue and most ethical behaviors were heteronomous, learned in the family, churches, or schools.

Today desire defines identity and relationships much more than duty, honesty rather than obedience is preferred as a virtue, and the most honest people are those who show themselves as they are and above all, they are as they wish to be.

Finally, most ethical behaviors are autonomous and the role of educational or religious institutions is usually belittled, if not considered indoctrination or imposition.

This makes convictions and relationships fluid, adhesions temporary, and interactions multiple and simultaneous, rather than unique or sequential.

Of course, the preceding description is a didactic contrast rather than a reflection of the multiple and heterogeneous reality in which we live.

The doctor–patient relationship is also crossed by this new liquid reality that Bauman describes: the doctor has ceased to be a demigod provided with all the knowledge of the traditional paternalistic relationship of medicine. Today the doctor–patient relationship is challenged by more empowered patients, often better informed and, above all, with different desires and needs for their lives.

These challenges require the doctor to recover the original meaning of his medical vocation, which is to care for and assist those who suffer.

An important group of our community suffers from conditions inherent to human nature and also suffers marginalization, denial, and exclusion from a society that rejects them, adding injustice and pain to their sufferings.

It is a human group that is excluded from clinical research trials [6, 11, 60, 93, 105–112], a community that often does not have access to information or health systems [75, 113–118].

On the other hand, it is a group open to actively participating [63, 119–121] if they are treated appropriately.

Therefore, I believe that it is time to understand individual responsibility in the integration, respect, and defense of the rights of the most vulnerable. Remembering that of Travis Manion: "If not me, then who," "If not here, then where"; "If not now, then when" as incentives for making correct [122–125] decisions.

Learning to communicate better with our patients is an exercise that has no medical contraindications: it is always good.

9.7 Teaching Exercises

1. Personal

   (a) Do I consider myself qualified to assist a member of the LGBTQ community?
   (b) Do I understand their medical needs and do I have the knowledge and skills to assist them?
   (c) Do I understand what "transition," "transman" or "transwoman" means?
   (d) Do I understand the importance of inquiring about someone's preferred pronouns and the pain I may cause them by using their "dead name"?
   (e) Have I read and understood the quality care standards necessary to competently assist members of the LGBTQ community?

2. In a group

   (a) Gather as a group and watch the documentary "Southern comfort" or the movie "Philadelphia."

      - Do you think that could happen in the institution where you work? If you think it couldn't happen, why not?
      - Have you implemented community training to assist patients from the LGBTQ community?
      - Do you know if there is a multidisciplinary team at the institution for the care of transgender patients?

   (b) Practice a role-play scenario in which you are consulted by an adolescent with gender identity problems and their parents. Analyze the way in which the doctor, the patient, or the parents communicate, mark the difficulties you observe and how you would think it appropriate to resolve them.
   (c) Is there a support group for members of the LGBTQ community in your hospital, parish, or other community? If so, try to invite one or many of them to talk about their work and health care difficulties.

References

1. Lambrou NH, Gleason CE, Obedin-Maliver J, et al. Subjective memory complaints associated with discrimination in healthcare settings among transgender and gender nonconforming older adults. Alzheimers Dementia. 2019;15:3–567. https://doi.org/10.1016/j.jalz.2019.06.3604.
2. Inman EM, Obedin-Maliver J, Ragosta S, et al. Reports of negative interactions with healthcare providers among transgender, nonbinary, and gender-expansive people assigned female at birth in the United States: results from an online, cross-sectional survey. Int J Environ Res Public Health. 2023;20(11):6007. https://doi.org/10.3390/ijerph20116007.
3. Clark KD, Lunn MR, Lev EM, et al. State-level policy environments, discrimination, and victimization among sexual and gender minority people. Int J Environ Res Public Health. 2022;19(16):9916. https://doi.org/10.3390/ijerph19169916.
4. Clark KD, Luong S, Lunn MR, et al. Healthcare mistreatment, state-level policy protections, and healthcare avoidance among gender minority people. Sex Res Soc Policy. 2022;19(4):1717. https://doi.org/10.1007/s13178-022-00748-1.
5. Flentje A, Clark KD, Cicero E, et al. Minority stress, structural stigma, and physical health among sexual and gender minority individuals: examining the relative strength of the relationships. Ann Behav Med. 2022;56(6):573–91. https://doi.org/10.1093/abm/kaab051.
6. Suen LW, Lunn MR, Katuzny K, et al. What sexual and gender minority people want researchers to know about sexual orientation and gender identity questions: a qualitative study. Arch Sex Behav. 2020;49(7):2301–18. https://doi.org/10.1007/s10508-020-01810-y.
7. Light A, Obedin-Maliver J. Opening the ob/gyn door for sexual and gender minority patients. Contemp Ob Gyn. 2019;64(1).
8. Mann A, Chan A, Rohatgi A, Caesar MA, Obedin-Maliver J, Kapp DS. Comparison of depressive symptoms and inflammation between sexual minorities and heterosexuals using NHANES study of 8538 participants. Sci Rep. 2022;12(1):3792. https://doi.org/10.1038/s41598-022-07702-6.
9. Obedin-Maliver J, Lisha N, Breyer BN, Subak LL, Huang AJ. More similarities than differences? An exploratory analysis comparing the sexual complaints, sexual experiences, and genitourinary health of older sexual minority and sexual majority adults. J Sex Med. 2019;16(3):347–50. https://doi.org/10.1016/j.jsxm.2019.01.308.
10. Lipkin P, Monseur B, Mayo JA, et al. Effect of prior training on reproductive endocrinology and infertility specialists' knowledge, skills, attitudes and behaviors regarding the care of transgender and gender diverse individuals. Fertil Steril. 2022;118(5):E49–50. https://doi.org/10.1016/j.fertnstert.2022.09.307.
11. Clark KD, Capriotti MR, Obedin-Maliver J, Lunn MR, Lubensky ME, Flentje A. Supporting sexual and gender minority health: research priorities from mental health professionals. J Gay Lesbian Ment Health. 2020;24(2):205–21. https://doi.org/10.1080/19359705.2019.1700865.
12. Streed CG, Lunn MR, Siegel J, Obedin-Maliver J. Meeting the patient care, education, and research missions: academic medical centers must comprehensively address sexual and gender minority health. Acad Med. 2021;96(6):822. https://doi.org/10.1097/ACM.0000000000003703.
13. Lunn MR, Obedin-Maliver J, Bibbins-Domingo K. Estimating the prevalence of sexual minority adolescents. J Am Med Assoc. 2017;317(16):1691. https://doi.org/10.1001/jama.2017.2918.
14. Moseson H, Zazanis N, Goldberg E, et al. The imperative for transgender and gender nonbinary inclusion: beyond women's health. Obstet Gynecol. 2020;135(5):1059. https://doi.org/10.1097/AOG.0000000000003816.

15. Obedin-Maliver J. Time to change: supporting sexual and gender minority people—an underserved, understudied cancer risk population. J Natl Compr Canc Netw. 2017;15(11):1305. https://doi.org/10.6004/jnccn.2017.7050.

16. Adams N, Hitomi M, Moody C. Varied reports of adult transgender suicidality: synthesizing and describing the peer-reviewed and gray literature. Transgend Health. 2017;2(1):60–75. https://doi.org/10.1089/trgh.2016.0036.

17. Casanova-Perez R, Apodaca C, Bascom E, et al. Broken down by bias: healthcare biases experienced by BIPOC and LGBTQ+ patients. AMIA Annu Symp Proc. 2021;2021:275–84.

18. Apodaca C, Casanova-Perez R, Bascom E, et al. Maybe they had a bad day: how LGBTQ and BIPOC patients react to bias in healthcare and struggle to speak out. J Am Med Inform Assoc. 2022;29(12):2075–82. https://doi.org/10.1093/jamia/ocac142.

19. McGarity-Palmer R, Saw A. Transgender clients' travel distance to preferred health care: a clinic-specific study. Transgend Health. 2022;7(3):282–6. https://doi.org/10.1089/trgh.2020.0101.

20. Hermaszewska S, Sweeney A, Camminga B, Botelle R, Elliott K, Sin J. Lived experiences of transgender forced migrants and their mental health outcomes: systematic review and meta-ethnography. BJPsych Open. 2022;8(3):e91. https://doi.org/10.1192/bjo.2022.51.

21. Coleman E, Radix AE, Bouman WP, et al. Standards of care for the health of transgender and gender diverse people, version 8. Int J Transgend Health. 2022;23(S1):S1–259. https://doi.org/10.1080/26895269.2022.2100644.

22. Martin JSJ. Building a bridge. How the Catholic Church and the LGBT community can enter into a relationship of respect, compassion and sensibility. 2nd ed. New York, NY: HarperCollins Publishers; 2018.

23. Mumford K, Fraser L, Knudson G. What the past suggests about when a diagnostic label is oppressive. AMA J Ethics. 2023;25:E446–51.

24. Lee H, Schabath MB, Curci MB, et al. Ask and tell: the importance of the collection of sexual orientation and gender identity data to improve the quality of cancer care for sexual and gender minorities. J Oncol Pract. 2017;13:542. https://doi.org/10.1200/JOP.

25. Suen LW, Lunn MR, Sevelius JM, et al. Do ask, tell, and show: contextual factors affecting sexual orientation and gender identity disclosure for sexual and gender minority people. LGBT Health. 2022;9(2):73–80. https://doi.org/10.1089/lgbt.2021.0159.

26. Cathcart-Rake EJ, Lightner DJ, Quevedo FJ, Ertz DC, Jatoi A. Cancer in transgender patients: one case in 385,820 is indicative of a paucity of data. J Oncol Pract. 2018;14(4):270–2. https://doi.org/10.1200/JOP.2017.027714.

27. Alpert AB, Renee Brewer J, Adams S, et al. Addressing barriers to clinical trial participation for transgender people with cancer to improve access and generate data. J Clin Oncol. 2023;41(10):1825–9. https://doi.org/10.1200/JCO.22.01174.

28. Hostetter CR, Call J, Gerke DR, Holloway BT, Walls NE, Greenfield JC. "We are doing the absolute most that we can, and no one is listening": barriers and facilitators to health literacy within transgender and nonbinary communities. Int J Environ Res Public Health. 2022;19(3):1229. https://doi.org/10.3390/ijerph19031229.

29. Dawson DB, White DL, Chiao E, et al. Mental and physical health correlates of tobacco use among transgender veterans of the Iraq and Afghanistan conflicts. Transgend Health. 2021;6(5):290–5. https://doi.org/10.1089/trgh.2020.0051.

30. Ramanadhan S, Salvia M, Hanby E, et al. "We're always an afterthought"—designing tobacco control campaigns for dissemination with and to LGBTQ +—serving community organizations: a thematic analysis. Cancer Causes Control. 2023;34(8):673–82. https://doi.org/10.1007/s10552-023-01706-x.

31. Portillo-Romero AJ, Allen-Leigh B, Nyitray AG, et al. Sex work and high-risk anal human papillomavirus infection among transgender women: the Condesa study. Transgend Health. 2021;6(6):315–24. https://doi.org/10.1089/trgh.2020.0075.

32. Lurain K. Treating cancer in people with HIV. J Clin Oncol. 2023;41(21):3682–8. https://doi. org/10.1200/jco.23.00737.

33. Alpert A, Kamen C, Schabath MB, Hamel L, Seay J, Quinn GP. What exactly are we measuring? Evaluating sexual and gender minority cultural humility training for oncology care clinicians. J Clin Oncol. 2020;38(23):2605–9. https://doi.org/10.1200/JCO.19.03300.

34. Harden RMG, Downie WW, Stevenson M, Wilson GM. Assessment of clinical competence using objective structured examination. Br Med J. 1975;1(5955):447–51. https://doi. org/10.1136/bmj.1.5955.447.

35. Matthew K, Marshall D, Shaw R, Tripp D. 2003 OSCE handbook. The world according to Kelly, Marshall, Shaw and Tripp; 2003.

36. Fornells-Vallés JM. The ABC of miniCEX. Educ Med. 2009;12(2):83–9.

37. Mini Mini-CEX. Competence descriptors; 2014.

38. Debra Pugh MFM, Sydney Smee P. Guidelines for the development of objective structured clinical examination (OSCE) cases; 2013.

39. Urbina J, Monks SM. Validating assessment tools in simulation. In: StatPearls. Treasure Island, FL: StatPearls Publishing; 2020. p. 1–9. http://www.ncbi.nlm.nih.gov/ pubmed/32809366.

40. Reddy S, Vijayakumar S. Evaluating clinical skills of radiation oncology residents: parts I and II. Int J Cancer. 2000;90(1):1–12. https://doi.org/10.1002/(SICI)1097-0215(20000220)90:1<1::AID-IJC1>3.0.CO;2-W.

41. Felthun JZ, Taylor S, Shulruf B, Allen DW. Empirical analysis comparing the tele-objective structured clinical examination (teleOSCE) and the in-person assessment in Australia. J Educ Eval Health Prof. 2021;18:23. https://doi.org/10.3352/jeehp.2021.18.23.

42. Shaban S, Tariq I, Elzubeir M, Alsuwaidi AR, Basheer A, Magzoub M. Conducting online OSCEs aided by a novel time management web-based system. BMC Med Educ. 2021;21(1):1–11. https://doi.org/10.1186/s12909-021-02945-9.

43. Kenaga H, Markova T, Stansfield RB, Kumar S, Morris P. An objective structured clinical examination case for opioid management: standardized patient ratings of communication skills as a predictor of systems-based practice scores. J Patient Cent Res Rev. 2021;8(3):261–6. https://doi.org/10.17294/2330-0698.1800.

44. Sepp K, Volmer D. Use of face-to-face assessment methods in E-learning—an example of an objective structured clinical examination (OSCE) test. Pharmacy. 2021;9(3):144. https://doi. org/10.3390/pharmacy9030144.

45. Kennedy AB, Riyad CNY, Gunn LH, et al. More than their test scores: redefining success with multiple mini-interviews. Med Sci Educ. 2020;30(3):1049–60. https://doi.org/10.1007/ s40670-020-01013-z.

46. Garabed LR, Almarzouq A, Hu J, Andonian S, El-Sherbiny M, Fahmy N. Objective structured clinical examinations (OSCE) performance among Quebec urology residents: a retrospective study from 2008-2019. Can Urol Assoc J. 2020;14(9):E435–44.

47. Shen E, Cristiano JA, Ellis LR. The electronic health record objective structured clinical Examination Station: assessing student competency in patient notes and patient interaction. MedEdPORTAL. 2020;16:10998. https://doi.org/10.15766/mep_2374-8265.10998.

48. Ferreira ÉDMR, Pinto RZ, Arantes PMMH, et al. Stress, anxiety, self-efficacy, and the meanings that physical therapy students attribute to their experience with an objective structured clinical examination. BMC Med Educ. 2020;20(1):1–9. https://doi.org/10.1186/ s12909-020-02202-5.

49. Harky A, Karimaghaei D, Katmeh H, Hewage S. The impact of COVID-19 on medical examinations. Biomed Act. 2020;91(4):e2020135. https://doi.org/10.23750/abm.v91i4.10487.

50. Sartori DJ, Hayes RW, Horlick M, Adams JG, Zabar SR. The TeleHealth OSCE: preparing trainees to use telemedicine as a tool for transitions of care. J Grad Med Educ. 2020;12(6):764–8. https://doi.org/10.4300/JGME-D-20-00039.1.

51. Stalmach-Przygoda A, Nowakowski M, Kocurek A, et al. Perceptions of clinical teachers acting as examiners regarding the value of objective structured clinical examinations. Folia Med Cracov. 2020;60(2):109–21. https://doi.org/10.24425/fmc.2020.135017.
52. Traba C, Holland B, Laboy MC, Lamba S, Chen S. A multi-modal remote clinical skills mini-course utilizing a teaching TeleOSCE. Med Sci Educ. 2021;31(2):503–9. https://doi.org/10.1007/s40670-020-01201-x.
53. Gil Deza E, De Simone G, Garcia Gerardi CF, et al. Design and validation of an observational standard clinical examination (OSCE) for clinical oncology based on ASCO/ASH curricular milestones. J Clin Oncol. 2016;34(15 Suppl):18150. https://doi.org/10.1200/jco.2016.34.15_suppl.e.
54. Gercovich D, Gil Deza E, Hirsch H, et al. Evaluation of empathy in a structured observational examination of clinical skills (OSCE) in the career of oncology at Instituto Oncológico Henry Moore-Universidad del Salvador (HM-ONCOUSAL). J Clin Oncol. 2016;34(15 Suppl):18151. https://doi.org/10.1200/jco.2016.34.15_suppl.e.
55. Gil Deza E, Abal M, Gil Deza L, et al. Caring for transgender cancer patients: shortcomings of medical education. J Clin Oncol. 2020;38(15 Suppl):11002. https://doi.org/10.1200/JCO.2020.38.15_suppl.11002.
56. Marmot M. Premonition ignored. Lancet. 2021;398(10295):110–1. https://doi.org/10.1016/s0140-6736(21)01459-8.
57. Moreira AA, Bisesi A. Transgender day of visibility 2022: an interview with Adam Armada-Moreira and Ave Bisesi on trans experiences in STEM. Commun Biol. 2022;5(1):288. https://doi.org/10.1038/s42003-022-03247-6.
58. Scheidell JD, Kapadia F, Turpin RE, et al. Incarceration, social support networks, and health among black sexual minority men and transgender women: evidence from the HPTN 061 study. Int J Environ Res Public Health. 2022;19(19):12064. https://doi.org/10.3390/ijerph191912064.
59. Falck F, Bränström R. The significance of structural stigma toward transgender people in health care encounters across Europe: health care access, gender identity disclosure, and discrimination in health care as a function of national legislation and public attitudes. BMC Public Health. 2023;23(1):1031. https://doi.org/10.1186/s12889-023-15856-9.
60. Round R, Gokool N, Manica G, Paschall L, Foulcer S. Improving access for and experience of transgender and non-binary patients in clinical research: insights from a transgender patient focus group and targeted literature reviews. Contemp Clin Trials. 2023;131:107243. https://doi.org/10.1016/j.cct.2023.107243.
61. Chaudhary S, Ray R, Glass BD. "I don't know much about providing pharmaceutical care to people who are transgender": a qualitative study of experiences and attitudes of pharmacists. Explor Res Clin Soc Pharm. 2023;9:100254. https://doi.org/10.1016/j.rcsop.2023.100254.
62. Langdon E, Kavanagh P, Bushell M. Exploring pharmacists' understanding and experience of providing LGBTI healthcare. Explor Res Clin Soc Pharm. 2022;6:100134. https://doi.org/10.1016/j.rcsop.2022.100134.
63. Hanby E, Gazarian PK, Potter J, Jones R, Elhassan N, Tan ASL. "I liked just that it was a communal thing": feasibility and acceptability of engaging with transgender and gender-diverse persons in a digital photovoice research study on commercial cigarette smoking risk and protective factors. Digit Health. 2023;9:20552076231169819. https://doi.org/10.1177/20552076231169819.
64. Lippe MP, Eyer JC, Roberts KE, et al. Affirmative palliative care for transgender and gender nonconforming individuals. Am J Nurs. 2023;123(4):48–53. https://doi.org/10.1097/01.NAJ.0000925508.62666.99.
65. Bristowe K, Timmins L, Braybrook D, et al. LGBT+ partner bereavement and appraisal of the Acceptance-Disclosure Model of LGBT+ bereavement: a qualitative interview study. Palliat Med. 2023;37(2):221–34. https://doi.org/10.1177/02692163221138620.

66. Adan M, Scribani M, Tallman N, Wolf-Gould C, Campo-Engelstein L, Gadomski A. Worry and wisdom: a qualitative study of transgender elders' perspectives on aging. Transgend Health. 2021;6(6):332–42. https://doi.org/10.1089/trgh.2020.0098.

67. Sequeira GM, Kahn NF, Bocek KM, et al. Pediatric primary care providers' perspectives on Telehealth platforms to support care for transgender and gender-diverse youths: exploratory qualitative study. JMIR Hum Factors. 2023;10:e39118. https://doi.org/10.2196/39118.

68. Silverberg R, Averkiou P, Servoss J, Eyez M, Martinez LC. Training Preclerkship medical students on history taking in transgender and gender nonconforming patients. Transgend Health. 2021;6(6):374–9. https://doi.org/10.1089/trgh.2020.0117.

69. Cooper K, Mandy W, Russell A, Butler C. Healthcare clinical perspectives on the intersection of autism and gender dysphoria. Autism. 2023;27(1):31–42. https://doi.org/10.1177/13623613221080315.

70. Keenan BP, Barr E, Gleeson E, Greenberg CC, Temkin SM. Structural sexism and cancer care: the effects on the patient and oncologist. Am Soc Clin Oncol Educ Book. 2023;43:e391516. https://doi.org/10.1200/EDBK_391516.

71. Summers ML. Using reflective practice to understand LGBTQ client needs. J Christ Nurs. 2017;34(4):242–5. https://doi.org/10.1097/CNJ.0000000000000361.

72. Morgan S, Davies S, Palmer S, Plaster M. Sex, drugs, and rock "n" roll: caring for adolescents and young adults with cancer. J Clin Oncol. 2010;28(32):4825–30. https://doi.org/10.1200/JCO.2009.22.5474.

73. Flentje A, Barger BT, Capriotti MR, et al. Screening gender minority people for harmful alcohol use. PLoS One. 2020;15(4):e0231022. https://doi.org/10.1371/journal.pone.0231022.

74. Weinand JD, Ehlinger EP, Conniff JF, Hayon RL, Kvach E. Supporting transgender and nonbinary residents. Transgend Health. 2019;4(1):222–5. https://doi.org/10.1089/trgh.2018.0074.

75. Light AD, Sevelius J, Obedin-Maliver J, Kerns J. Pregnancy after transitioning: the male-gendered experience with fertility, pregnancy, and birth outcomes. Fertil Steril. 2013;100(3):S406–7. https://doi.org/10.1016/j.fertnstert.2013.07.648.

76. Moseson H, Fix L, Ragosta S, et al. Abortion experiences and preferences of transgender, nonbinary, and gender-expansive people in the United States. Am J Obstet Gynecol. 2021;224(4):376.e1–11. https://doi.org/10.1016/j.ajog.2020.09.035.

77. Nosrati E, Marmot M. Punitive social policy: an upstream determinant of health. Lancet. 2019;394(10196):376–7. https://doi.org/10.1016/S0140-6736(19)31672-1.

78. Marmot M. The health gap: the challenge of an unequal world: the argument. Int J Epidemiol. 2017;46(4):1312–8. https://doi.org/10.1093/ije/dyx163.

79. Marmot M. Inclusion health: addressing the causes of the causes. Lancet. 2018;391(10117):186–8. https://doi.org/10.1016/S0140-6736(17)32848-9.

80. Marmot M, Bell R. Solutions for prevention and control of non-communicable diseases: social determinants and non-communicable diseases: time for integrated action. BMJ. 2019;364:l251.

81. Marmot M. Closing the gap in a generation. Health equity through action on the social determinants of health. Published online; 2008. https://doi.org/10.1080/17441692.2010.514617.

82. Marmot M. Just societies, health equity, and dignified lives: the PAHO equity commission. Lancet. 2018;392(10161):2247–50. https://doi.org/10.1016/S0140-6736(18)32349-3.

83. Wood AM, Kaptoge S, Butterworth A, et al. Risk thresholds for alcohol consumption: combined analysis of individual-participant data for 599 912 current drinkers in 83 prospective studies. Lancet. 2018;391(10129):1513–23. https://doi.org/10.1016/S0140-6736(18)30134-X.

84. Stringhini S, Carmeli C, Jokela M, et al. Socioeconomic status and the 25 × 25 risk factors as determinants of premature mortality: a multicohort study and meta-analysis of 1·7 million men and women. Lancet. 2017;389(10075):1229–37. https://doi.org/10.1016/S0140-6736(16)32380-7.

85. Nosrati E, Ash M, Marmot M, McKee M, King LP. The association between income and life expectancy revisited: deindustrialization, incarceration and the widening health gap. Int J Epidemiol. 2018;47(3):720–30. https://doi.org/10.1093/ije/dyx243.

86. Chung RYN, Marmot M, Mak JKL, et al. Deprivation is associated with anxiety and stress. A population-based longitudinal household survey among Chinese adults in Hong Kong. J Epidemiol Community Health. 2021;75(4):335. https://doi.org/10.1136/jech-2020-214728.

87. Bertossi Urzua C, Ruiz MA, Pajak A, et al. The prospective relationship between social cohesion and depressive symptoms among older adults from Central and Eastern Europe. J Epidemiol Community Health. 2019;73(2):117. https://doi.org/10.1136/jech-2018-211063.

88. Buddeberg E. Thinking the other, thinking otherwise: Levinas' conception of responsibility. Interdiscip Sci Rev. 2018;43(2):146–55. https://doi.org/10.1080/03080188.2018.1450927.

89. Dami ZA, Pandu I, Anakotta E, Sahureka A. The contribution of levinas' conception of responsibility to the ethical encounter counselor-counselee. Int J Soc Sci Hum. 2019;3(2). https://doi.org/10.29332/ijssh.vn2.291.

90. Benaroyo L. The significance of Emmanuel Levinas' ethics of responsibility for medical judgment. Med Health Care Philos. 2022;25(3):327. https://doi.org/10.1007/s11019-022-10077-0.

91. Hreško J. Jaspers' metaphysical guilt and levinas' infinite responsibility. Filosoficky Casopis. 2021;69(1). https://doi.org/10.46854/fc.2021.1r.35.

92. Lee JL, Huffman M, Rattray NA, et al. "I don't want to spend the rest of my life only going to a gender wellness clinic": healthcare experiences of patients of a comprehensive transgender clinic. J Gen Intern Med. 2022;37(13):3396–403. https://doi.org/10.1007/s11606-022-07408-5.

93. Bybee SG, Wilson CM. Why good cancer care means gender-affirming care for transgender individuals with gendered cancers: implications for research, policy, and practice. J Clin Oncol. 2023;41:3591–4. https://doi.org/10.1200/jco.22.01857.

94. Arthur EK, Glissmeyer G, Obedin-Maliver J, Rabelais E. A cancer equity and affirming care: an overview of disparities and practical approaches for the care of transgender, gender-nonconforming, and nonbinary people. Clin J Oncol Nurs. 2021;25(5):25–35. https://doi.org/10.1188/21.CJON.S.

95. Katz NT, Alpert AB, Aristizabal MP, et al. Partnering with patients and caregivers in cancer care: lessons from experiences with transgender, Hispanic, and pediatric populations. Am Soc Clin Oncol Educ Book. 2023;43:e397264. https://doi.org/10.1200/edbk_397264.

96. Katz A, Agrawal LS, Sirohi B. Sexuality after cancer as an unmet need: addressing disparities, achieving equality. Am Soc Clin Oncol Educ Book. 2022;42:11–7. https://doi.org/10.1200/edbk_100032.

97. Tarras ES, Alpert AB, Kennedy E, Sampson A, Sutter ME, Quinn GP. Protecting transgender and gender-diverse patients with cancer in a shifting political landscape. JCO Oncol Pract. 2020;16(6):287–8. https://doi.org/10.1200/jcoop.20.00011.

98. Rickman HP, Bauman Z. Hermeneutics and social science. Br J Sociol. 1980;31(1). https://doi.org/10.2307/590068.

99. Bauman Z, Dench G. Minorities in the open society: prisoners of ambivalence. Br J Sociol. 1989;40(4). https://doi.org/10.2307/590906.

100. Bauman Z. L'humanité eat project. Anthropol Soc. 2004;27(3). https://doi.org/10.7202/007921ar.

101. Bauman Z. Society enables and disables. Scand J Disabil Res. 2007;9(1):58–60. https://doi.org/10.1080/15017410500530068.

102. Bauman Z. Organization for liquid-modern times? Crit Sociol (Eugene). 2023;49(6). https://doi.org/10.1177/08969205231170923.

103. Jacobsen MH. Suffering in the sociology of Zygmunt Bauman. Qual Stud. 2021;6(1):68–90. https://doi.org/10.7146/qs.v6i1.124417.

104. Bauman Z. Wasted lives: modernity and its outcasts. New York: Wiley; 2017.

105. Ramirez AH, Sulieman L, Schlueter DJ, et al. The all of us research program: data quality, utility, and diversity. Patterns. 2022;3(8):100570. https://doi.org/10.1016/j.patter.2022.100570.

106. Berrahou IK, Snow A, Swanson M, Obedin-Maliver J. Representation of sexual and gender minority people in patient nondiscrimination policies of cancer centers in the United States. J Natl Compr Cancer Netw. 2022;20(3):253. https://doi.org/10.6004/JNCCN.2021.7078.

107. Altman MR, Cragg K, van Winkle T, et al. Birth includes us: development of a community-led survey to capture experiences of pregnancy care among LGBTQ2S+ families. Birth. 2023;50(1):109–19. https://doi.org/10.1111/birt.12704.

108. Kano M, Sanchez N, Tamí-Maury I, Solder B, Watt G, Chang S. Addressing cancer disparities in SGM populations: recommendations for a National Action Plan to increase SGM health equity through researcher and provider training and education. J Cancer Educ. 2020;35(1):44–53. https://doi.org/10.1007/s13187-018-1438-1.

109. Ghorbanian A, Aiello B, Staples J. Under-representation of transgender identities in research: the limitations of traditional quantitative survey data. Transgend Health. 2022;7(3):261–9. https://doi.org/10.1089/trgh.2020.0107.

110. Restar A, Jin H, Operario D. Gender-inclusive and gender-specific approaches in trans health research. Transgend Health. 2021;6(5):235–9. https://doi.org/10.1089/trgh.2020.0054.

111. Lyles CR, Lunn MR, Obedin-Maliver J, Bibbins-Domingo K. The new era of precision population health: insights for the all of us research program and beyond. J Transl Med. 2018;16(1):211. https://doi.org/10.1186/s12967-018-1585-5.

112. Jones NC, Reyes ME, Quinn GP, Schabath MB, Lee H, Lee Moffitt H. Survey of principal investigators in biobanking: knowledge, attitudes, and research behaviors about transgender and gender-diverse patients, vol. 16; 2023.

113. Moseson H, Fix L, Ragosta S, et al. P13 experiences of self-managed abortion among transgender, nonbinary, and gender expansive people in the US. Contraception. 2020;102(4):281. https://doi.org/10.1016/j.contraception.2020.07.032.

114. Moseson H, Fix L, Gerdts C, et al. Abortion attempts without clinical supervision among transgender, nonbinary and gender-expansive people in the United States. BMJ Sex Reprod Health. 2022;48(e1):e22. https://doi.org/10.1136/bmjsrh-2020-200966.

115. Light AD, Obedin-Maliver J, Sevelius JM, Kerns JL. Transgender men who experienced pregnancy after female-to-male gender transitioning. Obstet Gynecol. 2014;124(6):1120. https://doi.org/10.1097/AOG.0000000000000540.

116. Cipres D, Seidman D, Cloniger C, Nova C, O'Shea A, Obedin-Maliver J. Contraceptive use and pregnancy intentions among transgender men presenting to a clinic for sex workers and their families in San Francisco. Contraception. 2017;95(2):186. https://doi.org/10.1016/j.contraception.2016.09.005.

117. Maza M, Meléndez M, Herrera A, et al. Cervical cancer screening with human papillomavirus self-sampling among transgender men in El Salvador. LGBT Health. 2020;7(4):174. https://doi.org/10.1089/lgbt.2019.0202.

118. Cohen CM, Wentzensen N, Castle PE, et al. Racial and ethnic disparities in cervical cancer incidence, survival, and mortality by histologic subtype. J Clin Oncol. 2022;41:1059–68. https://doi.org/10.1200/JCO.22.

119. Lunn MR, Capriotti MR, Flentje A, et al. Using mobile technology to engage sexual and gender minorities in clinical research. PLoS One. 2019;14(5):e0216282. https://doi.org/10.1371/journal.pone.0216282.

120. Thompson HM, Clement AM, Ortiz R, et al. Community engagement to improve access to healthcare: a comparative case study to advance implementation science for transgender health equity. Int J Equity Health. 2022;21(1):104. https://doi.org/10.1186/s12939-022-01702-8.

121. Lunn MR, Lubensky M, Hunt C, et al. A digital health research platform for community engagement, recruitment, and retention of sexual and gender minority adults in a national longitudinal cohort study—the PRIDE study. J Am Med Inform Assoc. 2019;26(8–9):737. https://doi.org/10.1093/jamia/ocz082.

122. Green JL. If not me, then who? In: Decision point. New York: Routledge; 2021. https://doi.org/10.1201/b15975-8.
123. Richardson JE. 'If not me, then who?' Examining engagement with holocaust memorial day commemoration in Britain. Dapim Stud Holocaust. 2018;32(1):22–37. https://doi.org/10.1080/23256249.2018.1432253.
124. Sargeant S, Baird K, Sweeny A, Torpie T. "If not me, then who?": exploring the challenges experienced by front-line clinicians screening for, and communicating about, domestic violence in the emergency department. Violence Against Women. 2023;29(12–13):2508–26. https://doi.org/10.1177/10778012231186816.
125. Dryer C. If not me, then who? Teach Learn Nurs. 2017;12(1). https://doi.org/10.1016/j.teln.2016.09.006.

Chapter 10
Telehealth: The Pandemic Experience with Virtual Communication

10.1 Introduction

Interest in telemedicine dates back more than 70 years, [1, 2] in fact, the first published work dates back to the 1950s, according to what was reported by the Institute of Medicine of the United States Academies of Science [3, 4].

A search carried out in October 2023 in Pubmed, looking for the three key terms in this chapter: telehealth, telemedicine, and Patient Reported Outcome, regarding their presence in the titles of research papers produced the following results (Graphs 10.1, 10.2 and 10.3):

As we can see in the three preceding graphs, the first term that appears is telemedicine, followed by telehealth, which is a more comprehensive term, since it refers not only to the diagnosis and treatment of diseases but also to the prevention

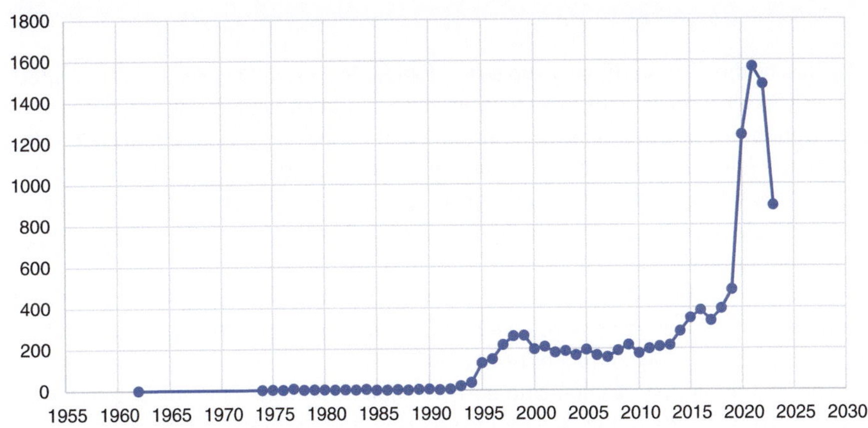

Graph 10.1 Frequency of titles with the word telemedicine in Pubmed

© The Author(s), under exclusive license to Springer Nature
Switzerland AG 2024
E. Gil Deza, *Improving Clinical Communication*,
https://doi.org/10.1007/978-3-031-62446-9_10

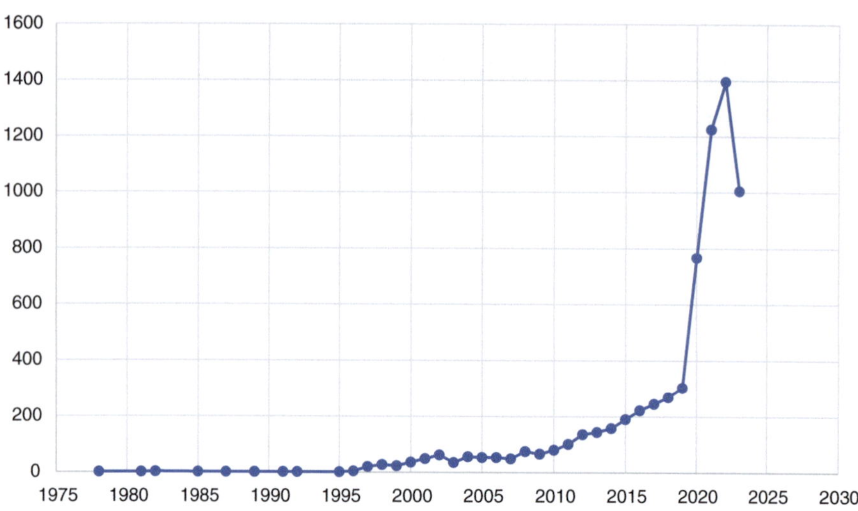

Graph 10.2   Frequency of titles with the word telehealth in Pubmed

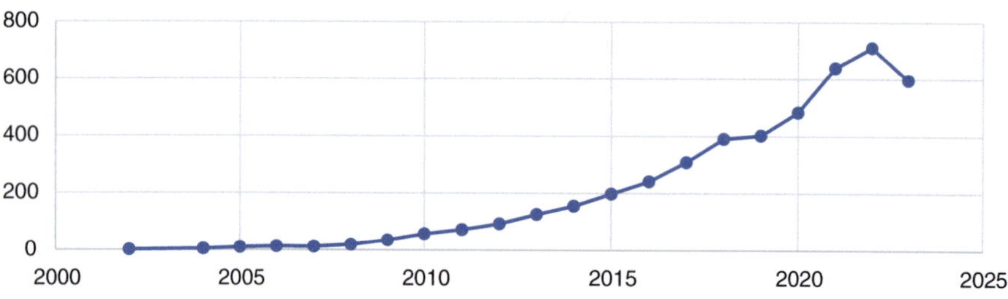

Graph 10.3   Frequency of the phrase "Patient Reported Outcome" in pubmed

and care of the disease. Finally the term "Patient Reported Outcome," which refers not only to what the patient reports about their health and quality of life, but also to data from home health monitoring, through cell phones or devices connected to the Internet, is shown in third place amongst the searched terms.

The second thing we can observe from the comparison of these three graphs is that both telemedicine and telehealth had a peak that grew five to ten times during the Covid-19 pandemic.

From the perspective of medicine, the Covid 19 pandemic, with the associated home isolation due to the risk of contagion and mortality prior to vaccination, acted as a catalyst for the development of telemedicine.

The best definition of telemedicine I was able to find was that of Shashi Gogia [2]: "(Telemedicine) is the use of information and communication technologies (ICTs) to deliver health services where there is physical separation between care providers and/or the recipients over both long and short distances. It is about *transmitting* voice, data, images, and information *rather than moving* care recipients, health professionals, or educators. It encompasses preventive as well as curative aspects of healthcare services for recipients. The interactions can be between care recipient(s), care providers or educators, and lately also computerized devices—standalone, as well as working through a mobile."

It seems to me that it is a definition that meets all the rules of being both specific and exhaustive:

(a) **It is a doctor–patient relationship in which there is a physical distance** (geographical: short or long; or temporal: synchronous or metachronous) between the patient and the doctor.
(b) **It is an interaction focused on communication**: oral or textual, with or without video.
(c) Voices, data, and images **are transmitted**.
(d) It is used in **prevention**, [5, 6] **curative treatments**, [7] **palliative** [8–10] treatments, and **research** [11].
(e) Both the symptoms reported by the patient [12, 13] and **the remote data** [14, 15] are recorded.
(f) **It enables the education** of patients [16, 17] and their families as well as **behavioral change** [18].

There are definitions that are very close to the concept of telemedicine while being distinct; one of them is **Telehealth**, which tries to cover topics that go beyond the doctor–patient relationship to incorporate administrative and educational aspects (both for prevention and health promotion) and the other is **eHealth or Digital Health**, which is a polysemous term that encompasses the interaction between medicine and informatics and covers all aspects of medical care, education, and provision of health services, especially through the Internet.

In this chapter, we will take all these terms as synonyms and use telemedicine as a general term and we will fundamentally deal with communication in the doctor–patient relationship which occurs electronically at a distance.

10.2   Brief History of Telemedicine

We could consider the history of telemedicine as an inevitable consequence of human progress, of the desire to transcend and overcome the limits of nature: from this perspective, the desire to see beyond our eyes and hear beyond our ears is an essential aspect of humanity.

Thus the oral word became written in order to more easily transcend time; and screams and smoke signals transformed into letters to more easily transcend space.

But in the nineteenth century, electricity transformed everything.

The telegraph was first used in the American Civil War to report casualties and request medical services in the mid-nineteenth century and in Australia in the early twentieth century to request assistance from air doctors to patients far from cities [2].

The telephone later supplanted them, with the first telemedicine intervention being requested by its own inventor, Alexander Graham Bell, in 1876, [19].

In the 1920s, television began to be used for diagnosis and consultation of patients. In fact, the University of Nebraska developed a teleconsultation for patients with neurological and psychiatric problems that was a pioneer in this field.

In the 1960s, satellites were the new revolution in telecommunications, and then at the end of the twentieth century, broadband Internet became available to the public, leading to its rapid development. Nowadays, 3G, 4G, 5G mobile devices and other alternatives, are the most current expression of that primordial desire to be able to communicate from a distance.

Telemedicine on Earth is a necessity, especially in underdeveloped, remote, and marginal communities, but when the space race began in the 1950s, it so happened that the most developed, fittest, most sophisticated and carefully selected people needed telemedicine (particularly psychological or psychiatric evaluations from thousands of miles away). Who are we talking about? Astronauts.

This meant that in the United States, India, China, and Russia, space agencies with formidable budgets allocated a significant portion of their money to the design of devices for real-time recording of body variables, location of ailments, image transmission and administration of drugs, and diverse therapies.

The initial models were also tested on earth in similarly isolated locations: residents living in areas with difficult access, workers at maritime oil rigs, high mountain climbers, and in prisons.

Another field of experimentation and development of telemedicine has been widespread crises such as the earthquake that devastated Armenia in 1988, the tsunami that hit Fukushima in 2011 or the recent Covid-19 pandemic worldwide, as well as in the different war conflicts in Croatia, Iraq, Afghanistan, and now in Ukraine that have proven its usefulness for medical assistance and logistics.

The development of robotics for the construction of space stations and the repair of satellites gave rise to surgical robots that are revolutionizing surgery.

Finally, we can see the development of telemedicine as the consequence of a formidable multimillion dollar business opportunity: there are more than 350,000 mobile health applications, which have been developed to assign appointments, remember medications, alert about the appearance of symptoms, help control the stress, record calories consumed, or encourage physical exercise, among many other things.

If we compare classical medicine, as practiced by William Osler and telemedicine, we would find a picture similar to that in Table 10.1:

That is why we should not think that there is a competition between the classical and the modern way of carrying out clinical practice, but rather we should focus on imagining how to integrate the best of both.

The disregard of the "medical touch" that is established in the clinical examination is a mistake that we must not fall into if we want to get the most out of the encounter with the patient and "technophobia" is another mistake that we must avoid if we want to interact using technology at our service and that of our patient.

Table 10.1 Comparison of classic medical consultation with modern teleconsultation

Synchronous	Synchronous or Metachronous
Not registered	Registered
Doctor and patient face to face	Doctor and patient in front of a screen
Anamnesis	Anamnesis
Inspection	Inspection
Palpation	No palpation
Olfaction	No smell
Percussion	No percussion
Auscultation	Auscultation
Blood pressure recording	Blood pressure recording
EKG	EKG
Study observation	Study observation
No GPS	GPS
No biochemical sensors	Multiple biochemical sensors in real time: Oxygen saturation——blood glucose——electrolytes——urine——various substances.
Communicate findings	Communicate findings
Assign forecasts and risks	Assign forecasts and risks
Evaluate therapeutic alternatives	Evaluate therapeutic alternatives
Not artificial intelligence	Artificial intelligence
Make decisions	Make decisions
Record in medical history	Record in medical history
Prescription of master recipes	Electronic prescription of commercial drugs.
Follow-up on subsequent queries	Home monitoring in real time through mobile devices.
Difficult access to the family doctor	Easy accessibility to the GP
Low medical burnout	High medical burnout

We will analyze what we learned in the Covid-19 pandemic about telemedicine and teleconsultations in clinical practice and in the educational field [20–26].

We will start with clinical practice.

10.2.1   Telemedicine and Teleconsultations in the Clinical Practice

The Covid-19 pandemic took us by surprise, not because there were no voices that warned about its risk but because those voices were not heard, and the first stage of fighting this condition was disorganized, improvised, and basically the only tool that worked worldwide was the mandatory isolation of the population.

In Argentina, we experienced one of the most extensive isolation periods, which began on March 20, 2020 and ended in September of that same year. For 6 months, the population (particularly the elderly) was isolated in their homes.

My own workplace, Instituto Oncológico Henry Moore, specializes in the outpatient care of cancer patients. We receive approximately 2500 new cases per year; we administer chemotherapy, immunotherapy, or hormone therapy treatments to approximately ten thousand patients and we have approximately the same number of follow-up patients.

We were therefore faced with the problem of providing care to some 25,000 people and, at the same time, protecting our staff.

How did we do it?

1. We separated our staff into two groups:

   (a) Older people and people with comorbidities (obesity, diabetes, hypertension, cardiovascular or tumor history) who only performed home administrative or medical support tasks.
   (b) The rest of the staff would perform mixed tasks; The assistance teams were divided into two shifts and each of them covered half the week on-site and the other half of the week with telecare.

       We provided the recommended protective material at each stage of the pandemic and only allowed family members to be present in consultations where the patient was incapable of attending alone.

2. We divided the Institute, which has three floors, into two service floors and a Backup floor in case a floor had to be closed.
3. Patients were divided into three groups:

   (a) Those who were undergoing treatment for a curable disease, whose in-person consultations had to remain unchanged.
   (b) Those who were receiving palliative care, where we optimized treatments to administer oral medication where possible, we increased time between doses as much as possible and whose in-person consultations were limited to the minimum necessary for proper care.
   (c) Those patients who were undergoing follow-up checks, where we established teleconsultation as the main form of care. Only in those cases in which it was essential to perform a clinical examination were patients called to the Institute.

The secretarial staff was also divided into two teams to work on alternate days. Two of the twelve secretaries were in charge of receiving in-person patients and the remaining ten were in charge of telephone attention to patients.

The nursing staff was divided into two shifts and the day hospital operation was reduced from 12 to 8 h.

We increased the number of telephone lines from ten to forty. We digitized the telephone exchange for patient telephone assistance. We increased the number of telephone operators from one to eight.

We updated computer technology so that everyone (doctors and administrators) could have remote access to medical records while maintaining confidentiality and security.

We optimized the broadband Internet service so that the access speed was as fast as possible and we provided all staff with 4G-capable mobile phones.

This allowed us to uninterruptedly assist the entire population in treatment and follow-up throughout the pandemic, while only having 22 confirmed cases of Covid-19 out of 141 employees, none of which were fatal.

The closure of the operating rooms and the delay in imaging diagnostic shifts reduced first-time cases by half, but in return, we had more cases of patients with advanced, young, and symptomatic cancers, so the treatment rate was maintained unaltered.

The training of the health team in telecare was protocolized and each of the people who had to interact with patients was evaluated and qualified for the task.

To do this we had to design and adapt virtual communication protocols.

10.3   Virtual Communication Protocols

Below I will transcribe the virtual care protocol that we follow at the institute:

The two access routes for patients were telephone or email.

Therefore, the patient's first point of contact was the telephone operator or one of the secretaries in charge of the email.

1. Telephone Attention Protocol

   (a) Greeting and personal introduction.

      - Good day/afternoon.
      - You are contacting the Henry Moore Institute.
      - My name is:……………………………….
      - Please provide me with the following information.

         – Name and surname.
         – ID number.
         – Telephone number of the person who is calling so that I can contact you again in case this call is disconnected.

      - "How can I help you?" (Reason you are communicating):

         – **If it is due to a case of Covid or probable Covid**:

         – Transfer patient to their Insurance's Covid health care or to the Covid unit from the city of Buenos Aires, who will determine the severity of the condition and whether or not it is necessary to hospitalize the patient (give the appropriate telephone numbers). Request the name of the family doctor and inform the doctor for follow-up on the case.

- **Covid oncological emergency**.
- Refer to the ER.
- **If you are a follow-up or first-time patient who requires clinical consultation**.
- Refer to secretary.
- **If it is a family member calling to report the death of the patient**.
  Refer to secretary

2. Secretarial Attention Protocol

   (a) **If it's a follow-up patient** that requires consultation.

   - Enter the database and identify the patient.
   - If the treating doctor is only teleworking because they are at risk, explain to the patient the situation and the reason why they will be referred to the care of another doctor on the team.
   - Ask if they use WhatsApp and have made video calls.
   - Assign a day and time for teleconsultation when we can contact them. Explain they should be in a private space and that the meeting will last thirty minutes.
   - Inform the name of the doctor who will contact them and the telephone number from which they will do so.

   (b) **If it's a first-time patient** that requires consultation.

   - Enter a new medical history into the database.
   - Request affiliation data for medical history.
   - Request personal phone number and email and that of a trusted family member.
   - Ask if they use WhatsApp and have made video calls.
   - Assign a day and time for teleconsultation in which we can contact them and have a private space for 30 min.
   - Inform the name of the doctor who will contact them and the telephone number from which they will do so.

   (c) **If it is a family member calling to report the death of the patient.**

   - Enter the database.
   - Register the death.
   - Inform the treating doctor.

3. Medical Teleconsultation Protocol

   (a) Establish communication with video call at the agreed time.

   - **Presentation and greeting.**
   - **Ask if the person feels comfortable and has the ability** to have this meeting.
   - **Ask if they are in a safe environment** where privacy and confidentiality are respected.

- **Ask if they wish to use a different phone or if they want to use a computer** (through Zoom, Google Meet, or a similar program).
- **Request an email** to be able to send a written recommendation, if necessary.
- **Establish a communication agenda**:

  - Current health status.
  - Previous illnesses.
  - Medication they are currently taking.
  - Based on the availability of vaccines, we asked about vaccination against covid specifically.
  - Pathological diagnosis of cancer.
  - Imaging studies that have been performed.
  - Reason for current inquiry.
  - Questions they want to ask.
  - Action plan.

    Further studies.
    Medical consultation: assign an in-person appointment if necessary.
    Treatments to be performed.

  - Next consultation to be carried out virtually: set date and time.
  - Leave a communication channel open that they can use (cell phone or doctor's email).
  - Check that all instructions have been understood.
  - Close the query.

- **How should the interview be carried out?**

  - Show understanding of patient and family communication difficulties.

    "I understand how difficult it is to be able to communicate this way."
    "I would like to be able to be there physically to assist you."
    "It is also very difficult for us not to be able to hug and physically examine the patient."
    "These devices are a blessing but they do not replace face- to-face meetings."

  - Look at the camera of your mobile device or computer, not at the screen.

    The equivalent of looking into the eyes of the patient in the in-person consultation is looking into the camera lens.
    Be confident and composed, i.e., stay still and move slowly.
    Inform the patient if you are going to change position or move to reach an object.
    When you listen carefully, if you nod or shake your head, do so very obviously, or it will not be perceived by the patient.

– Speak slowly and show empathy with the patient.

> "I'm here to help you, take all the time you need."
> "I hear anxiety or fear in your voice."
> "I get the impression that this is very difficult for you and your family."

– Restate the salient points of the patient's narrative to ensure that you have correctly understood what the patient or family member has stated.

> "Let's see if I understood properly (relate what you understood...)"
> "From what I understand the sequence was..."
> "If I understood correctly, what you are most interested in is...?
> "Do you have any other questions or other topics that you would like to discuss at this time?"

– Constantly check that the patient or family member understands what you say.

> "Please, if there is anything you don't understand, let's go over it."
> "Is there any point you would like us to look at again?"
> "Although I am going to send them to your email, if you are so kind, can you read me the instructions I gave you?"

– When communicating your conclusions, express them in a language that is understandable and appropriate for each patient.

> If what you are going to communicate is bad news, warn the patient in advance and make sure that they are in a position to listen to it.

> > "What I have to tell you is delicate: do you want us to talk now or do you want us to do it another time? Is there anyone with you at home or near you who can accompany you?"
> > "Unfortunately, at this time, the treatment would present a great risk to you" or similar phrases should mark the context of the pandemic and the risk of complications with a health system that can collapse.

> If a treatment is indicated, the objective of the treatment must be clearly explained:

> > "The treatment that I indicate is intended to cure the disease and therefore we must do it in the following way."
> > "Even though we cannot cure the disease, treatment can help us to significantly prolong survival."
> > "The purpose of the treatment is to try to alleviate the symptoms caused by the disease, which is why we indicate it in this way at this time."

The expected toxicity must be highlighted and the patient's behavior in the event of any adverse effect must be anticipated (at least for the most frequent symptoms):

Nausea and vomiting.
Diarrhea.
Fever.
Mouth sores.
Shortness of breath.

– Close the query.

Explain that the time has come to end the consultation.
Thank the patient for the willingness to teleconsult.
Be happy with the work you were able to do together.
Express the hope or desire that the problems can be resolved and that we can be physically present again.
Repeat your phone or email so the patient can contact you.
Say goodbye.

These were the protocols that we implemented and with which we carried out more than 15,000 virtual consultations during the pandemic.

The most important complications were related to technology (connection difficulties, choppy conversations, interrupted connections), especially from mobile devices; there were fewer problems with connections when using computers, although it should be noted they were used less than phones.

The learning curve was relatively quick and, after 2 weeks of practice, all doctors and administrators showed they were consistently applying the aforementioned protocols.

For most patients, teleconsultation was "the safest way to communicate, but it does not replace a face-to-face meeting." Virtually everyone expressed it that way.

A clear advantage was being able to record what happened to the patient during home follow-up, both after antitumor treatment and in palliative care [13, 14, 27–29].

When it comes to the acceptance of these tools, there are three variables that we must consider [30–38]:

1. Young patients were more satisfied than older patients (probably because they were used to this form of communication pre-pandemic).
2. Patients from provinces other than Buenos Aires and those who lived further away from the city center were more satisfied than patients who lived closer to the center.
3. Control patients were more satisfied with virtual consultations than patients currently receiving treatment.

10.3.1 *Virtual Classes and Exams in Medical Teaching*

Most universities were closed during the Covid-19 pandemic, and student internships were likewise cancelled, especially since young doctors were usually called to work in Covid emergency rooms, which made them a tremendous risk to cancer patients.

Therefore, teaching activity had to be redesigned for the new virtual standard, at least in two aspects: teaching and evaluations [15, 16, 39–60].

In the case of teaching, professors were trained in the use of virtual platforms to organize classes in such a way to ensure active student participation.

The creation of a quiet area at home for the purpose of teaching classes was recommended, as well as the use of virtual backgrounds or a white background while teaching.

Communication with the students was protocolized, with the first class oriented only to the use of their preferred tool (Zoom, Google Meet, or Blackboard) as follows:

1. **Establish individual communication with each of the participants at the beginning of the class**:

   (a) Presentation:

   - Name.
   - Age.
   - Preferred pronoun.
   - Nickname.
   - Hobby.
   - Cell phone number.
   - Email.

   (b) **Recommend a safe place in the home for class participation** where the background is a wall or is virtual or white.
   (c) Find out what network connection capacity you have and whether it needs to be optimized.
   (d) Although it is recommended that the camera remains on during class, if it is intermittent you can turn it off.

2. **Show understanding** of the difficulties in using the tool and virtual classes.

   (a) "I understand how difficult it is to be able to communicate this way."
   (b) "I would like to be able to be physically in front of you in person."
   (c) "It is also difficult for us not to be able to teach normally."
   (d) "These devices are a blessing but they do not replace in-person classes."

3. **Review the tool's use with your students**:

   (a) Check the microphone and camera buttons.
   (b) Practice using chat to ask or answer.

(c) Practice screen sharing for presentations.
(d) Practice how to upload a presentation.

4. **Speak slowly and show empathy** with the student.

(a) "I'm here to help you, take the time you need."

5. **Create an email or WhatsApp group** for group communications.
6. **Explain how the classes will be taught** and attendance will be recorded.
7. **Explain how you will carry out the subject's final exam**:

(a) Questionnaires.
(b) Final group work.
(c) Individual final work.

8. **End the class** [17].

(b) Thank the students for their participation.
(c) Be happy with the work you were able to do together.
(d) Express the hope or desire that the problems can be resolved and that we can be physically present again.
(e) Repeat your phone or email so they can contact you.
(f) Say goodbye.

To ensure student participation, we chose four fundamental strategies:

(a) **Design the class as an exercise in finding the answer to a particular problem**. The answer or answers had to be given at the end of a discussion cycle between students in response to the different questions posed by the teacher.
(b) **Short presentations by students** on the topics to be developed in class. These were used for individual evaluations that were then integrated at the end of the class.
(c) **Debates of positions found among students**. Which facilitated the sharing of ideas.
(d) **Metacognitive questionnaires and post-class reflection tasks**.

Using these protocols and techniques, more than 5000 hours of classes were taught during the pandemic.

There was a learning curve of approximately ten encounters until the teacher was comfortable with their preferred tool.

The students showed a faster adaptation than the teachers and the possibility of sharing the content of the classes, recording them and being able to view them asynchronously and their active participation during the teaching of the subjects, allowed them to become friends with this teaching modality [61–64].

We all learned from this situation. In some cases, we incorporated this practice and maintained it in athenaeums, bibliographic discussions, or research designs, but above all, we revalued the personal teacher–student encounter that allows a much deeper interaction than the virtual one.

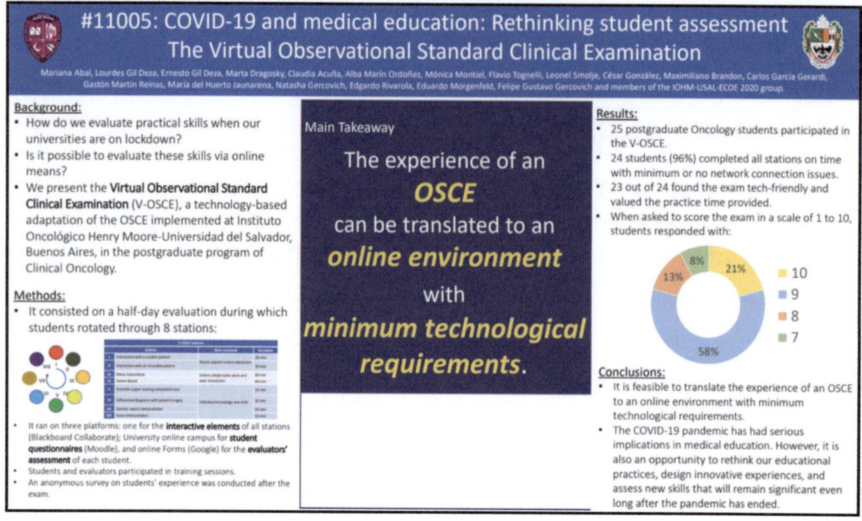

Fig. 10.1 Virtual OSCE poster at ASCO meeting 2021

One of the most important challenges we faced was the transformation of the OSCE (Observational Standard Clinical Examination) into a Virtual OSCE.

Its design and implementation were presented at the American Society Congress of Clinical Oncology (ASCO)) in 2021 as a poster (Fig. 10.1).

By redesigning the exam, it was not only feasible to implement it virtually but also to evaluate communication skills in telemedicine.

Clearly this form of communication through computer systems between two natural intelligences, that of the doctor and that of the patient, poses the enormous challenge of the possibility of the patient interacting with an artificial intelligence without being able to distinguish it from human intelligence.

This challenge leads us to have to analyze the role of artificial intelligence in current medicine and the role of medical humanism in the new reality of the twenty-first century.

10.4 Artificial Intelligence, Telemedicine, and Medical Humanism

In order to analyze the impact of artificial intelligence (AI) on modern medicine, we must begin with the story of Alan (Turing) and Eliza.

Turing was a computer genius who, from a very young age, became interested in cryptography and especially in the possibility of mathematically analyzing language.

This allowed him to design a machine capable of deciphering the encryption method of another machine, called "enigma," which was used to encrypt the messages that the Nazis sent to their combat units, especially naval ones.

"Enigma" was a servo-electric rotor machine, patented in 1918 and marketed from 1923 to encrypt commercial transactions, it was adopted by the German navy in 1926 and later by the other German military forces. The machine designed for commercial purposes used three rotors, the military ones between five and seven rotors, so they had hundreds of thousands of possible combinations.

We must understand that the German submarine force, the so-called U-boats, was one of the most effective elements in the fight for control of the sea, and therefore, for war supplies in the Second World War.

Intercepting their communications and deciphering the orders they received saved countless lives and shortened the duration of the war by several years.

This was possible thanks to the genius of Alan Turing who understood that only a machine could defeat another machine and to the Nazi obedience who signed all the reports with the greeting "Heil Hitler." Knowing what to search for allowed them to find it.

Eliza's story [65–70] was the first intersection of a computer program (artificial intelligence that emulated Carl Rogers' psychoanalytic empathy), telemedicine, and medical humanism.

"Eliza" was a computer program designed by Joseph Wizenbaum of MIT in the 1960s and was the first conversational bot on medical aspects, in this case, it emulated a consultation with a psychiatrist.

The "conversation" was started by a human and the program selected some key words and responded with a question or comment, giving the interlocutor the sensation of an empathetic response.

We can see a copy of a dialogue with Eliza extracted from the article by Benton et al. [71] or in the web.

Eliza's success was extraordinary, the interlocutor quickly forgot that he was "talking" to a machine, that "he was not thinking what he was saying" but was running an algorithm that emulated an interaction.

It is something similar [71, 72] to what happens with ChatGPT, which is **G**enerative, **P**retrained artificial intelligence based on **Transformers**.

It is not our intention to delve into what artificial intelligence is, [73–76] we simply want to highlight that the use of transformers [75] means that it can give a different value to each term according to the linguistic context in which it is expressed and that allows it to interpret the meaning of a phrase with increasing precision (distinguishing the literal from the ironic, humorous, reflective, etc.).

This gives you much greater subtlety and allows you to find more appropriate responses to the listener.

On the other hand, being pretrained [77] with billions of terabytes of writings, speeches, works of art and all kinds of human interventions, its repertoire is increasingly broader.

It is not uncommon for the interaction to use words like "please" or "thank you" from the human to the machine, in a similar way to what we would use with another human.

On the other hand, the performance of the first artificial intelligences was between bad and modest, but the most modern ones show, in the medical field, a performance similar to that of a doctor with an above average GPA, which makes them very good.

This is so important that we must accept that today artificial intelligence is the eighth epistemic order: patients use it to inform themselves, educate themselves, and make decisions.

We currently use artificial intelligence in medicine to improve pathologists' diagnoses; discern the drivers of a tumor in molecular pathology; help radiologists identify tiny lesions; plan the best route to robotically remove an organ; embolize an aneurysm or design a drug. We must now also add that our patients can freely ask private questions and often find a correct answer with the use of AI.

What then is the role of the doctor in these situations?

We must incorporate this tool into our clinical practice, understanding that it will allow us to individualize with increasing precision the most effective treatment for the patient's pathology, but our role will be to do something beyond individualizing it, personalizing it.

What is the difference between individualizing and personalizing?

Individualization is finding the specific differences in a certain disease that make it more susceptible to being treated with a certain substance or through a certain sequence.

What are you most sensitive to? In what dose? Managed in what way? For how long? Where in the world?

These are answers that artificial intelligence will allow us to obtain in microseconds. Of course, it will have all the biases that current publications have, that is, it will tend to prioritize the most recent and most expensive, over the old and cheap, but it is the same thing that happens with current medical natural intelligence: the influence of marketing will also affect artificial intelligence.

So what does it mean to personalize?

Personalizing is knowing our patient, their values, fears, desires, and hopes. What makes them unique in our eyes? What distinguishes them from others, why do they want to be treated and for what purpose?

For artificial intelligence, each patient will be another case of a certain ailment, for the doctor each patient must be a unique person affected by a certain ailment.

If we as doctors do not know our patient, their environment, their desires, and their fears, then we will not be able to provide something that no other intelligence can do: prudent advice to a suffering patient.

Artificial intelligence will allow us to better aim increasingly powerful weapons, medical humanity will tell us when we should shoot and when we should refrain from doing so.

No medication is more powerful than that which is administered by a conscientious physician to an unsuspecting patient.

This encounter between trust and awareness is the foundation of the doctor–patient relationship, which is essentially therapeutic in itself.

We can imagine something similar in the field of bioethics.

It is not complex to design an algorithm that optimizes cost/effectiveness to levels of great sophistication.

Now, is cost/effectiveness or cost/efficiency the most humane way to manage values?

Algorithmic bioethics will allow us to analyze a problem from a principalist perspective, it will even allow us to allocate resources in a more balanced and transparent way, but it will always be insufficient to address bioethical problems if we lose sight of the uniqueness of the people involved and the context in which they occur.

That is where listening, dialogue, and deliberation allow us to find an optimal path where the least number of values are harmed or the greatest number of them are promoted.

We can use our trusted moral compass to help us reflect and navigate this new, AI fueled map, but the decision will always be real, because no matter how clear the map is, it is still only a representation of reality, not reality itself.

Not incorporating artificial intelligence into our practice is a mistake of the same magnitude as incorporating it without proper critical thought.

For the good of our patients, we must do it in a proactive and prudent way.

10.5 Teaching Exercises

1. Personal

    (a) Do you have experience in telemedicine?
    (b) Do you follow a certain communication protocol?
    (c) What do you find most difficult in virtual communication?
    (d) Do you use artificial intelligence in your daily life? Could you indicate the fields in which you use it?
    (e) Do you use artificial intelligence in your professional life? Could you indicate in what situations you use it?
    (f) Do your patients use artificial intelligence? How do you feel about it?
    (g) Do you feel like artificial intelligence competes with any of your domains?
    (h) Do you recognize the difference between individualizing a treatment and personalizing a treatment?

2. Group

    (a) Design a teleconsultation protocol for first-time patients who call your institution.
    (b) Design a bot service protocol for assigning queries in your service.

(c) Get together in a group and ask a scientific question, such as the efficacy of a given drug or treatments for a given disease. Then do a search on Pubmed or a similar database and select the answer that you consider the most appropriate.

   • Do the same exercise by asking ChatGPT. Notice the differences.

      – Ask the program to optimize the question or refine the answers.
      – How many steps did it take?
      – How long did it take you?
      – What is the most notable difference between the first and the second way of seeking the truth?

(d) Select one person in the group whom everyone considers to be the greatest expert on a topic and ask him or her to design the index of a book on that topic in ten chapters. Note how long it takes and what topics they cover.

   • Ask Chat GPT or similar to design an index of ten chapters on the same topic. Observe the time it takes and the topics it covers.

(e) With the group, design a seven-slide presentation for a ten-minute class on a certain topic.

   • Ask Chat GPT or similar to design the same.

(f) Take a scientific text and translate it as a group into your language. Notice how long it took.

   • Take the same text and use a translator like Google and see how long it took and the differences with the group-produced text.

References

1. Frehse AE. Overview and history of telehealth in telemedicine: overview and application in pulmonary, critical care, and sleep medicine. 2021. https://doi.org/10.1007/978-3-030-64050-7_1.
2. Gogia S. Rationale, history, and basics of telehealth. In: Fundamentals of telemedicine and telehealth; 2019. https://doi.org/10.1016/B978-0-12-814309-4.00002-1.
3. Masys DR. Telemedicine: a guide to assessing telecommunications in health care. J Am Med Inform Assoc. 1997;4:2. https://doi.org/10.1136/jamia.1997.0040136.
4. Field MJ. Telemedicine: a guide to assessing telecommunications in healthcare. J Digit Imaging. 1997;10(3 SUPPL. 1) https://doi.org/10.1007/bf03168648.
5. Hubschman-Shahar LE. Lactation telehealth in primary care: a systematic review. Breastfeed Med. 2022;17:1. https://doi.org/10.1089/bfm.2021.0105.
6. Kalb LG, Kramer JM, Goode TD, et al. Evaluation of telemental health services for people with intellectual and developmental disabilities: protocol for a randomized non-inferiority trial. BMC Health Serv Res. 2023;23:1. https://doi.org/10.1186/s12913-023-09663-6.
7. Kloosterman EM, Rosman JZ, Berkowitz EJ, Rosenbaum M, Wettenstein Z. Remote-control interrogation, testing, and reprogramming of cardiac implantable electronic devices with tele-

health protocol for the Management of Patients at home: the DOMUM REMOTUS study. J Innov Card Rhythm Manag. 2023;14:2. https://doi.org/10.19102/icrm.2023.14024.

8. Santos DS, Batistelli CRS, Lara MMDS, Ferreira EDS, Moreira TR, Cotta RMM. The effectiveness of the use of telehealth programs in the care of individuals with hypertension and, or diabetes mellitus: systematic review and meta-analysis. Diabetol Metab Syndr. 2022;14:1. https://doi.org/10.1186/s13098-022-00846-5.

9. Cho Y, Yang R, Gong Y, Jiang Y. Use of electronic communication with clinicians among cancer survivors: health information National Trend Survey in 2019 and 2020. Telemed e-Health. 2023;29(6) https://doi.org/10.1089/tmj.2022.0203.

10. Ostan R, Varani S, Giannelli A, et al. Distance monitoring of advanced cancer patients with impaired cardiac and respiratory function assisted at home: a study protocol in Italy. J Clin Med. 2023;12:5. https://doi.org/10.3390/jcm12051922.

11. Petrova EV, Avadhanula V, Michel S, Gincoo KE, Piedra PA, Anandasabapathy S. Remote laboratory management: respiratory virus diagnostics. J Vis Exp. 2019;2019:146. https://doi.org/10.3791/59188.

12. Vercell A, Gasteiger N, Yorke J, Dowding D. Patient-facing cancer mobile apps that enable patient reported outcome data to be collected: a systematic review of content, functionality, quality, and ability to integrate with electronic health records. Int J Med Inform. 2023:170, 104931. https://doi.org/10.1016/j.ijmedinf.2022.104931.

13. Chung AE, Basch EM. Incorporating the patient's voice into electronic health records through patient-reported outcomes as the "review of systems.". J Am Med Inform Assoc. 2015;22:4. https://doi.org/10.1093/jamia/ocu007.

14. Prinsen CAC, Mokkink LB, Bouter LM, et al. COSMIN guideline for systematic reviews of patient-reported outcome measures. Qual Life Res. 2018;27:5. https://doi.org/10.1007/s11136-018-1798-3.

15. Klonoff DC, Shang T, Zhang JY, Cengiz E, Mehta C, Kerr D. Digital connectivity: the sixth vital sign. J Diabetes Sci Technol. 2022;16:5. https://doi.org/10.1177/19322968211015241.

16. Cooke A, Castellanos S, Enriquez C, et al. Telehealth for management of chronic non-cancer pain and opioid use disorder in safety net primary care. BMC Health Serv Res. 2023;23(1) https://doi.org/10.1186/s12913-023-09330-w.

17. Zhou C, Pavlakos R, Clark M, Jue VI, Clinard VB. Pharmacy telehealth services: perspectives from an Academic Medical Center. J Pharm Pract. 2023;36(2) https://doi.org/10.1177/08971900211030652.

18. Snoswell CL, Haydon HM, Kelly JT, Thomas EE, Caffery LJ, Smith AC. How do consumers prefer their care delivered: in-person, telephone or videoconference? J Telemed Telecare. 2023. Published online; https://doi.org/10.1177/1357633X231160333.

19. Aronson SH. The lancet on the telephone 1876–1975. Med Hist. 1977;21(1) https://doi.org/10.1017/S0025727300037182.

20. Monaghesh E, Hajizadeh A. The role of telehealth during COVID-19 outbreak: a systematic review based on current evidence. BMC Public Health. 2020;20(1) https://doi.org/10.1186/s12889-020-09301-4.

21. Wosik J, Fudim M, Cameron B, et al. Telehealth transformation: COVID-19 and the rise of virtual care. J Am Med Inform Assoc. 2020;(6):27. https://doi.org/10.1093/jamia/ocaa067.

22. Chi NC, Demiris G. A systematic review of telehealth tools and interventions to support family caregivers. J Telemed Telecare. 2015;21(1) https://doi.org/10.1177/1357633X14562734.

23. Keenan AJ, Cert G, Tsourtos G, Tieman J. The value of applying ethical principles in telehealth practices: systematic review. J Med Internet Res. 2021;23(3) https://doi.org/10.2196/25698.

24. Snoswell CL, Stringer H, Taylor ML, Caffery LJ, Smith AC. An overview of the effect of telehealth on mortality: a systematic review of meta-analyses. J Telemed Telecare. 2021 . Published online; https://doi.org/10.1177/1357633X211023700.

25. Valentine AZ, Hall SS, Young E, et al. Implementation of telehealth services to assess, monitor, and treat neurodevelopmental disorders: systematic review. J Med Internet Res. 2021;23(1) https://doi.org/10.2196/22619.

26. Lundereng ED, Nes AAG, Holmen H, et al. Health care professionals' experiences and perspectives on using telehealth for home-based palliative care: scoping review. J Med Internet Res. 2023:25. https://doi.org/10.2196/43429.

27. Churruca K, Pomare C, Ellis LA, et al. Patient-reported outcome measures (PROMs): a review of generic and condition-specific measures and a discussion of trends and issues. Health Expect. 2021;24(4) https://doi.org/10.1111/hex.13254.

28. Wiering B, de Boer D, Delnoij D. Patient involvement in the development of patient-reported outcome measures: a scoping review. Health Expect. 2017;20(1) https://doi.org/10.1111/hex.12442.

29. Meirte J, Hellemans N, Anthonissen M, et al. Benefits and disadvantages of electronic patient-reported outcome measures: systematic review. JMIR Perioper Med. 2020;3(1) https://doi.org/10.2196/15588.

30. Edirippulige S, Armfield NR. Education and training to support the use of clinical telehealth: a review of the literature. J Telemed Telecare. 2016;23(2) https://doi.org/10.1177/1357633X16632968.

31. Snoswell CL, Chelberg G, De Guzman KR, et al. The clinical effectiveness of telehealth: a systematic review of meta-analyses from 2010 to 2019. J Telemed Telecare. Published online. 2021; https://doi.org/10.1177/1357633x211022907.

32. Jennett PA, Affleck Hall L, Hailey D, et al. The socio-economic impact of telehealth: a systematic review. J Telemed Telecare. 2003;9(6) https://doi.org/10.1258/135763303771005207.

33. Cox A, Lucas G, Marcu A, et al. Cancer survivors' experience with telehealth: a systematic review and thematic synthesis. J Med Internet Res. 2017;19(1) https://doi.org/10.2196/jmir.6575.

34. Peters GM, Kooij L, Lenferink A, Van Harten WH, Doggen CJM. The effect of telehealth on hospital services use: systematic review and meta-analysis. J Med Internet Res. 2021;23(9) https://doi.org/10.2196/25195.

35. Totten AM, Womack DM, Griffin JC, et al. Telehealth-guided provider-to-provider communication to improve rural health: a systematic review. J Telemed Telecare. 2022; https://doi.org/10.1177/1357633X221139892. Published online

36. Kidd L, Cayless S, Johnston B, Wengstrom Y. Telehealth in palliative care in the UK: a review of the evidence. J Telemed Telecare. 2010;16(7) https://doi.org/10.1258/jtt.2010.091108.

37. Kamei T, Kanamori T, Yamamoto Y, Edirippulige S. The use of wearable devices in chronic disease management to enhance adherence and improve telehealth outcomes: a systematic review and meta-analysis. J Telemed Telecare. 2022;28(5) https://doi.org/10.1177/1357633X20937573.

38. Doraiswamy S, Abraham A, Mamtani R, Cheema S. Use of telehealth during the COVID-19 pandemic: scoping review. J Med Internet Res. 2020;22(12) https://doi.org/10.2196/24087.

39. Eckhoff DO, Diaz DA, Anderson M. Using simulation to teach intraprofessional telehealth communication. Clin Simul Nurs. 2022:67. https://doi.org/10.1016/j.ecns.2022.03.006.

40. Kamalova L, Gaifullina R, Umbetova MZ, Novgorodtseva IV. Telehealth communication strategies of medical students in the context of the COVID-19 pandemic. Educ Self Dev. 2022;17(3) https://doi.org/10.26907/esd.17.3.18.

41. Wright HH, O'Shea MC, Sekula J, Mitchell LJ. Assessment of communication skills using telehealth: considerations for educators. Front Med (Lausanne). 2022;9. https://doi.org/10.3389/fmed.2022.841309.

42. Street RL, Treiman K, Kranzler EC, et al. Oncology patients' communication experiences during COVID-19: comparing telehealth consultations to in-person visits. Support Care Cancer. 2022;30(6) https://doi.org/10.1007/s00520-022-06897-8.

43. Weaver MS, Lukowski J, Wichman B, Navaneethan H, Fisher AL, Neumann ML. Human connection and technology connectivity: a systematic review of available telehealth survey instruments. J Pain Symptom Manag. 2021;61(5) https://doi.org/10.1016/j.jpainsymman.2020.10.010.

44. van Galen LS, Wang CJ, Nanayakkara PWB, Paranjape K, Kramer MHH, Car J. Telehealth requires expansion of physicians' communication competencies training. Med Teach. 2019;41(6) https://doi.org/10.1080/0142159X.2018.1481284.

45. Simacek J, Elmquist M, Dimian AF, Reichle J. Current trends in telehealth applications to deliver social communication interventions for young children with or at risk for autism spectrum disorder. Curr Dev Disord Rep. 2021;8(1) https://doi.org/10.1007/s40474-020-00214-w.

46. Hajjar L, Kragen B. Timely communication through telehealth: added value for a caregiver during COVID-19. Front Public Health. 2021:9. https://doi.org/10.3389/fpubh.2021.755391.

47. Lama Y, Davidoff AJ, Vanderpool RC, Jensen RE. Telehealth availability and use of related technologies among Medicare-enrolled cancer survivors: cross-sectional findings from the onset of the COVID-19 pandemic. J Med Internet Res. 2022;24(1) https://doi.org/10.2196/34616.

48. Craig EA, Dounavi K, Ferguson J. Effectiveness of a brief functional analysis and functional communication training conducted through telehealth. J Dev Phys Disabil. 2023;35(2) https://doi.org/10.1007/s10882-022-09857-6.

49. Rietdijk R, Power E, Attard M, Heard R, Togher L. A clinical trial investigating telehealth and in-person social communication skills training for people with traumatic Brain injury: participant-reported communication outcomes. J Head Trauma Rehabil. 2020;35(4) https://doi.org/10.1097/HTR.0000000000000554.

50. Weaver MS, Neumann ML, Navaneethan H, Robinson JE, Hinds PS. Human touch via touchscreen: rural nurses' experiential perspectives on telehealth use in pediatric hospice care. J Pain Symptom Manag. 2020;60(5) https://doi.org/10.1016/j.jpainsymman.2020.06.003.

51. Soltwisch M, Howden E. Clinician-led telehealth follow-up communications: a potential solution for primary care. Consultant. 2022;62(9) https://doi.org/10.25270/con.2022.04.00001.

52. Rivet EB, Edwards C, Lange P, Haynes S, Feldman M, Cholyway R. Telehealth training for surgeons to empathetically deliver bad news via video-mediated communication. Am Surg. 2023;89(3) https://doi.org/10.1177/00031348211030458.

53. Duane JN, Blanch-Hartigan D, Sanders JJ, et al. Environmental considerations for effective telehealth encounters: a narrative review and implications for best practice. Telemed e-Health. 2022;28(3) https://doi.org/10.1089/tmj.2021.0074.

54. Rietdijk R, Power E, Brunner M, Togher L. Protocol for a clinical trial of telehealth-based social communication skills training for people with traumatic brain injury and their communication partners. Brain Impairment. 2019. Published online; https://doi.org/10.1017/BrImp.2019.9.

55. Colucci M, Baldo V, Baldovin T, Bertoncello C. A "matter of communication": a new classification to compare and evaluate telehealth and telemedicine interventions and understand their effectiveness as a communication process. Health Informatics J. 2019;25(2) https://doi.org/10.1177/1460458217747109.

56. Wittenberg E, Goldsmith JV, Chen C, Prince-Paul M, Johnson RR. Opportunities to improve COVID-19 provider communication resources: a systematic review. Patient Educ Couns. 2021;104(3) https://doi.org/10.1016/j.pec.2020.12.031.

57. Shirvani MM, Rezaee N, Nasirodin Tabatabaei SM, Navidian A. The effect of telehealth communication on anxiety, depression, and visits of family members of COVID-19 patients admitted to intensive care units. Med Surg Nurs J. 2023;11(4) https://doi.org/10.5812/msnj-136064.

58. van Houwelingen CTM, Moerman AH, Ettema RGA, Kort HSM, ten Cate O. Competencies required for nursing telehealth activities: a Delphi-study. Nurse Educ Today. 2016:39. https://doi.org/10.1016/j.nedt.2015.12.025.

59. Skelly K, Thompson JA, Chu K, et al. Teachers' perspectives on communication in the context of supervising learners during telehealth encounters. Qual Health Commun. 2023;2(1) https://doi.org/10.7146/qhc.v2i1.132129.

60. Tarbi EC, Durieux BN, Brain JM, et al. Measuring palliative care communication via telehealth: a pilot study. J Pain Symptom Manag. 2023;66(1) https://doi.org/10.1016/j.jpainsymman.2023.04.001.

61. Hindman D, Windish D, Michtalik H, Bertram A, Prichett L, Pahwa A. An educational needs assessment of telehealth in primary care among US internal medicine residents. South Med J. 2023;116(6) https://doi.org/10.14423/SMJ.0000000000001568.
62. Bajra R, Frazier W, Graves L, et al. Feasibility and acceptability of a US National Telemedicine Curriculum for medical students and residents: multi-institutional cross-sectional study. JMIR Med Educ. 2023:9. https://doi.org/10.2196/43190.
63. Demiris G, Edison K, Schopp LH. Shaping the future: needs and expectations of telehealth professionals. Telemed e-Health. 2004;10(SUPPL. 2) https://doi.org/10.1089/tmj.2004.10.s-60.
64. Cardile D, Corallo F, Cappadona I, et al. Auditing the audits: a systematic review on different procedures in telemedicine. Int J Environ Res Public Health. 2023;20(5) https://doi.org/10.3390/ijerph20054484.
65. Weizenbaum J. ELIZA—A Computer program for the study of natural language communication between man and machine. Commun ACM. 1983;26(1) https://doi.org/10.1145/357980.357991.
66. Shah H, Warwick K, Vallverdú J, Wu D. Can machines talk? Comparison of Eliza with modern dialogue systems. Comput Human Behav. 2016:58. https://doi.org/10.1016/j.chb.2016.01.004.
67. Bassett C. The computational therapeutic: exploring Weizenbaum's ELIZA as a history of the present. AI Soc. 2019;34(4) https://doi.org/10.1007/s00146-018-0825-9.
68. Rajaraman V. From ELIZA to ChatGPT. Resonance. 2023;28:6. https://doi.org/10.1007/s12045-023-1620-6.
69. Affsprung D. The ELIZA defect. 2023; https://doi.org/10.1145/3600211.3604744.
70. Natale S. If software is narrative: Joseph Weizenbaum, artificial intelligence and the biographies of ELIZA. New Media Soc. 2019;21(3) https://doi.org/10.1177/1461444818804980.
71. Benton MC. Evaluating quality of chatbots and intelligent conversational agents; 2017. https://www.researchgate.net/publication/316184347
72. Kirakowski J, O'Donnell P, Yiu A. The perception of artificial intelligence as "human" by computer users. In: Lecture notes in computer science (including subseries lecture notes in artificial intelligence and lecture notes in bioinformatics), vol. 4552. LNCS; 2007. https://doi.org/10.1007/978-3-540-73110-8_40.
73. Le Cun Y. Learning process in an asymmetric threshold network. Disordered Systems and Biological Organization; 1986. https://doi.org/10.1007/978-3-642-82657-3_24.
74. Sermanet P, Cun YL, Krizhevsky A, et al. Regression methods for localization. Comput Vis Pattern Recognit Workshop. 2014;518(5)
75. Conneau A, Schwenk H, Cun YL, Barrault L. Very deep convolutional networks for text classification. In: *15th Conference of the European Chapter of the Association for Computational Linguistics, EACL 2017—Proceedings of Conference.* Vol 2.; 2017. doi:10.18653/v1/e17-1104.
76. Lepetit V. Yann Le Cun, Turing prize 2018: profound ideas. Bulletin 1024. 2019;14 https://doi.org/10.48556/sif.1024.14.99.
77. Bottou L, Le Cun Y. Large scale online learning. Advances in Neural Information Processing Systems; 2004.

Chapter 11
Communication and Burnout Prevention

11.1 Introduction

The history of Burnout syndrome, defined as personal exhaustion resulting from work stress, can be traced back to the Bible itself: in chapter 18 of the book of Exodus, Moses' father-in-law recommends that he organize and delegate tasks, as otherwise he would be exhausted (Exodus chapter 18, 17–18).

The first medical description of what we know today as Burnout syndrome can be seen in George Beard's publication [1] in the precursor to the New England Journal of Medicine, which we can see in the following Fig. 11.1.

THE

BOSTON MEDICAL AND SURGICAL JOURNAL.

NEW SERIES.] THURSDAY, APRIL 29, 1869. [VOL. III.—No. 13.

Original Communications.

NEURASTHENIA, OR NERVOUS EXHAUS-
TION.

By GEORGE BEARD, M.D., Lecturer on Nervous Diseases in the University of New York.

I AM to speak to-night of a *condition* of the system that is, perhaps, more frequently than any other, in our time at least, the cause and effect of disease.

I refer to *neurasthenia*, or exhaustion of the nervous system.

in the habit of employing the term *neurasthenia* to express the morbid state that is commonly indicated by the indefinite phrase nervous exhaustion.

This nomenclature would seem to be justified by philological analogy, by scientific convenience, and by actual necessity.

The derivation of the term *neurasthenia* is sufficiently obvious. It comes from the Greek νευρον, " a nerve," *a*, privative, and σθενος, " strength; " and, therefore, being literally interpreted signifies want of strength in the nerve.

The character of this malady, if I be al-

Fig. 11.1 Original article by Beard in the Boston Medical and Surgical Journal

© The Author(s), under exclusive license to Springer Nature Switzerland AG 2024

E. Gil Deza, *Improving Clinical Communication*,
https://doi.org/10.1007/978-3-031-62446-9_11

Let us remember that Beard's description is greatly influenced by the experience of the United States Civil War that had ended a few years before and by the vitalist ideas of the time period, which held that "vital force" defined not only anatomical structure but also the correct function of organs [2].

Hence the large number of tonics, many of them harmless, many of them dangerous, that were used to treat these conditions.

In the history of medicine, many changes of great magnitude are the consequence of observations sent to prestigious journals in the form of letters or short writings: the description of Korotkoff sounds to non-invasively determine blood pressure through [3] auscultation in 1905, Hans Selye's letter to Nature [4–6] for the first description of stress as a cause of disease on July 4, 1936 and Charles Perou's letter [7] to Nature on August 17, 2000 on the different molecular types in breast cancer, are three outstanding examples of small publications that generated a revolution in medical ideas.

I say this simply to highlight that there are many who publish tons of papers without use or meaning, and there are others who in four lines of writing change the history of science and health, because they modify our way of detecting or looking at a disease.

Hans Selye had that virtue, he was the first who helped us see what it was that diseases had in common.

Until that moment, most doctors were looking for a small difference that could give their own name to a symptom, syndrome, or semiological maneuver. Medicine was overflowing with eponyms, each one of them implied a small difference.

Selye looked at the common effects of all diseases and described stress as a syndrome of adaptation to all of them, a common reaction to an aggression of any nature, acute or chronic.

Starting in the 1950s, more and more causes of stress were detected and in the 1970s, [8] Herbert Freudenberger described Burnout as the syndrome resulting from work-related stress in health personnel.

Maslach later designed the most widely used instrument for its detection and treatment [9, 10].

11.2 What is Burnout Syndrome in the Health Team?

It is a state of progressive health impairment due to caring for a fellow human being.

It is related to the perception of suffering while at the same being aware of the personal or communal limitation of alleviating it.

This leads to the loss of incentive to continue performing the task, which becomes routine, mechanical, distant, and accompanied by the feeling of uselessness.

The professional perceives his role as that of an actor in a bad play; he does not want to leave the stage, but is dissatisfied with the script and his performance.

This leads to several symptoms, including depersonalization, isolation, shame, depression, loss of joy, lack of communication, increase in the use of toxic substances (alcohol, tobacco, sedatives, and illegal drugs), absenteeism, job abandonment, family crisis, and suicide.

This doesn't happen overnight. It is a process characterized by the silencing of emotions and relationships.

If we had to describe burnout in the health team, we would do so using Maslach's description: "The exhaustion dimension was also described as wearing out, loss of energy, depletion, debilitation, and fatigue. The cynicism dimension was originally called depersonalization (given the nature of human services occupations), but was also described as negative or inappropriate attitudes towards clients, irritability, loss of idealism, and withdrawal. The ineffectiveness dimension was originally called reduced personal accomplishment, and was also described as reduced productivity or capability, low morale, and an inability to cope." [9].

These three elements: exhaustion, cynicism, and lack of commitment, we will analyze below.

11.2.1   Exhaustion Syndrome Appears First

What does being exhausted mean?

According to the National Board of Health and Welfare in Sweden (Table 11.1).

Table 11.1   Diagnostic criteria for exhaustion disorder [11]

(a) Physical and mental symptoms of exhaustion during at least 2 weeks. The symptoms have developed in response to one or more identifiable stressors, which have been present for at least 6 months

(b) Markedly reduced mental energy, manifested by reduced initiative, lack of endurance, or increased time needed for recovery after mental efforts

(c) At least four of the following symptoms have been present most of the day, nearly every day, during the same 2-week period:
1. Persistent complaints of impaired memory and concentration
2. Markedly reduced capacity to tolerate demands or to perform under time pressure
3. Emotional instability or irritability
4. Insomnia or hypersomnia
5. Persistent complaints of physical fatigue and lack of endurance
6. Physical symptoms such as muscular pain, chest pain, palpitations, gastrointestinal problems, vertigo, or increased sensitivity to sounds

(d) The symptoms cause clinically significant distress or impairment in social, occupational, or other important areas of functioning

(e) The symptoms are not due to the direct physiological effects of a substance (e.g., abuse of a drug or medication) or a general medical condition (e.g., hypothyroidism, diabetes, infectious disease)

(f) If criteria for major depression, dysthymia, or generalized anxiety disorder are met simultaneously, exhaustion disorder is set as an additional specification to any such diagnosis

As we see, this syndrome has several physical, mental, emotional, and relational components.

All of them must be long-lasting, being present for at least 2 weeks in order to be considered as components of burnout.

It is very reasonable that many of them affect us occasionally at some point, if only for a short time.

Among the physical symptoms are persistent fatigue, even before starting a task, persistent muscle pain, palpitations, gastrointestinal disorders, vertigo, or increased sensitivity to sounds, especially high-pitched ones. All of these, without us being able to attribute them to any disease or medication that we are taking or have recently stopped taking.

Among the mental symptoms are lack of initiative, attention, commitment, or the need to recover after an effort such as paying attention, reading a manuscript, or a medical history.

Among the mood symptoms are loss of memory or concentration. Emotional instability. Insomnia or hypersomnia. Rapid fatigue or lack of consistency. Depression or anxiety.

Among the relationship symptoms are irritability and intolerance to work demands or time pressure, all of which increases conflict in the team.

11.2.2   Cynicism and Detachment

As a consequence of exhaustion, the doctor, nurse, psychologist, or administrator (or any of the members of the health team) distances themselves from the person they must care for. Their task seems to be minor, performed in a stereotyped, mechanized way, and no longer provides satisfaction. It may even come to be regarded as despicable.

The feeling arises that anyone could do the task, or that the task could be done in any way the professional desires.

Patients are seen as cases, things, or numbers. The medical task is seen as a deceptive performance, a fraud.

11.2.3   Ineffectiveness and Lack of Accomplishment

These feelings continue to deepen and those affected begin to abandon their obligations, delegating tasks they shouldn't, and not showing up for work.

It is a vicious circle in which the feeling that work is useless leads to doing worse work and therefore creates as a self-fulfilling prophecy.

There is a direct relationship between burnout syndrome and work, family and personal conflict.

From this perspective, burnout is "contagious" because as it generates conflict in the team, it generates greater stress that exponentially increases conflict.

There is also a direct correlation between burnout and physical health. This relationship is complex—people affected by chronic situations (obesity, hypertension, diabetes) are more likely to suffer from Burnout and Burnout worsens chronic disease conditions.

Therefore, one of the most important responsibilities of the team leader or coordinator is to detect what is happening among members of their team.

Every time there is conflict, there is an opportunity to evaluate what is happening to each of us and what is happening to the relationship between us all.

That is, facing the burnout of one of the team members as a symptom of an illness that affects the team and is manifested by its most sensitive members.

The important thing about the topic we're discussing in this chapter is that the most important tool to be able to deal with this problem is the word.

In order to put into words what happens to us, it is the task of the team coordinators to approach those who begin to isolate themselves, it is the task of their colleagues to ask if they can help them with something and it is the task of those who begin to feel affected by their work as a caregiver to ask themselves: *What's wrong with me? What triggered this crisis? What are the alternatives I see to get out of it? Am I taking care of my life? Have I abandoned my duties?*

Putting into words the feelings and emotions that affect us, as well as having an environment in which one is listened to, is the way to prevent and treat Burnout syndrome.

11.3   Why Is it Difficult for us to Accept that We Are Stressed and that we May be Suffering from this Syndrome?

In my experience, and after an exhaustive review of published papers on the matter, there are two barriers that prevent us from recognizing burnout: difficulty in recognizing our [12–36] own vulnerability and a resistance to seeing medicine as a cause of illness.

Talking about our vulnerability is facing our fears.

In my personal case, I have four big fears: the fear of causing harm to someone in my family (in the case of Covid, the fear of infecting them), the fear of making a mistake, the fear of madness, and the fear of death.

When we face our fears, they lose their strength to the extent that we are able to contemplate them and discover what lies beneath: the love for those around us, the value of truth, the light of reason, and the desire to live.

It is very difficult to love and not fear that something undesirable will happen to those you love; to cultivate the search for truth and not be afraid to make mistakes; to strive to exercise order, logic, memory and not fear chaos; it is very difficult to be grateful for the life you have and enjoy living it and not fear losing it.

In some way, the work we do in healthcare, our choice of practicing medicine and the specialty that each person practices are also manifestations of the fear that we want to combat.

Being able to talk about it with other team members allows you to share these ideas and feelings.

We often see that when this communication happens, we have a lot more in common than we think and many of us are experiencing the same anguish. That is why, sometimes, the voice of the first person to put their troubles into words is also the voice of many who feel the same, but have not yet found the words to express it.

Secondly, it is difficult to recognize that the art and science of healing is a cause of illness for some people.

We don't talk about the risk of contracting an infection when treating a patient, even though Hepatitis, HIV, tuberculosis, SARS, and Covid have been responsible for the deaths of numerous doctors and nurses.

We don't talk about the burden caused by the exercise of our profession.

In part, this is related to the bureaucratic overload of healthcare work, as more and more forms, orders, prescriptions, summaries have to be filled out in order to move the wheels of the health industry machine.

We don't talk about the impact on our health of being witnesses, often helpless ones, of the suffering of a human being.

We don't talk about the conversations with our patients that continue to repeat in our minds long after they have left.

We don't talk about the pleading look of those who ask for one more minute, something we cannot give them.

We don't talk about the intimate feeling that if a particular case had occurred just a few months later, at the time when the cure appeared, perhaps the patient would have been saved.

We don't talk about the moral burden of having to make decisions about who to save because the limitations of the health system do not allow us to save everyone.

We don't talk about the faces of patients that overlap with the faces of our relatives during rest hours.

We don't talk about how we are where no one wants to be, listening to what no one wants to hear, doing what few are willing to do.

We don't talk about the effort it takes to return to the superficial problems of everyday life after having dived into the waters of existential problems.

We don't talk about the silence and deflection we use with our loved ones when they ask us how our day was.

We don't talk about the sorrow we feel when a patient dies, even if they do so relieved and peaceful.

11.4   Medicine Is the Cause of Illness, Fatigue, and Burnout

We may know it better today than we did yesterday, but all great doctors have had their dark nights, their times of discouragement, their moments of great sorrow.

But perhaps the most important evidence of the impact that the practice of medicine has on the healthcare team's own health can be seen in three easily measurable facts: absenteeism, job abandonment, and the rate of medical suicides [37–44].

Absenteeism precedes abandonment, and this may be the last resort before taking one's own life.

When we analyze suicide among doctors, what the different studies carried out show is that male doctors have a suicide rate that is 40% higher than men in other professions, which rises to 130% higher than women in other professions for female doctors.

The difference between doctors and other professions, and between genders, is based on three crucial elements:

(a) Doctors know how to commit suicide in a more efficient manner.
(b) Female doctors suffer discrimination at work, receiving less pay than their male counterparts and having to demonstrate greater talent and commitment to advance.
(c) Female doctors suffer from sexual harassment on many occasions.

These last two reasons should lead us male doctors to deep reflection, since we are often the cause of the suffering of our female colleagues.

This emotional impact is linked to the fact that two orders of problems are mixed in the medical task: (a) solving the puzzle that is a disease (pathology). For this purpose, we have data collection and we can establish an algorithm that solves them; but we also have to glimpse the mysteries of illness: here data is no longer helpful, and in an increasingly secularized world, many times the doctor is the repository of patients' existential anguish. In this task, we have no more tools than our own brain, our own heart, and our own experience, all of them fallible and fragile tools.

One of the usual problems in doctors' marriages is silence, especially on the male part of the equation, when faced with the usual question from the spouse: How was it today? The answer is limited to a four-letter word "good."

What does the word good summarize?

All the emotions, experiences, and challenges to which we are exposed.

We usually don't have a record of what that means.

That's why for one day, I recorded the most important emotions related to my work. After seeing the list and the reasons for them, it seemed to me that the figure that best represents them is lhat of a roller coaster.

They go up, they go down, they turn, they speed up, they slow down, they turn you upside down, in short it is a dynamic that defies the laws of physics and mental health.

The rollercoaster of emotions that I recorded is the following one. I share it with you because I am sure that if you try the same exercise, you will see something very similar.

Fasten your seat belt and join me on the tour:

1. **Be careful to try not to cause harm when communicating the diagnosis.** When we are going to communicate a diagnosis, doctors are afraid of generating in our patient an emotional reaction that we cannot control. The patient is as afraid to listen to us as the doctor is to say what needs to be said.

2. **Accompany the patient in the therapeutic decision.** When we present therapeutic options, we try to show a panorama that covers the most tolerable (but usually also less effective) to the most intolerable (due to toxicity, complexity of implementation, or cost——but which are usually more effective), trying to allow the patient to exercise their freedom and select the one that best suits their values, even if many times it is not the one we personally prefer. This leaves us with a complex feeling: although we think that we have done our job well and the patient has chosen freely, we also believe that they have made a suboptimal choice.

3. **Joy at the end of the treatment.** The completion of the treatment is a very special moment, especially when it is a treatment carried out preventively (adjuvant); however, it is also the moment when the ship leaves the port. The treatment gives a feeling of security, that something is being done against the potential disease, and yet, at the end of it, there is a feeling of helplessness, where we ask ourselves *Now what?* Therefore, joy and uncertainty are mixed in equal parts.

4. **Gratitude for the healing.** When time passes (the most common limit is five years, but it can vary between two and ten) and the patient once again has the same cancer risk as the population of the same age without evidence of disease, we consider that it has been cured. That is the moment in which the patient is discharged from oncological follow-up to enter the common clinical surveillance of the community. It is a moment of completion and detachment, which all oncologists are grateful for, although not without some regret at stopping regularly seeing a person for whom we feel affection. We long for them to never have to see us again but we are sad to stop seeing them nonetheless.

5. **Outrage at discrimination and ignorance.** Many times we see patients who have lost their chances of a cure, and this can be for a variety of reasons: because the cancer wasn't discovered early enough, because they were unaware of what was happening to them, or worse still, because the health system has put up so many barriers that the poorest and most vulnerable couldn't get access to the treatment: they live in remote areas, they suffer from transportation problems, appointments are delayed for months, lack of basic diagnostic instruments, bureaucratic indifference, lack of solidarity and exploitation. More than once one wishes that it were mandatory for politicians, judges, and other public ser-

vants that they and their families receive care only in state-operated and funded hospitals. I am sure that there would be a substantial improvement in care if this was the case. Cancer is a disease less deadly than ignorance and much less deadly than indifference.

6. **Compassion in the face of injustices suffered.** When one records the medical history of patients, one not only records the history of the illness they are suffering from, but the history of their life. The stories of some of our patients are stories of great pain and suffering. One of my patients underwent 36 operations for spina bifida and had to catheterize her bladder by herself at the tender age of three, in kindergarten. Another was kidnapped. Another suffered domestic violence. One of my patients came from Syria fleeing a massacre in which his entire family died. Another was a survivor of a Nazi death camp. Each encounter with a person allows us to glimpse life stories that are sometimes a synthesis of the inhumanity of our century.

7. **Fear of follow-up studies**. Patients fear that they are not being adequately studied and fear that the studies will report bad news. We also have the same fear. Today we have increasingly sophisticated methods to scrutinize a person's body, we can cut it into one-millimeter slices from the skull to the feet and we can do it assisted by artificial intelligence, which without any emotional affectation, will compare the structures with millions of images in seconds and will detect anomalies with unprecedented precision. That will translate into bad news. Sometimes ignorance truly is bliss. That's why doctors are often bad patients. A healthy person, today, is a poorly studied patient. It is important to do follow-up studies that are necessary and useful, but not doing them if they are unnecessary or useless is just as, if not more, important. Curiosity is not a useful reason to carry them out.

8. **Understand the patient's disappointment at the impact of recurrence.** The diagnosis is bad news, the recurrence of illness in someone who was in control is devastating. The patient not only relives the anguish of the first diagnosis but also feels that everything they've done is useless, that the trust placed in the medical word has been misplaced, that the pacts he made with life, God, or with themselves have been violated. Disease recurrence is a much greater crisis than the onset of the disease. That is why in certain conditions it is very important to prepare the patient, especially in the case of breast conservation, especially after preoperative chemotherapy treatment (neoadjuvant). It is important for the patient to know that we try to preserve the breast, that most of the time it is possible but that, if the disease returns and we must remove the breast, that does not mean that their prognosis necessarily worsens. It is different when the recurrence is distant, which would be a metastasis, since this implies that a focus of seeded tumor, probably before the primary one could be detected, has survived the treatments that we implement. The breakdown of trust that occurs at that moment requires understanding and humility on the part of the doctor to rebuild the bridge.

9. **Tolerance toward treatments without scientific evidence**. A large number of patients resort to treatments without scientific evidence: diets, folk remedies, traditional medicines, homeopathy, witches, charlatans, and an extensive list of others. They are medicines based on belief and testimonies, most of them are harmless, some only seek an economic transaction between the one who deceives and the one who wants to be deceived, but others are dangerous. From my perspective, credulity is a right and therefore I do not judge that aspect of these practices; but security is a duty and therefore I do judge them in this regard. If any of them are unsafe, I talk to my patient about the risk they are running and the evidence I have of the damage or the suspicion I have of it. We must refrain from judging the beliefs of others, because, ultimately, many of us who are vehemently sure of some fact today will tomorrow discover that it was a simple belief. Caring without judging is an art that is learned and which we must practice daily.

10. **Confronting our limitations by exhausting antitumor treatments**. Every time a patient worsens and an illness affects their health and compromises their life despite the treatments we institute, we feel that we have failed, that something has failed, that we have reached a limit. This causes a lot of pain; dealing with that limitation is a daily task for oncologists. We also get excited about new things, we also get hopeful when a new product is launched or a new discovery is made. One of the first, if not the first learning in palliative care, is that there is an insurmountable limit that is beyond our desires and our capabilities.

11. **Confrontation with uncertainty regarding the progression of the disease**. Dealing with uncertainty does not only mean not knowing the time of death, today it also means not being sure of the responses of tumors to new therapies. Before we said: "when a patient has three months of life expectancy and there is no effective treatment, they should be referred to the palliative care service." Today we say palliative care must be implemented from the moment of diagnosis and tumors must be exhaustively analyzed from a molecular point of view to see if there is a tool in practice or in research that we can use. This means that each case presents us with more doubts than certainties.

12. **Acceptance of anguish in the face of death**. Death, the mere idea of one's own death or that of a loved person, generates anguish. It is probably the anguish that underlies all and any loss in our lives. The fear of disappearing, the ignorance of what comes after. There we place our Faith. Even agnostics and atheists believe that after our death there is nothing. But it is still a belief, as valid as those who believe that there is something or someone. When we accompany someone to death, most of the moments of death are peaceful but the agony is distressing. Talking to a patient about death, about their wishes and beliefs is very motivating for the doctor as well, since the patient is akin to a mirror that gives us back our humanity.

13. **Openness to existential dilemmas.** In an increasingly secularized world, the doctor is often the repository of a person's existential problems and dilemmas. What do we know about what can happen to their life? Should you continue with your tasks or leave them to give more time and attention to your home? What do we think about them marrying the person who accompanied them during these years, now that our patient thinks they have little time left? Is having religious feelings genuine or a simple childhood regression? Should the patient communicate with that relative, whom you haven't seen in so long, now that you know they are going to die? Should the patient be cremated or follow some other burial method? None of us has the correct answer and many of these problems can be solved in more than one way, but we are only asked for an attitude: listening and eventually an opinion, which must be at the same time prudent and respectful.

14. **Humility in the face of undeserved thanks**. Many patients and their families are grateful, and they express it with words, gestures, writings, and gifts. The worst thing a member of the healthcare team can believe is that they are deserved and fair. It is a show of affection, not justice. What most people thank us for is our presence, not the success of our actions.

15. **Serenity in the face of undeserved aggression**. Some people or their family members attack us, with words, gestures, or actions. We live in an increasingly violent society and the anonymity provided by social networks causes many people to express their pain at the death of a loved one, such as anger at the impotence of the health team, the health system, or the treating professional. Most of these attacks do not consider that behind them, there is a person or a family, who many times, in an unfair and undeserved way, suffer these insults or damage to their property or person. Also when this happens, we must suffer them with serenity, seeking the advice of peers or eventually legal advice, but understanding that reacting violently to the injustice suffered can trigger even more undesirable consequences.

16. **Guilt for the mistakes made**. We all make mistakes, those who believe they don't make them are simply ignorant. The effort must be made to reduce them to a minimum, but knowing that some will inevitably occur. Attention cannot be absolute, memory fails, the finger touches a key different from the one desired, distraction leads us to do what we do not want. The best system is one that encourages review of what others do. You build a trustworthy team when all members know that if they detect an error and correct it, we all benefit. That doesn't mean you don't feel responsibility and guilt when you make a mistake.

17. **Remorse in the face of personal incapacity**. As we gain experience and age, there are certain tasks that we do better and others that, unfortunately, we do worse, certain maneuvers that when we were residents we could do by heart and now our memory fails us. One of the advantages of working in teams where there are several generations is that the younger ones do with greater agility, speed, and confidence the things that we older people do worse. These feelings

are complex because, on the one hand, it mixes gratitude and pride at seeing another younger member of our team do something they excel at, yet, on the other, there is remorse and regret at not being able to do it ourselves.

18. **Shame in the face of ignorance**. The speed with which knowledge is produced and the volume of it (something that will increase with artificial intelligence) makes it impossible to be updated instantly even in very limited specialties. In the discussions of cases in committees, one is amazed at the speed of information research of the youngest people and the quality of information they are capable of processing. Again the feeling is complex, on the one hand, admiration, and on the other, shame at our own limitations.

19. **Surprise at an unexpected evolution**. When we share the cases of the week, we often also update past cases and all experienced doctors witness cases that have an unexpectedly good evolution. Treatments that one began with low expectations of success and yet achieve excellent results. That is a reason for great joy and a strong incentive to continue the task.

20. **Grieving the mistreatment of a colleague**. Also, in these group meetings, we often hear the pain of a colleague who has been mistreated. In general, these attacks are seen more toward young people and often women. This generates enormous regret, since one is aware of the effort and commitment that many of them put into their work and how much the lack of respect and abuse to which they are subjected affects them. All of us, but especially the older ones, must fight so that the violence and lack of respect that are so often seen on the street do not make it into our institutions.

21. **Envy of other people's success**. In these meetings, we also share the successes, the lucidity of the idea, the clarity of the experiment, the forcefulness of the demonstration; all of this is wonderful and enriching, but although it is an execrable feeling, envy surrounds each congratulation on the success of the other.

22. **Pain at the contempt of others**. One is always very careful when giving power to another's word. The opinions of others should not affect us, but they always do in some way, especially when they are accompanied by contempt.

    Most medical residencies encourage competition among peers through the "no" game.

    (a) In principle the other "IS NOT RIGHT."
    (b) If he is right, it is "OBVIOUS AND ANCIENT" knowledge, which is why you didn't bother to mention it.
    (c) If it is not old or obvious then "IT WAS NOT TESTED."
    (d) If it was tested, it was not with a "DOUBLE-BLIND RANDOMIZED STUDY."
    (e) If it was a randomized double-blind study, "IT WAS NOT PUBLISHED IN ENGLISH."
    (f) If it was published in English, "IT WAS NOT PUBLISHED IN THE NEW ENGLAND."
    (g) If it was published in the New England, "YOU JUST DISCOVERED THE ONE WHO STOLE YOUR LAST ISSUE" and it is better to be ignorant than a criminal.

Knowing how to play it means that you suffered from it or exercised it. In any case, when the other considers that what you know or learned is not valuable, it causes pain and sorrow.

23. **Admiration for the wisdom of others**. Sharing clinical cases and patient care experience allows you to enrich yourself with the knowledge of others and that allows you to discover wisdom in the questions and answers they give to their patients, their families, or other team members. This generates a feeling of admiration for the wisdom and kindness with which some people are capable of dealing with very delicate and complex topics.

    In fact, the oncopediatrics team led by Dr. Blanca Diez at Fleni institute wrote the following:

Talking with Children Is...

- To listen carefully, that is, to be aware of the characteristic of their cognitive development and their previous experiences.
- To never lie.
- To use understandable terms, not euphemisms or empty phrases.
- Never to contradict and always to respect their beliefs and family customs.
    During a guided visualization, 3-year-old Javier, suffering from a neuroblastoma in its final stage, imagined traveling through space to a castle. When asked who was with him, he immediately answered: Zorro! It was this film character that he choose to be his imaginary companion during his last days.
- To talk to the parents in the presence of the child, avoiding the famous conspiracy of silence.
- To always use the therapeutical triad in communication: empathy, honesty, and warmth. [45].

    There is no nobler or harder duty than caring for a dying child.

24. **Vertigo in the face of risk**. There are situations that necessarily escape what is protocolized, what is standard, what is known. There we resort to improvisation, extrapolation, experience, and desires. Unlike a research protocol, where the risk that the patient runs will serve the search for truth, in the case of treatments outside of research trials, when there are no standard resources left, these seek to offer the patient a treatment that we want them to benefit from, without knowing if they will or not. In some ways, it's like a trapeze artist's jump without a net, and that always makes you dizzy.

25. **Hope in the face of the inevitable**. Even when we know that the patient is incurable, that we have done everything we know to improve their condition, even when we know that they will inevitably die, we have hope. Hope that it won't be today. Hope that it won't be painful. Hope that it will be peaceful. Hope that the family will accept it with serenity. Hope that their life has not been in vain. Hope for oncologists is a muscle that is exercised daily. It may not be an optimistic hope, but it is still hope.

26. **Resignation in the face of loss**. One of the forms of detachment is resignation. When a patient dies, you review everything you have done and the relationship you managed to build. As a member of the health team, you learn a lot from each patient, each patient is an expert in their life and there are patients' lives that are very rich and varied. I have had the opportunity to meet professionals

from various fields, politicians, gamblers, traffickers, smugglers, low and high-ranking prostitutes, painters, dancers, actors, generals, priests, and bishops. All of them, without fail, in the privacy of the office and naked of tinsel and uniforms, had lives in which they had been able to solve very serious problems with creativity, although not always legally. The feeling one gets is that when they leave this life the world is a little sadder. Resignation is a feeling that mixes gratitude and joy at having been able to meet them and the pain of never seeing them again.

27. **Reaffirmation in the senses**. At the end of the day, after traveling this path of emotions and feelings, one remembers Nietsche's phrase: *"He who has a why to live for can bear almost any how."* and remembers again the hopes with which this path of medicine began. The desires and hopes with which we underwent our residency and the professional path that we have developed.

28. **Understanding in the face of inexperience**. Many times one witnesses the excessive expectations, the unequal struggles and the hopes against all hope of the youngest. And it's OK. The advantage of teams in which there are young and old is that the force of hope and the restraint of experience often work to balance the scales in decision-making.

29. **Consolation in the face of hopelessness.** Many expectations are not met and many hopes are not realized. That is where we older people have to practice the art of consolation. One has expectations and hopes not because they all come true but because some are fulfilled. If treatment is not started with hope, it will surely be quickly abandoned. If a treatment is not indicated with expectations of success, you are doing the wrong thing. Unfortunately, expectations and hopes are not enough, though I wish they were.

30. **Love of art**. At the end of the day, when I begin the journey home and remember this roller coaster of fear, care, accompaniment, joy, indignation, sadness, shame, surprise, understanding, consolation, and so many others, I rediscover the value of love for our art. The art of accompanying, caring, and healing allows us to daily take the pulse of the feelings, emotions, and choices essential for a life, lived to the fullest until the last moment. That is what the doctors who preceded us have experienced over time and those who come after us will experience.

11.5   Learn to Work with Stress

What we must learn is to manage the stressors of the work of the health team and, above all, how communication training helps us in three crucial aspects: commitment to work, the work team, and satisfaction with work [46–99].

11.5.1   Commitment to Work *Must be Human and Professional, which for me Is Summarized in Two Words:* Here *and* Now

Here represents the human aspect, we must strive to be fully present with the person we are with while doing what we are doing. This sounds easy, but it requires training and commitment. If I am seeing a patient, I make sure the phone does not ring, the secretary filters any incoming messages (which I will respond to between consultations) and if there is an emergency they must knock on the door. When I am with a patient, I am completely focused on them. That reflects the human commitment to the other person.

Now represents the professional aspect. My attention is encompassed by the patient's problem. I try not to get distracted or worry. When my time with the patient ends, I record what I observed, communicated, indicated, or requested and then try to forget them for the moment.

I need five minutes of restoration between patient and patient. I cannot start the consultation with the next patient while worrying about the previous consultation, it is not fair to the patient I am currently with. It's not **professional**.

What is the restoration like? First, I do a mental summary of what happened to see if I forgot anything. Secondly, I try to relax for a minute or two using breathing techniques. Then I ask my secretary to pass the messages to me and I respond to them. Next, I wash my hands and call the next patient. This is my usual routine until my office work ends.

I do something similar in case meetings, paper readings, dissertations, and other such activities. I try to be present humanly and professionally in each of them.

11.5.2   The Work Team

One of the most important tasks of those of us who have a responsibility in managing others is the hermeneutics of work teams.

What is happening on the team?

This often manifests itself in the non-verbal language of its members. Do they arrive on time? Where do they sit? How do they treat each other? How do they react to comments? How do they pose the problems? Who starts talking? How do they respond to you?

Here again, listening skills are crucial.

Before responding, the person in charge must ensure that they have adequately understood the problem: understand before judging.

When faced with a common problem, follow the rule of the monk who wrote the first rule for Christian monks, Abbot Saint Benedict: let the youngest, the newest, the most inexperienced begin to speak.

Having the youngest start has several advantages: first, it trains new arrivals in the practice of deliberation, second, creative solutions may appear that are not influenced by past experiences, and third, it leaves more time for reflection for the older members of the team.

If you lead the meeting, speak at the end, summarize the positions and eventually limit the problem to two or three solutions, so the debate can be much more constrained.

If you cannot reach a unanimous solution, request a vote, in which everyone can freely adhere to a proposal.

Remember that many times what is sought in a team meeting is not necessarily a solution, but rather an attitude of listening and understanding.

Be scrupulously respectful of people and stern with arguments.

Understand the difference between delegating a task and delegating a responsibility.

In the first case, you consider that the person is capable of performing a task and can be rated on their performance.

When you delegate a responsibility, on the other hand, you are prioritizing a person within the team to lead a certain process.

If you delegate a task, your responsibility as a boss is to make sure it is carried out properly.

If you delegate a responsibility, you must refrain from intervening as a boss, the tasks must be delegated by the responsible person, otherwise it will never allow you to grow.

11.5.3 Satisfaction with Work

One of the main causes of frustration and stress in work teams is the lack of recognition when a task is performed.

Knowing how to recognize the work of others helps reduce the stress of the task. This means recognizing both effort and success.

Not every effort is successful, but it is the path to success.

Not all cardiopulmonary resuscitation brings the patient out of arrest.

Not all chemotherapy cures cancer.

Not all research ends in a publication.

Not every publication ends in a prize.

The effort we put every day to improve a little is part of the professional work of all team members and it is good to recognize it.

It's part of the satisfaction of the job.

As a counterpart, successism, which considers that only achievements should be considered, has two unpleasant consequences:

(a) It leads to excessive pride, of those who record only triumphs, and maniacally deny errors, or despise small progress.

(b) It ends up destroying teams, since unhealthy competition is established between its members, instead of a collaborative task.

Building a work environment in which everyone is recognized for their contribution and the conviction that the team's achievement is superior to individual achievement is also the responsibility of the bosses or coordinators of the work groups.

11.6 Self-Care a Key Element in Preventing Burnout

Given that stress is part of our daily lives and learning to deal with it is one of the tasks we must address, what are the instruments to do it?

Self-care [100–108].

Self-care is a key point of medical health. The crucial components of self-care are caring for physical and mental health and caring for personal, family, and social relationships.

Caring for physical health consists of adapting work to our possibilities and not allowing ourselves to be destroyed by it.

All effective strategies for avoiding burnout and preventing exhaustion and abandonment of tasks are focused on three strategies: limiting work hours, regulating our weight, and increasing physical activity. They are the things that we all know we should do, but few do.

Limiting working hours is feasible, but the drawback is the impact this has on the family economy.

One of the most frequent causes of job dissatisfaction is economic [109–111]. This is particularly true in countries with economic instability and lack of career or professional development.

However, the success of this achievement lies in the negotiation of the employment contract, for which most doctors have not received any training.

Some outstanding points of that negotiation are the following:

(a) Know exactly what remuneration will be received and the description of tasks that one must perform.

(b) When one is looking for a job and is inexperienced in the subject, that is, part of the payment is to obtain knowledge, one must make it clear and establish a moment of renegotiation at the moment when the learning curve has ended. Because from that moment on, a part of the "salary" disappears.

(c) When one is sought after and is an expert on a topic, they have greater freedom of negotiation, but if part of their task is to teach another to carry out a practice, when the learner obtains the knowledge, the salary is usually renegotiated.

(d) The best negotiation is the one you do the day before starting work.

(e) Unionization and public employment have some advantages over private employment in that many labor "rights" are agreed upon without one having to personally renegotiate their salary, but in stable economic systems, they tend to be jobs with lower salaries than in the private sector.

(f) In the private sector, you have greater freedom of negotiation, but what you achieve depends on your personal ability. This usually always generates some tension, especially if there is no transparent remuneration policy, between what some doctors receive in relation to others, or doctors in relation to the rest of the health team personnel (nurses, psychologists or administrative staff).

The truth is that there is a training deficit in the negotiation of working conditions, both at undergraduate and graduate level.

Unfortunately, most of us learn alone, late, and poorly how to negotiate the best working conditions for ourselves and our team.

The second point of self-care is physical and mental health.

Taking care of physical health is something that we doctors usually neglect. It is that we are better at advising than giving examples, or as the Spanish saying goes: "In a blacksmith's house, people use wooden knives."

We must recognize that the diseases related to stress are those of civilization: obesity, hypertension, diabetes, and cancer.

This is based on chronic stress along with a sedentary lifestyle.

We have a genomic profile that was developed for long periods of famine, seeking food through gathering and hunting, in small nomadic communities.

We live in big cities, most trips in big cities are made in public or private vehicles and delivery is just around the corner from where we live.

Many of us spend 8 h sitting in front of a computer.

It is a problem of evolutionary medicine, which all of us understand perfectly to explain to a patient, but we do not apply it to ourselves.

Clearly weight control and physical activity have enormous benefits on health, quality of life, and longevity.

Finally, self-care is taking care of relationships.

People are relational beings.

First of all with ourselves. What Julian Marías called the constitutive "sameness" of the human person.

The cause of greater burnout in relation to our values and beliefs is the so-called "moral distress." [112–114].

In these situations, there is a conflict between what we think should be done in a certain way and the way something is being done with a patient [115–123].

It may be related to a treatment, a diagnostic or therapeutic procedure, or the way of communicating an event.

Objectively, it has been studied more in nursing than among doctors and when one tries to evaluate it, for example, through instruments such as the "moral distress scale," what one observes is that it is about evaluating the impact it has on us in three main spheres:

11.6.1   What We Are Witnesses of

Especially when we know that something is being done without the patient having given consent, or something that the patient would refuse if they knew the expectations or experience with which it was being done.

Some examples of this include:

- Doctors who carry out resuscitation maneuvers on dying patients when they know they will serve no purpose just to comply with a formality.
- The inclusion of patients in clinical trials without valid consent.
- Diagnostic or therapeutic procedures whose purpose is not to benefit the patient but to practice defensive medicine and avoid possible litigation.
- Procedures whose purpose is the training of health personnel and not for the benefit of the patient.
- Use of ineffective doses or drugs for a patient.
- Refusing to use opioid medication in a patient with advanced cancer pain in palliative treatments for fear that the patient will become addicted or the sedation could be seen as the cause of death.
- Restriction of access to medication or expensive procedures.
- Use of medication of dubious or expired origin.

11.6.2   That of Which We Are Instruments

Compliance with orders that we consider inappropriate for the patient's health.

The obligation to remain silent under penalty of losing our job if we disclose something that is incorrect.

Artificially keeping a patient ventilated because no one wants to make the decision to remove life support even in cases with no possibility of recovery.

Failure to respect the do not resuscitate orders signed by the patient.

Carrying out procedures or care for which we do not feel qualified.

11.6.3   The Quality of the Work our Colleagues Do

Working with colleagues who are not qualified to carry out the task they perform.

Assisting a doctor who does not provide adequate care to a patient.

Work with less colleagues than those required to ensure safety.

All this generates stress and burnout, because, when faced with these problems, one often chooses to remain silent, but the pressure accumulates until it explodes.

These moral conflicts are always serious, because they affect one's very being, putting in conflict what we're doing with what we **wish** we were doing.

That distance between the expectations with which one embraced a vocation or started a job and reality is cause for depression and anxiety. The greater the distance, the greater the depression and anxiety it generates in the person, because we can deceive almost everyone, except ourselves.

Only we know how many times we have acted correctly or incorrectly and our conscience, if we have not disensitised it, tells us what we do wrong.

The second area of relationship is **intimacy**.

Intimacy is the place where we unmask ourselves. It is the area where we can take off the mask (that every person wears and presents themselves with) and show the hidden face of who we are.

Marriage is often one of the most suffering relationships for doctors. The divorce rate among health professionals is very high.

This is not only because doctors and nurses spend many hours of the day away from home but also because when they return home they are generally mute.

To this we must add alcoholism, as well as addiction to sedatives and other drugs, which is more common among doctors than among other professions.

The third area is that of relationships with other people, especially in the workplace.

Personal care, careful speech, avoiding gossip, insults, contempt, moderation in behavior, are all key elements to building a healthy work environment.

Avoiding unnecessary friction and discomfort in others, is an effort by the entire team so that the workplace in which so many hours and so many emotions are shared can be a pleasant, clean, cared for place, in which one wants to be with their companions.

11.7 The Word is the Means to Deal with Burnout

Again, communication training and practice help us deal with burnout [46–48].

Not only because training in communication with the patient allows us to face different scenarios with greater efficacy but because the word allows us to identify in ourselves the feelings and emotions that show that we are isolating ourselves, that we are overwhelmed, exhausted, resentful, far from our usual commitment, that we are being affected by the task.

Putting these emotions into words is a task of reflection and internal dialogue.

What do I feel? What is generating these emotions? How can we manage them?

These words allow us to share our feelings with our family, our therapist, and at work.

In some way, naming what happens to us allows us to look at the problem more objectively and in a way, to measure it more clearly.

Sharing what we feel and what happens to us with our colleagues is also giving others the opportunity to speak. It shouldn't be a surprise that many are going through the same thing and the problem does not become apparent until someone begins to speak.

That way, speaking is an opportunity for the entire group.

Highlighting moral distress also requires words.

An important point of this topic is training in the deliberative method of analysis of ethical situations.

Facing problems requires not falling into the temptation to think only of dilemmas. Problems allow us to analyze different aspects of a specific situation; reducing problems to dilemmas means that there are only two sides and two possible solutions.

Real situations are rarely dilemmas, almost all are complex problems.

Explaining what makes us uncomfortable, what we think is a mistake, or what we understand to be incorrect gives other people the opportunity to explain themselves, so that we can understand another point of view, to see the problem from another perspective.

It allows us to explore different possible solutions and to see which of them damages the least values or optimizes the most values.

It may not change our way of seeing the problem, it may not change what we have solved, but at least we will have made an attempt to solve it in the best possible way and not just the only way we have been able to imagine.

Practicing medicine is increasingly challenging, requiring more and more institutional and team commitment to patient care.

It is a task that can seriously affect our health and our relationships, so we must carry it out carefully, respecting our limits and sharing our problems and solutions.

In the next chapter, I will share with you what my personal communications kit is, some things may be useful to you.

11.7.1 Teaching Exercises

1. Personal

    (a) Have you ever suffered burnout?
    (b) Have you had feelings related to exhaustion, cynicism, or distance from your commitments?
    (c) Have you had moral distress in your practice?
    (d) How did you handle it?
    (e) What response did you have from your colleagues?
    (f) What response did you have from the authority or institution?
    (g) Do you take care of your physical and mental health?
    (h) Do you do a physical activity?

    (i) Do you practice any type of meditation?

    (j) Do you have any hobbies?

2. Group Activities

    (a) Do you periodically hold team meetings aimed at seeing how work affects each person?

    (b) If a colleague begins to show signs of stress, what is the group's reaction? What is the coordinator's reaction?

    (c) Is there a protocol for handling a medical error if it occurs?

    (d) How have they resolved moral problems, if they ever had any?

    (e) Is the workplace (or class) climate pleasant and safe? Are there ways to improve it?

    (f) Have you and your group had training in moral deliberation? Do you have the feeling that some moral problems are reduced to dilemmas and the richness is lost in seeking different solutions?

    (g) Are there any extra-curricular activities that you do as a team?

References

1. Beard G. Neurasthenia, or nervous exhaustion. Boston Med Surg J. 1869;III(13):217–21.
2. Lipsitt DR. Is Today's 21st century burnout 19th century's neurasthenia? J Nerv Ment Dis. 2019;207(9):773–7. https://doi.org/10.1097/NMD.0000000000001014.
3. Korotkoff N. To the question of methods of determining blood pressure. Rep Imp Milit Med Acad. 1905:2.
4. Selye H. Stress and the general adaptation syndrome. Br Med J. 1950;1(4667) https://doi.org/10.1136/bmj.1.4667.1383.
5. Chrousos GP. Stressors, stress, and neuroendocrine integration of the adaptive response the 1997 hans selye memorial lecture. Ann N Y Acad Sci. 1998:851. https://doi.org/10.1111/j.1749-6632.1998.tb09006.x.
6. Rochette L, Dogon G, Vergely C. Stress: eight decades after its definition by Hans Selye: "stress is the spice of life.". Brain Sci. 2023;13:2. https://doi.org/10.3390/brainsci13020310.
7. Perou CM, Sørile T, Eisen MB, et al. Molecular portraits of human breast tumours. Nature. 2000;406(6797) https://doi.org/10.1038/35021093.
8. Freudenberger HJ, Staff burn-out. Journal of Social Issues. 1974;90(1).
9. Maslach C, Leiter MP. Understanding the burnout experience: recent research and its implications for psychiatry. World Psychiatry. 2016;15(2):103–11. https://doi.org/10.1002/wps.20311.
10. Maslach C, Jackson SE. The measurement of experienced burnout. J Organ Behav. 1981;2:99–113.
11. Lindsäter E, Svärdman F, Rosquist P, et al. Characterization of exhaustion disorder and identification of outcomes that matter to patients: qualitative content analysis of a Swedish national online survey. Stress Health. 2023;1 https://doi.org/10.1002/smi.3224. Published online October
12. Kim BM, Hur M. Effects of generational gap on job burnout within firefighting organizations: focusing on the mediating effect of generational conflict and communication skills. Fire Sci Eng. 2023;37(3) https://doi.org/10.7731/kifse.f5a90859.

13. Bunjak A, Černe M, Nagy N, Bruch H. Job demands and burnout: the multilevel boundary conditions of collective trust and competitive pressure. Hum Relat. 2023;76(5) https://doi.org/10.1177/00187267211059826.

14. Khan MT, Mitchell N, Assifi MM, Chung M, Wright GP. Surgeon burnout and usage of personal communication devices: examining the technology "empowerment/enslavement paradox.". J Surg Res. 2023;285 https://doi.org/10.1016/j.jss.2022.12.023.

15. Marra DEC, Simons MU, Schwartz ES, Marston EA, Hoelzle JB. Burnt out: rate of burnout in neuropsychology survey respondents during the COVID-19 pandemic, brief communication. Arch Clin Neuropsychol. 2023;38(2) https://doi.org/10.1093/arclin/acac081.

16. Yu J, Soh KL, He L, Wang P, Soh KG, Cao Y. The experiences and needs of hospice care nurses facing burnout: a scoping review. Am J Hosp Palliat Med. 2023;40(9) https://doi.org/10.1177/10499091221141063.

17. Saravanan P, Nisar T, Zhang Q, Masud F, Sasangohar F. Occupational stress and burnout among intensive care unit nurses during the pandemic: a prospective longitudinal study of nurses in COVID and non-COVID units. Front Psych. 2023:14. https://doi.org/10.3389/fpsyt.2023.1129268.

18. Setyaningrum RP, Muafi M. Managing job burnout from workplace telepressure: a three way interaction. SA J Hum Resour Manag. 2023:21. https://doi.org/10.4102/sajhrm.v21i0.2151.

19. Wiji Astuti IS, Kuntoro, Qomaruddin MB, et al. How nursing staffs deal with burnout syndrome through job satisfaction and self-efficacy: the fight or flight mechanism. J Public Health Afr. 2023;14(S2) https://doi.org/10.4081/jphia.2023.2551.

20. Bahr TJ, Ginsburg S, Wright JG, Shachak A. Technostress as source of physician burnout: an exploration of the associations between technology usage and physician burnout. Int J Med Inform. 2023:177. https://doi.org/10.1016/j.ijmedinf.2023.105147.

21. Rahman R, Ross AM, Huang D, Kirkbride G, Chesna S, Rosenblatt C. Predictors of burnout, compassion fatigue, and compassion satisfaction experienced by community health workers offering maternal and infant services in New York state. J Community Psychol. 2023;51(4) https://doi.org/10.1002/jcop.22967.

22. Amick AE, Schrepel C, Bann M, et al. From battles to burnout: investigating the role of interphysician conflict in physician burnout. Acad Med. 2023;98(9) https://doi.org/10.1097/ACM.0000000000005226.

23. Mikkelson AC, Hesse C. Conceptualizing and validating organizational communication patterns and their associations with employee outcomes. Int J Bus Commun. 2023;60(1) https://doi.org/10.1177/2329488420932299.

24. Hilty DM, Groshong LW, Coleman M, et al. Best practices for technology in clinical social work and mental health professions to promote well-being and prevent fatigue. Clin Soc Work J. 2023;51(3) https://doi.org/10.1007/s10615-023-00865-3.

25. Sullivan AB, Hersh CM, Rensel M, Benzil D. Leadership inequity, burnout, and lower engagement of women in medicine. J Health Serv Psychol. 2023;49(1) https://doi.org/10.1007/s42843-023-00078-9.

26. Hendrikx K, Van Ruysseveldt J, Proost K, van der Lee S. "Out of office": availability norms and feeling burned out during the COVID-19 pandemic: the mediating role of autonomy and telepressure. Front Psychol. 2023:14. https://doi.org/10.3389/fpsyg.2023.1063020.

27. Emold C, Schneider N, Meller I, Yagil Y. Communication skills, working environment and burnout among oncology nurses. Eur J Oncol Nurs. 2011;15(4) https://doi.org/10.1016/j.ejon.2010.08.001.

28. Alabi RO, Hietanen P, Elmusrati M, Youssef O, Almangush A, Mäkitie AA. Mitigating burnout in an oncological unit: a scoping review. Front Public Health. 2021:9. https://doi.org/10.3389/fpubh.2021.677915.

29. Abusanad A, Bensalem A, Shash E, et al. Prevalence and risk factors of burnout among female oncologists from the Middle East and North Africa. Front Psychol. 2022:13. https://doi.org/10.3389/fpsyg.2022.845024.

30. Kutluturkan S, Sozeri E, Uysal N, Bay F. Resilience and burnout status among nurses working in oncology. Ann General Psychiatry. 2016;15(1) https://doi.org/10.1186/s12991-016-0121-3.

31. LeNoble CA, Pegram R, Shuffler ML, Fuqua T, Wiper DW. To address burnout in oncology, we must look to teams: reflections on an organizational science approach. J Oncol Pract. 2020;16(4) https://doi.org/10.1200/JOP.19.00631.

32. Bar-Sela G, Lulav-Grinwald D, Mitnik I. "Balint group" meetings for oncology residents as a tool to improve therapeutic communication skills and reduce burnout level. J Cancer Educ. 2012;27(4) https://doi.org/10.1007/s13187-012-0407-3.

33. Abusanad A, Bensalem A, Shash E, et al. Burnout in oncology: magnitude, risk factors and screening among professionals from Middle East and North Africa (BOMENA study). Psychooncology. 2021;30(5) https://doi.org/10.1002/pon.5624.

34. Sisk BA, Schulz G, Kaye EC, Baker JN, Mack JW, DuBois JM. Conflicting goals and obligations: tensions affecting communication in pediatric oncology. Patient Educ Couns. 2022;105(1) https://doi.org/10.1016/j.pec.2021.05.003.

35. Taleghani F, Ashouri E, Saburi M. Empathy, burnout, demographic variables and their relationships in oncology nurses. Iran J Nurs Midwifery Res. 2017;22(1) https://doi.org/10.4103/ijnmr.IJNMR-66-16.

36. Gibson C, O'Connor M, White R, Baxi S, Halkett G. Burnout or fade away; experiences of health professionals caring for patients with head and neck cancer. Eur J Oncol Nurs. 2021:50. https://doi.org/10.1016/j.ejon.2020.101881.

37. Zimmermann C, Strohmaier S, Niederkrotenthaler T, Thau K, Schernhammer E. Suicide mortality among physicians, dentists, veterinarians, and pharmacists as well as other high-skilled occupations in Austria from 1986 through 2020. Psychiatry Res. 2023:323. https://doi.org/10.1016/j.psychres.2023.115170.

38. Duarte D, El-Hagrassy MM, Couto TCE, Gurgel W, Fregni F, Correa H. Male and female physician suicidality: a systematic review and meta-analysis. JAMA Psychiatry. 2020;77(6) https://doi.org/10.1001/jamapsychiatry.2020.0011.

39. Laboe CW, Jain A, Bodicherla KP, Pathak M. Physician suicide in the era of the COVID-19 pandemic. Cureus. 2021; https://doi.org/10.7759/cureus.19313. Published online

40. Anderson P Physicians experience highest suicide rate of any profession; https://www.medscape.com/viewarticle/896257.2018.

41. Jeelani R, Lieberman D, Chen SH. Is patient advocacy the solution to physician burnout? Semin Reprod Med. 2019;37(5–6) https://doi.org/10.1055/s-0040-1713428.

42. Schernhammer E. Taking their own lives—the high rate of physician suicide. N Engl J Med. 2005;352(24) https://doi.org/10.1056/nejmp058014.

43. Schernhammer ES, Colditz GA. Suicide rates among physicians: a quantitative and gender assessment (meta-analysis). Am J Psychiatry. 2004;161(12) https://doi.org/10.1176/appi.ajp.161.12.2295.

44. Dyrbye LN, Thomas MR, Massie FS, et al. Burnout and suicidal ideation among U.S. medical students. Ann Intern Med. 2008;149(5) https://doi.org/10.7326/0003-4819-149-5-200809020-00008.

45. Surbone A, Zwitter M, Rajer M, Stiefel R. Introduction communication: back to the human side of medicine. New Challenges in Communication with Cancer Patients 1, 2013:vii–xiv. doi:https://doi.org/10.1007/978-1-4614-3369-9. Published online January.

46. Wert K, Donaldson AM, Dinh TA, et al. Communication training helps to reduce burnout during COVID-19 pandemic. Health Serv Res Manag Epidemiol. 2023:10. https://doi.org/10.1177/23333928221148079.

47. Bry A, Wigert H, Bry K. Need and benefit of communication training for NICU nurses. PEC Innov. 2023:2. https://doi.org/10.1016/j.pecinn.2023.100137.

48. Ivančević S, Maričić M, Vlastelica T. Communication and academic burnout: the effects of social support and participation in decision-making. Communications. 2023; https://doi.org/10.1515/commun-2022-0095. Published online

49. Luhombo KK, Omondi DO, Aswani DR. Assessing internal communication and teacher burnout: an empirical study of school administrators in select public high schools in Kakamega County, Kenya. J Humanities Educ Dev. 2023;5(2) https://doi.org/10.22161/jhed.5.2.4.
50. Ellis LA, Tran Y, Pomare C, et al. Hospital organizational change: the importance of teamwork culture, communication, and change readiness. Front Public Health. 2023:11. https://doi.org/10.3389/fpubh.2023.1089252.
51. Funding E, Viftrup DT, Knudsen MB, Haunstrup LM, Tolver A, Clemmensen SN. Impact of training in serious illness communication and work life balance on physicians' self-efficacy, clinical practice and perception of roles. Adv Med Educ Pract. 2023:14. https://doi.org/10.2147/AMEP.S406570.
52. Wittenberg E, Reb A, Kanter E. Communicating with patients and families around difficult topics in cancer care using the COMFORT communication curriculum. Semin Oncol Nurs. 2018;34(3) https://doi.org/10.1016/j.soncn.2018.06.007.
53. Back AL, Arnold RM, Baile WF, Tulsky JA, Fryer-Edwards K. Approaching difficult communication tasks in oncology. CA Cancer J Clin. 2005;55(3) https://doi.org/10.3322/canjclin.55.3.164.
54. Wang Y, Feng W. Cancer-related psychosocial challenges. Gen Psychiatr. 2022;35:5. https://doi.org/10.1136/gpsych-2022-100871.
55. Hlubocky FJ, Rose M, Epstein RM. Mastering resilience in oncology: learn to thrive in the face of burnout. Am Soc Clin Oncol Educ Book; 2017.;(37). https://doi.org/10.1200/edbk_173874.
56. Wittenberg-Lyles E, Goldsmith J, Reno J. Perceived benefits and challenges of an oncology nurse support group. Clin J Oncol Nurs. 2014;18(4) https://doi.org/10.1188/14.CJON.E71-E76.
57. Font A, Corti V, Berger R. Burnout in healthcare professionals in oncology. Procedia Econ Financ. 2015:23. https://doi.org/10.1016/s2212-5671(15)00320-2.
58. De Vries AMM, De Roten Y, Meystre C, Passchier J, Despland JN, Stiefel F. Clinician characteristics, communication, and patient outcome in oncology: a systematic review. Psychooncology. 2014;23(4) https://doi.org/10.1002/pon.3445.
59. Fu W, Agarwal A, Chow E, Henry B. The impact of breaking bad news on oncologist burnout and how communication skills can help: a scoping review. J Pain Manag. 2017;10(1)
60. Russkikh SV, Moskvicheva LI, Tarasenko EA, et al. Measures to increase job satisfaction of oncologists at outpatient cancer centers. Public Health Life Environ. 2023;31(7) https://doi.org/10.35627/2219-5238/2023-31-7-15-25.
61. Singh A, Xiao L, O'Brien BJ, et al. Burnout among early-career medical oncologists: a single-institution experience. J Clin Oncol. 2022;40(16_suppl) https://doi.org/10.1200/jco.2022.40.16_suppl.11015.
62. Moadel AB, Papalezova K, Milner G, Gipson-Fine A, Kalnicki S. A systemic look at professional burnout and well-being within an urban cancer center as a roadmap to recovery. J Clin Oncol. 2022;40(16_suppl) https://doi.org/10.1200/jco.2022.40.16_suppl.11017.
63. Hergaux P, Bauchetet C, Préaubert-Sicaud C, et al. Accompanying the end of life and bereavement in oncology: ateam affair. What can we expect from the guidelines? Bull Cancer. 2022;109(6) https://doi.org/10.1016/j.bulcan.2022.01.012.
64. Appleton L, Poole H, Watmough S, Ramos-Silva A. Psychological wellbeing in professionals working in the cancer setting: the impact of the covid-19 pandemic. Support Care Cancer. 2022;30. ((Appleton L.; Watmough S.) Clatterbridge Cancer Centre NHS Foundation Trust, United Kingdom(Poole H.; Ramos-Silva A.) Liverpool John Moores University, United Kingdom)
65. Feldman DB, O'Rourke MA, Corn BW, et al. Development and validation of the self-efficacy for medical communication scale. J Clin Oncol. 2021;39(15_suppl) https://doi.org/10.1200/jco.2021.39.15_suppl.12124.

66. Vitinius F, Stock S, Wunsch A, et al. Fostering communicative competence and performance of physicians (KPAP study protocol)-multimodal assessment of long term effects of a communication trainings programme (funded by German cancer aid). Oncol Res Treat. 2020;43(Supplement 1)
67. Rogers SC, Walker AR, Otterson GA, Dettorre J. The experience of first-year hematology and oncology fellows after implementing a wellness chief fellow at an academic cancer center. J Clin Oncol. 2020;38(15_suppl) https://doi.org/10.1200/jco.2020.38.15_suppl.11017.
68. Colombat P, Dauchy S, Machavoine JL. Burnout syndrome in oncology and hematology healthcare professionnals. Hématologie. 2019;21(5) https://doi.org/10.1684/hma.2015.1066.
69. Ashton K. Bullying, burnout, and boundaries: navigating the ethical challenges of interdisciplinary teamwork. Psychooncology. 2019;28(Supplement 1)
70. Forbat L, Barclay S. Reducing healthcare conflict: outcomes from using the conflict management framework what is already known on this topic? Arch Dis Child. 2019;104
71. Gerhart JI, Sanchez Varela V, Burns JW. Brief training on patient anger increases oncology providers' self-efficacy in communicating with angry patients. J Pain Symptom Manag. 2017;54(3) https://doi.org/10.1016/j.jpainsymman.2017.07.039.
72. Seungmin C, Wayne F, Arnav A et al. The impact of breaking bad news on oncologist burnout and how communication skills can help: A scoping review. J Pain Manag. 2016;10
73. Anis H. Building capacity: a psycho-oncology training program for a multi-disciplinary team. Pediatr Blood Cancer. 2016;63. ((Anis H.) CanKids. Kidscan, Paediatric Psycho-Oncology Program, New Delhi, India)
74. Machavoine JL. Medical doctors and caregivers' burnout in oncology: psychodynamic approach in institution. Psycho-Oncologie. 2015;9(1)
75. Fujimori M, Uchitomi Y. Effect of communication skills training program for oncologists on their burnout and psychiatric disorder. Psychooncology. 2015;24
76. Butow P, Brown R, Aldridge J, et al. Can consultation skills training change doctors' behaviour to increase involvement of patients in making decisions about standard treatment and clinical trials: a randomized controlled trial. Health Expect. 2015;18(6) https://doi.org/10.1111/hex.12229.
77. Emanuel LL, Johnson R. Truth telling and consent. In: Oxford textbook of palliative medicine; 2015. https://doi.org/10.1093/med/9780199656097.003.0104.
78. Rangachari D, Donehower RC. Across the cancer continuum: a communication skills curriculum for oncology fellows. J Clin Oncol. 2014;32(15_suppl) https://doi.org/10.1200/jco.2014.32.15_suppl.e20556.
79. Tanriverdi O. A medical oncologist's perspective on communication skills and burnout syndrome with psycho-oncological approach (to die with each patient one more time: the fate of the oncologists). Med Oncol. 2013;30(2) https://doi.org/10.1007/s12032-013-0530-y.
80. Die Trill M. Physicians' emotions in the cancer setting: A basic guide to improving well-being and doctor-patient communication. In: New challenges in communication with cancer patients. 2013. https://doi.org/10.1007/978-1-4614-3369-9_18.
81. Bernard M, De Roten Y, Despland JN, Stiefel F. Oncology clinicians' defenses and adherence to communication skills training with simulated patients: an exploratory study. J Cancer Educ. 2012;27 https://doi.org/10.1007/s13187-012-0366-8.
82. Estryn-Behar M, Lassauniere JM, Fry C, de Bonnieres A, SESMAT C. Does interdisciplinarity reduce suffering at work? Comparison of carers (doctors and nurses) working in palliative care, oncology/haematology and geriatric care. Med Palliat. 2012;11(2)
83. Turner J, Kelly B, Girgis A. Supporting oncology health professionals: a review. Psycho-Oncologie. 2011;5(2) https://doi.org/10.1007/s11839-011-0320-8.
84. Kovács M, Kovács E, Hegedus K. Is emotional dissonance more prevalent in oncology care? Emotion work, burnout and coping. Psychooncology. 2010;19(8) https://doi.org/10.1002/pon.1631.

85. Butow P, Cockburn J, Girgis A, et al. Increasing oncologists' skills in eliciting and responding to emotional cues: evaluation of a communication skills training program. Psychooncology. 2008;17(3) https://doi.org/10.1002/pon.1217.
86. Armstrong J, Holland J. Surviving the stresses of clinical oncology by improving communication. Oncology. 2004;18(3)
87. Penson RT, Dignan FL, Canellos GP, Picard CL, Lynch TJ. Burnout: caring for the caregivers. Oncologist. 2000;5(5) https://doi.org/10.1634/theoncologist.2000-0425.
88. Fallowfield L, Jenkins V. Effective communication skills are the key to good cancer care. Eur J Cancer. 1999;35(11) https://doi.org/10.1016/S0959-8049(99)00212-9.
89. Felton JS. Burnout as a clinical entity—its importance in health care workers. Occup Med (Chic Ill). 1998;48(4) https://doi.org/10.1093/occmed/48.4.237.
90. Graham J, Ramirez AJ, Cull A, et al. Job stress and satisfaction among palliative physicians. Palliat Med. 1996;10(3)
91. Molyneux C. Burnout. Wounds UK. 2022;18:3. https://doi.org/10.4018/ijsem.2020070102.
92. Edú-valsania S, Laguía A, Moriano JA. Burnout: a review of theory and measurement. Int J Environ Res Public Health. 2022;19(3) https://doi.org/10.3390/ijerph19031780.
93. Brockner J, van Dijke M. Work engagement and burnout in anticipation of physically returning to work: the interactive effect of imminence of return and self-affirmation. J Exp Soc Psychol. 2024:110. https://doi.org/10.1016/j.jesp.2023.104527.
94. Ramirez AJ, Graham J, Richards MA, Cull A, Gregory WM. Mental health of hospital consultants: the effects of stress and satisfaction at work. Lancet. 1996;347(9003):724–8. https://doi.org/10.1016/s0140-6736(96)90077-x.
95. Sibille K, Greene A, Bush JP. Preparing physicians for the 21st century: targeting communication skills and the promotion of health behavior change. Ann Behav Sci Med Educ. 2010;16(1):7–13. https://doi.org/10.1007/bf03355111.
96. Surbone A. Cultural aspects of communication in cancer care. Support Care Cancer. 2008;16(3):235–40. https://doi.org/10.1007/s00520-007-0366-0.
97. Baider L, Surbone A. Cancer and the family: the silent words of truth. J Clin Oncol. 2010;28(7):1269–72. https://doi.org/10.1200/JCO.2009.25.1223.
98. Surbone A. Telling the truth to patients with cancer: what is the truth? Lancet Oncol. 2006;7(11):944–50. https://doi.org/10.1016/S1470-2045(06)70941-X.
99. Galeazzi O. Truth, disease, and prognosis. An historical-anthropological analysis. Ann N Y Acad Sci. 1997;809:40–55. https://doi.org/10.1111/j.1749-6632.1997.tb48067.x. PMID: 9103555.
100. Alexander GK, Rollins K, Walker D, Wong L, Pennings J. Yoga for self-care and burnout prevention among nurses. Workplace Health Saf. 2015;63(10) https://doi.org/10.1177/2165079915596102.
101. Velez-Cruz RJ, Holstun VP. Pandemic impact on higher education faculty self-care, burnout, and compassion satisfaction. J Humanist Couns. 2022;61(2) https://doi.org/10.1002/johc.12174.
102. Rupert PA, Pakenham KI. Self-care and burnout: a proactive values-based perspective. In: Comprehensive clinical psychology, second edition, vol. 2; 2022. https://doi.org/10.1016/B978-0-12-818697-8.00102-3.
103. Krasner MS, Epstein RM, Beckman H, et al. Association of an educational program in mindful communication with burnout, empathy, and attitudes among primary care physicians. JAMA. 2009;302(12) https://doi.org/10.1001/jama.2009.1384.
104. Kearney MK, Weininger RB, Vachon MLS, Harrison RL, Mount BM. Self-care of physicians caring for patients at the end of life "being connected···a key to my survival.". JAMA. 2009;301(11) https://doi.org/10.1001/jama.2009.352.
105. De Vibe M, Solhaug I, Tyssen R, et al. Mindfulness training for stress management: a randomised controlled study of medical and psychology students. BMC Med Educ. 2013;13(1) https://doi.org/10.1186/1472-6920-13-107.

106. Gopal R, Glasheen JJ, Miyoshi TJ, Prochazka AV. Burnout and internal medicine resident work-hour restrictions. Arch Intern Med. 2005;165(22) https://doi.org/10.1001/archinte.165.22.2595.

107. Shanafelt TD, Oreskovich MR, Dyrbye LN, et al. Avoiding burnout: the personal health habits and wellness practices of US surgeons. Ann Surg. 2012;255(4) https://doi.org/10.1097/SLA.0b013e31824b2fa0.

108. Sansó N, Galiana L, Oliver A, Pascual A, Sinclair S, Benito E. Palliative care professionals' inner life: exploring the relationships among awareness, self-care, and compassion satisfaction and fatigue, burnout, and coping with death. J Pain Symptom Manag. 2015;50(2) https://doi.org/10.1016/j.jpainsymman.2015.02.013.

109. Cruess RL, Cruess SR. Commentary: professionalism, unionization, and physicians' strikes. Acad Med. 2011;86(5) https://doi.org/10.1097/ACM.0b013e318212a93d.

110. Salib S, Valencia V, Moreno A. And now, please sign on the dotted line: teaching residents about professional life after residency. South Med J. 2018;111(5) https://doi.org/10.14423/SMJ.0000000000000804.

111. BMA. Doctors and the European working time directive. British Medical Association.

112. McCracken C, McAndrew NS, Schroeter K, Klink K. Moral distress: a qualitative study of experiences among oncology team members. Clin J Oncol Nurs. 2021;25(4) https://doi.org/10.1188/21.CJON.E35-E43.

113. Eche IJ, Phillips CS, Alcindor N, Mazzola E. A systematic review and meta-analytic evaluation of moral distress in oncology nursing. Cancer Nurs. 2023;46(2) https://doi.org/10.1097/NCC.0000000000001075.

114. DeBoer RJ, Mutoniwase E, Nguyen C, et al. Moral distress and resilience associated with cancer care priority setting in a resource-limited context. Oncologist. 2021;26(7) https://doi.org/10.1002/onco.13818.

115. Whitehead PB, Herbertson RK, Hamric AB, Epstein EG, Fisher JM. Moral distress among healthcare professionals: report of an institution-wide survey. J Nurs Scholarsh. 2015;47(2) https://doi.org/10.1111/jnu.12115.

116. Cohen TR, Wolf ST, Panter AT, Insko CA. Introducing the GASP scale: a new measure of guilt and shame proneness. J Pers Soc Psychol. 2011;100(5) https://doi.org/10.1037/a0022641.

117. Kälvemark S, Höglund AT, Hansson MG, Westerholm P, Arnetz B. Living with conflicts-ethical dilemmas and moral distress in the health care system. Soc Sci Med. 2004;58(6) https://doi.org/10.1016/S0277-9536(03)00279-X.

118. Epstein EG, Hamric AB. Moral distress, moral residue, and the crescendo effect. J Clin Ethics. 2009;20(4) https://doi.org/10.1086/jce200920406.

119. Morley G, Ives J, Bradbury-Jones C, Irvine F. What is 'moral distress'? A narrative synthesis of the literature. Nurs Ethics. 2019;26(3) https://doi.org/10.1177/0969733017724354.

120. Vig EK. As the pandemic recedes, will moral distress continue to surge? Am J Hospice Palliat Med. 2022;39(4) https://doi.org/10.1177/10499091211030456.

121. Lake ET, Narva AM, Holland S, et al. Hospital nurses' moral distress and mental health during COVID-19. J Adv Nurs. 2022;78(3) https://doi.org/10.1111/jan.15013.

122. Kherbache A, Mertens E, Denier Y. Moral distress in medicine: an ethical analysis. J Health Psychol. 2022;27(8) https://doi.org/10.1177/13591053211014586.

123. Morley G, Bradbury-Jones C, Ives J. The moral distress model: an empirically informed guide for moral distress interventions. J Clin Nurs. 2022;31(9–10) https://doi.org/10.1111/jocn.15988.

Chapter 12
A Personal Communication Kit

12.1 Introduction

The doctor–patient relationship ultimately remains an interpersonal and intimate encounter, no matter how much technology may influence it today. It takes place between two people, in a limited time and in a small space.

There, in that moment, the essence of that relationship re-emerges: the patient's trust placed in the knowledge and experience of the doctor, alongside the doctor's conscience, who puts their entire being and knowledge at the service of the patient.

It is the fusion of that trust and that awareness that makes this encounter, fleeting and transitory, transform into a therapeutic encounter that the patient treasures in their memory, being able to remember the transformative words that helped them live better even years later.

These words, figures, and images constitute the material with which each of the doctors or the other members of the team fill their kit with useful questions and answers for future patients [1–4].

I'll share mine with you now.

12.2 Uniqueness of the Person: Why Is this Patient Important to Me?

Each person is unique and irreplaceable.

We repeat this ad nauseam.

In fact, this idea is so important that we talk about personalized treatments in reference to individualized treatments against molecular targets detected in a tumor [5–8].

E. Gil Deza, *Improving Clinical Communication*,
https://doi.org/10.1007/978-3-031-62446-9_12

This is technically a misuse of the term, since the tumor is not a *person*, it has no personality, no values, no desires, and no meaning for its life.

Personalizing diagnosis and treatment begins with a series of simple questions: Why is this person unique? What's special about them? What does the illness they suffer from mean to them? Why do they think it occurred? Why now? What are they afraid will happen? What do they expect to happen? What do they want to take away from this consultation? How can I be useful to them?

As you see, this series of questions begins with the details that make this person unique:

Are the conditions of their birth what makes them original?

I have had patients who grew up believing they were their grandmother's children all their lives and treating their mother like another sister; children born when their mothers were kidnapped or in torture camps; children born as a result of rape; children born in a rich family that became poor or born in a poor family that became rich; the daughter of a catholic bishop who'd hung up his habits; another was born on the ship on which they escaped from the Nazis, with no other family than her father and mother; adopted; abandoned; accepted; beloved; cared for; attacked; children who were born the day a brother died in an accident. *"I have been the daughter of my mother's tears all my life,"* a patient told me; another was an only child, the sixth and last in a long line that had lived in the same house since the times of her great-great-grandmother. She'd had no children and was menopausal, so the line ended with her.

Is it maybe the conditions of their upbringing or education?

Boarding school children in Europe who only saw their family on vacation; the children of artists who were among their father's paintings since they could crawl and led a bohemian life; children educated by English governesses, who completed primary and secondary school without ever having had a school friend or another teacher; children of immigrants who came alone with their parents escaping the persecution of Christians in Syria; teenagers who left home at the age of 15 and since then learned to live alone on the streets; locksmiths trained by thieves; smugglers who began to ply their trade at the age 16. As the saying goes *"There is room for everyone in the vineyard of the Lord."*

Is it your work that makes you unique?

Nuns; priests; the captain of the last sailing merchant ship in our country; a polo player; a painter; an actor; protocol experts; an art dealer; an anthropologist; a museum designer; an antique car mechanic; a chef; a governess; a maid. The ways in which people make a living are so varied.

Is it their relationships?

A minister's mother; a judge; a journalist; a college professor's daughter; a friend's sister; the matriarch of a gypsy family; the wife of a high-ranking military man; the clinic director's friend; a disaster victim's mother.

Is it their gifts?

I had a patient from outside Buenos Aires, more than 15 years ago, who brought me a sausage that I had never seen before: it was a salami that had cheese inside. From then on I always recognized him as "salami and cheese," and every time we saw each other the password was just that, "salami and cheese." His name was Carlos, but even today, when I speak to his wife, we recognize each other by the same password.

Is it their looks?

"Ginger" is a redhead who has hair like fire and is a ray of sunshine with her children and husband; "Skinny" was always skinny and her only concern was to not gain weight; "Big guy" was two meters ten centimeters tall and weighed 180 kilos, and all of that mass was heart; "Count," was called that because all his life he dressed like an English count, I never saw a wrinkled shirt on him. Unique and unforgettable.

Is it the circumstances of the disease?

One of my patients was a doctor who was diagnosed with a brain tumor 2 weeks after graduating. Another was diagnosed with cervical cancer 3 months into her first pregnancy. Yet another was diagnosed with colon cancer 2 days before her *quinceañera* party. And another patient was diagnosed with breast cancer 2 months after getting married. Life surprises you in very special circumstances.

Is it their life story? Their way of speaking? Their religion? Their hobby? Their politics?

What makes the patient original, unique, unforgettable?

One of my flaws is that I can't put names to faces until I've seen someone three or four times. That is why I need to identify what makes my patients unique and different from everyone else. That uniqueness is what I associate with each patient's condition and it's how I remember their medical history and all the choices we've made along the way.

I tell my patients this the first time we meet and I explain why I need to identify them with something that makes them unique [9–12].

But I'll go one step further, in this era of so many *-omics*: genomics, proteomics, transcriptomics, we need *personomics*: the personalization of words and treatments, adapting what we say and when we say it to the values and desires of the patient [13–15].

12.3 The Value of Ignorance

There are patients who frequently maintain that they "want to know everything."

When that conversation takes place, I tell them that I am going to answer honestly everything they want to know, but luckily I don't know everything.

A large part of our happiness consists of not knowing. And one of the things we don't know is how long we are going to live.

One can believe, imagine, sense, or wish for a limit to our life.

But it is still a projection——one of the many possible projections——and life defies perfectly designed trajectories.

Just as one does not place microphones or hidden cameras to monitor the person one loves, since part of one's happiness is trust, one is also careful not to scrutinize what is happening with one's health too much and much less consider the medical prognosis as an absolute truth [16–20].

What is interesting about this patient's need to "know everything" is *why* they need to know that "truth" and *what* they want to do with it.

Suppose for a moment that we could predict with complete accuracy how many heartbeats you've left. What use would that be?

I hazard to guess no one wants such an accurate forecast. Imagine for a moment that you could know that you have 40,633,721 heartbeats left (which is more or less a year). By reading this line, you already lost one. Would you continue reading?

If that were true, I think the vast majority would throw the book away immediately.

Therefore we can say *"we want to know everything,"* but not with such accuracy.

Ok, what is the order of inaccuracy you tolerate? A day? A week? A month? A year? Five years?

It depends on the cause and age, you could say.

But you most likely want to know everything about the diagnosis and treatment, not so much the prognosis.

But we have to ask again, what of uncertainty are you comfortable with, because most diagnoses, even those based on pathological anatomy, have a level of error and uncertainty. What level is that? Well, in principle, the one in which it would be as dangerous to continue seeking the diagnosis as the consequences of not starting treatment.

And regarding the treatments?

We always have a level of uncertainty that has to do with the individual. Everything we know about treatments (which decreases if the patient is a woman, or worse, a child) is based on the evidence of what happens in the populations included in studies.

The more similar the patient is to the people included in the study, the more likely it is that... well, nothing is more likely. The evolution of an individual cannot be inferred from the probabilities of a population.

That is to say, all our evidence allows us to know how we should treat a population of people similar to those studied, so that similar average results are obtained in both groups, but we do not know at all what will happen to our individual patient.

What does this mean?

It means it is important to understand that knowing does not always improve our quality of life; many times we act based on a series of beliefs that work for us.

We believe that the diagnosis is accurate, at least up to an acceptable level of security.

We believe that the treatment we will do is appropriate for our patient.

We believe that if we act this way, you are more likely to benefit.

Above all, we firmly believe that our patient is special.

Since all doctors firmly believe that each of our patients is special, we could call this a widespread illusion.

Many joys are based on hopes founded on an illusion. The good thing is that sometimes they come true.

12.4   The Power of Placebo

We already saw the power of the placebo when we talked about the power of the medical word, but I often use it to demonstrate the power of the drugs we use today.

The placebo is very powerful, it is capable of lowering the blood pressure of hypertensive patients, reduce blood glucose in diabetics, and relieve pain for cancer patients. And this is generally in the order of 30%, that is, one in three patients benefits just by believing that what they receive can help them [21–25].

The power of belief is tremendous and is one of the wonders of the human person.

Now imagine the power of drugs that have been consistently and independently shown to be superior to placebo.

It is interesting to think that the placebo effect must be present in both groups of patients: it is acting alone in those who receive just the placebo, but it is also accompanying the pharmacological efficacy in those who received an actual drug.

Believing that one can benefit from the medication one is receiving is always beneficial, which is why no doctor should prescribe something he or she does not believe in and no patient should receive something he or she is not convinced will benefit them.

To reinforce this concept, I tell you the story of an "unpublished work" that a researcher from a North American company told us.

The story, which was shared with us at a symposium in Argentina 40 years ago, goes more or less like this: this group studied chemotherapy vs. placebo in a tumor called myeloma many years ago and demonstrated that chemotherapy allowed patients to live longer than those who had only received placebo.

Several years later, he studied the dose intensity of chemotherapy and its impact on survival. It showed that those who had received 80% of the dose lived longer than those who received 60% of the dose and these longer than those who had received 40% of the dose. Laying the foundation for dose intensity as a predictor of treatment benefit.

A few years later, someone thought of studying the dose intensity of the placebo. This led to several arguments, since the placebo does not have active ingredients, therefore it has no dose and consequently it has no dose intensity, but they eventually decided to study it.

And they showed that those who had received 80% of the placebo lived longer than those who received 60% and longer than those who had received 40%.

It should be clarified that those who received 80% of the placebo lived less than those who received 80% of the chemotherapy, but *longer* than those who received 60% of the chemotherapy.

Now, if they do not measure dose intensity, because there is no dose, what intensity do they measure? One can answer this in several ways: (a) the concept of dose intensity measures the patient's adherence and this reflects their general condition; (b) The concept of dose intensity is complex and includes the patient's belief and tolerance is greater in those who believe more in efficacy; (c) With the placebo, the intensity of belief is measured and this impacts survival.

In short, there are several interpretations. But they never published it as far as I know, and I have searched for it extensively.

The truth is that when I tell this to my patients, I reaffirm: "I believe that what I am telling you is going to be useful to you. Otherwise I wouldn't suggest it."

12.5   The Gift of Freedom

A cancer diagnosis is always bad news.

Bad news has the peculiarity of generating turbulence, turbulence disrupts the things that we thought we had figured out a while ago.

That said, it is clear that bad news is never good news, redundant as it sounds.

Now, bad news that disrupts our entire structure allows us to reevaluate how we are living and, more importantly, how we want to live the time we have left.

And that is something that a cancer diagnosis can help bring about. Make all the necessary transformations to live as well as possible for as long as possible.

That is what the exercise of freedom consists of.

Are you living how you want? Doing what you want? The way you want? With the people you love?

Awesome, there is nothing you should change. You are living freely and fully.

But what if that isn't the case? If you're free, yet also inside a cage? Can you do some of (but not all) the things you want? Neither freely nor fully?

If that's true, then you will never have so much strength to be able to change, to be able to choose, to be able to carry out your project, as in this moment.

The vast majority of our lives we live conditioned by a past that we cannot change and by a future that we cannot foresee, as Jon Kabat Zinn maintained [26, 27].

These two anchors condition our decisions for most of our lives. When a crisis occurs that questions our certainties, we can free ourselves from both restrictions and focus on the present.

That is the challenge of freedom, choosing what to do in the present, genuinely, making the effort to leave the past in the past and the future in the future.

Here and now.

At this very moment.

Just for today.

Exercise freedom.

What do you choose to do? That defines you, no matter what happens.

12.6   The Value of the Voyage

A very old way of seeing life is as a journey [28–31].

What happens, I explain to my patients, is that our modern way of traveling is totally different from the way we used to travel.

Today we have a very efficient way of traveling, we live in cities, so each address is established precisely, we know with certainty where we want to go, and we have GPS, Waze, or similar apps which tell us which routes we take. They will save time, money, or both.

If we travel between cities the same thing happens: buses, trains, planes, or boats take us with greater or lesser speed to our destination, but always quickly when compared to our ancestors.

But the truth is that we are descendants of nomads from the jungles, savannahs, deserts, or seas.

The route was made as we walked or sailed, we knew with certainty the place and time of departure, we were not so sure of the place or day of arrival, nor if we were going to find what we were looking for at all.

That transformed each trip into an adventure and more than one discovery (like the entire American continent) was made by accident.

Life is much more like the trips of our ancestors than modern trips and after a diagnosis like cancer it is good to remember that.

When I say this, I often give the paradigmatic example of the best travel book I know: the book of Exodus.

I imagine that book told by two girls who left Egypt when they were 6 years old. Sarah and Esther. The joy of departure was indescribable, they would be free, they would cross the Red Sea and enter the promised land.

Throughout the trip, Sarah and Esther have grown: they underwent the Bat Mitzvah, they got married, they had children. They have set up and taken down the tents numerous times: 40 years, 14,600 days and nights have passed.

There I ask my patients to imagine day 14,599.

Can you imagine?

Sarah and Esther stirring the stew, chatting among themselves. Solomon and Bathsheba have already given them grandchildren. What will their names be? If it's a boy, will they still be uncircumcised? Isn't it time to forget old quarrels?

They are getting older.

Throughout their lives Moses has gone from being a great national hero to a poor, disoriented old man.

The land promised to their parents, who died in the desert, is further away every day. When are we going to arrive?

Nobody knows. No one knows that tomorrow will be the day they will reach the land flowing with milk and honey.

Nobody knows what is going to happen because that day is exactly the same as any other day.

This is how you live and build life, step by step. That is why it is important to enjoy the trip again and recover the adventurous spirit of those who knew where they wanted to go, but did not know exactly how they would do it or what surprises, good or bad, each day held for them.

A diagnosis that confronts us with our worst fears and our vulnerability may well be transformative in the way we live the rest of our lives.

This frequently leads us to the problem of time or the paradox of infinities.

12.7   The Paradox of Infinities

The problem of time management is a problem that affects us all, whether we're healthy or sick.

What happens is that when we are sick or diagnosed with a serious illness that can cost us our lives, our awareness of the way we manage our time gets brought into sharper focus.

Patients often ask us how much time they have left, the answer is simple: *infinite. What do you mean, infinite?* The patients usually respond.

How much time do you have until tomorrow? Until next year? Ten years? The heat death of the universe? You can divide time into infinite periods, the same we can with numbers.

That is the paradox of infinities. One infinity can be greater than another, but both are *infinite.*

A circle is made up of infinite points and each point of a circle corresponds exactly to another, even if it is contained in the first. The circumference of a circle that has a diameter of 1 cm can be contained in that of another, larger circle of two centimeters in diameter and yet *both have an infinite number of points* [32–34].

These mathematical ideas about the study of space also apply to the study of existential time.

When you feel like you don't have time, the answer we have to look for is what is it you need that time *for* and try to bring that future as close as possible.

If one learns that the distance to tomorrow is an infinity of possibilities as rich and varied as the distance to a day a year or ten from now, then one can live each day as a small circumference that adds another centimeter to the diameter of our life.

That often leads to another variant of that theme, which is how many lives does a person have?

12.8   How Many Lives Does Man Have?

When we get to this point, I often turn to a story attributed to a Zen master, which I read when I was younger.

I have to be honest here, I must paraphrase the story somewhat as my memory isn't what it used to be:

A disciple asked his teacher: *How many lives does a person have?*
The teacher meditated for a while before answering and then told the student:
There are people who live only one life: they are born one day and die after a while, living only one life.
There are people who live each age as a life. They are those people who when they are children are adorable children and at every age they are fully what they should be, when they are old they are also adorably old.

There are those who live each year as a different life. They have different purposes, goals, achievements and learning each year. Many move jobs or homes and establish different relationships every year. They seem superficial, but perhaps they are just living in a different year.

There are those who live each season of the year as a life.

There are those who live each week as a life in itself.

There are those who live each day as a full life that begins when they open their eyes and lasts until they go to the world of dreams.

There are, finally, those who are capable of living a full life with every breath.

I think it must be difficult to live each breath as a life in itself, but I really like the idea that life is more than a unit, but that we can learn every day how to live better.

One of the most beautiful ways to live better is to remove the weight that overwhelms us from the injustices we suffer or inflict.

That leads us to forgiveness and reconciliation.

12.9 Forgiveness and Reconciliation

Forgiveness and reconciliation are concepts that are frequently confused. One of the men who has studied this problem in greater depth is Everett Worthington [35–42] and their studies have been applied especially in palliative care [43–46].

Worthington's story is extremely interesting because he is a graduate in nuclear engineering who later studied psychology and specialized in the field of forgiveness.

He has worked intensively in Ireland, South Africa, and many other countries plagued by violence between citizens.

He has deeply studied the role of forgiveness in marital relationships.

And furthermore, being an expert on the topic of forgiveness, he had to face the murderers of his elderly mother, who, before killing her, raped her.

So, here we have a person trained in what we would call *hard sciences* who dedicated himself to the study of psychology and had to apply all the theory that he had developed on himself.

His works are extremely interesting and I urge my readers to read his texts, which have helped me a lot in dealing with personal matters.

What do I tell my patients?

One way to live lighter is to take out of the backpack those weights that we have been carrying throughout our lives.

Let's start by taking away the weight of the injustices suffered: the role of forgiveness.

Worthington maintains that forgiveness is something one gives to oneself. Start by leaving in the past what is in the past. They deceived you, they don't continue to deceive you. They lied to you, they don't continue to lie to you. They hit you, they don't keep hitting you. They raped you, they don't continue to rape you.

That is to say, forgiveness is a choice about how you want to live in the present and the future: do you want to allow the past to continue guiding your life? Or on the contrary, you live your life aware of what happened but putting a limit on the damage that has been done to you.

The most difficult things to forgive are not those that have been done to us, but rather those that have been done to a loved one.

This is where justice plays a key role in the health of the population. In a country where there is justice, it is easier to forgive, without justice it is a much more difficult prospect.

But we said forgiveness is something we give to ourselves, that is why you can forgive someone who does not want to be forgiven because they think they did nothing wrong. You can forgive someone who died and therefore will not receive our forgiveness.

Forgiveness is born in the person who has been offended and limits the damage that the offender does to us. That makes our lives freer and healthier.

Reconciliation, on the other hand, is born in the offender. It begins with the awareness of the damage they've caused before they humbly approach the offended party to express their regret for what has happened.

Reconciliation seeks nothing and expects nothing.

It might be given or not, depending on the understanding and generosity of the one who was harmed.

Reconciliation does not *repair* an injustice. Furthermore, justice can be the area in which the aggressor can reflect on the damage he has caused.

It is good to understand the play of these four concepts: forgiveness, reconciliation, justice, and coexistence. Because they are independent concepts: the first is born in the offended party, the second in the offender, the third is a legal concept, and the fourth is the proximity, advisable or not, between the offended party and the offender.

Some people can forgive, be forgiven, and reconcile and yet it might be best if they're not near each other.

The truth is that, many times, the diagnosis of an incurable disease, the awareness of the limited time in life and the desire to live more fully in the present and the future (however much of a future we may have), is a strong stimulus to forgive and reconcile with those who offended us or whom we have offended.

12.10   Problem Hierarchy

In order to live in the fullest and happiest way, we must abandon our preoccupations. In Spanish, as in English, it is one of the most instructive words, as it is formed by the prefix *"pre"* which means *everything we do before* and *"occupations"* which is the *task or activity that we must carry out.*

In other words, worrying is everything we do before we actually start working.

These concerns are usually invasions from the past that we cannot change or the future we cannot foresee, instead of getting busy, which is what the present time calls us to do.

One of the wisest ways to use our time is to take care to live fully in the present, to leave in the past what has already been and leave to the future what can happen.

I'm old now. I'm already retired. I'm already sick. Will I see them grow? Will I live another Christmas? Will they remember me? Will I suffer?

There are several formidable writings, but none of the ones I have read have managed to surpass Ecclesiastes in the third chapter, verses 1 to 11 [47]:

A Time for Everything
3 There is a time for everything,
and a season for every activity under the heavens:
² a time to be born and a time to die,
a time to plant and a time to uproot,
³ a time to kill and a time to heal,
a time to tear down and a time to build,
⁴ a time to weep and a time to laugh,
a time to mourn and a time to dance,
⁵ a time to scatter stones and a time to gather them,
a time to embrace and a time to refrain from embracing,
⁶ a time to search and a time to give up,
a time to keep and a time to throw away,
⁷ a time to tear and a time to mend,
a time to be silent and a time to speak,
⁸ a time to love and a time to hate,
a time for war and a time for peace.

It is not known who is the author of Ecclesiastes, it is attributed to Solomon (like the book of Proverbs) and probably written in 950 BC.

It is a beautiful call to enjoy every occasion, those of peace as well as those of restlessness; those of success and those of failure; those of sowing as well as those of harvesting. Because time is the only thing we have.

It is also a call to attention. To be deeply attentive to what we're living through, in a world that increasingly seeks our distraction and absorbs our time. Get out of that condition in which we are led and take the direction of our life and focus on our time to what life demands of us.

The clarity and success of the author's word is so profound that he says in the second verse: "there is a time to be born and a time to die."

We should take birth and death not as designs but as tasks we are summoned to undertake. There is a personal and mysterious way of doing them, we are not aware of the first and but we *are* aware of the second.

They are so closely related that we can create our birth at the time of our dying, by saying goodbye, abandoning, delegating, ordering, closing, finishing, changing, concluding.

But we should not die early, we should wait for the time to do so.

One way to do this is to make a graph, with the Y-axis grading the problems from unimportant to extremely important and the X-axis grading the problems between those that are not urgent and those that are urgent.

There would be four spaces like this:

1. Unimportant urgent.
2. Extremely important urgent.
3. Neither urgent nor important.
4. Important but not urgent.

According to many wise men, we should not spend time on those who are not urgent or important.

We should focus on the urgent and important ones immediately.

We should only pay a minimum of attention to the urgent ones that are not important.

Instead, we should spend most of our time on important things that are not urgent: family, friends, education, the enrichment of our spirit.

Another way to objectify how we act is to focus on the following topic.

12.11   The Problem List

This is an exercise that I instruct my patients to do personally and intimately.

First, take a piece of paper and make a list of all your problems. Absolutely all that you can remember, from the most important to the simplest.

Then I ask them to order them according to a temporal criterion described by Jon Kabat-Zinn's [48]:

(a) On the left, write all those problems that are in the past.
(b) In the middle, write all those problems that are in the present.
(c) On the right, write all those problems that are in the future.

If one is human, then out of every ten problems that afflict us, five are in a past that cannot be changed, four in a future that cannot be foreseen, and one in the present. This last one is the only one we can actually deal with.

This exercise helps put in perspective how we are using our time, since 90% of us are plagued by problems from either the past or future. It also helps reduce the number of problems we need to pay attention to.

It is true that we should not need the diagnosis of a serious illness to make this task a daily exercise, but it is no less true that many times the strength and stimulus to carry it out come from an unpleasant and unexpected situation.

There is another task that is crucial to undertake as young as possible.

12.12   Choosing a Star

I often tell my patients a story that originated in a desert town. The author is anonymous, though probably Arabic. My grandfather, who was also a doctor, told it to me when I was 10 years old.

The story goes like this:

There are times in life when you wake up in the middle of the desert.
You don't know where to go.
Wherever you look, there is only sand, dunes, on the entire horizon, in all directions.
In that case, you should set up your tent and wait for the darkest night.
On that night, you must look at the sky and choose a star.
You star.
You must follow her, without a moment's hesitation. No matter where it takes you, you must let yourself be guided by it and follow it tirelessly every night.
You may be lucky and choose a star that will get you out of the desert quickly. You may be unlucky and choose a star that slowly takes you out of the desert, even taking you deeper into the desert before you get out.
It doesn't matter, good or bad luck does not depend on you.
But what you should never do is change stars, because you will only go around in circles and you will never leave the desert.

Each and every one of us has our star, intimate, unique, the one that we must follow at all costs, lest we lose ourselves.

When assaulted by loneliness, pain, or anguish, that is when we must look at it more clearly and follow its path with greater determination.

For this, it is convenient to distribute our emotions, which is the next topic.

12.13   The Emotions Portfolio

For me there are two big bad words: success and failure. Few words have caused quite as much pain.

What is success? What is failure? How many of your successes led to your failure and how many failures fostered your successes?

When one is faced with a chronic illness that endangers one's life and the quality of said life, one can make the mistake of thinking that its evolution can only be healing or death.

The danger of thinking that way is that we end up dismissing all the small steps that improve our quality of life that don't result in full recovery.

We have made a bet and gone all in: if we win, we take it all...but if we lose, it's all gone. There is no nuance to be had.

At a meeting for nursing professionals during the Chemotherapy Congress Foundation, I heard Dr. Anthony Back [49]talk about the *emotions portfolio*.

The idea is as simple as it is brilliant.

Just as it is inadvisable to bet everything on a single investment or stock, it is useful to see if we can diversify our emotions portfolio.

It is reasonable to bet that one will be cured, and it is possible to win...but what happens if one is not cured, if the treatment manages to prolong life but not cure the disease, or if it does not prolong life but manages to mitigate the symptoms and improve the quality of life?

How would we enjoy those achievements, which seem minor compared to healing, if we only hope to be cured?

Would the treatment be worth it?

What would we do if our symptoms improved or tumor growth stopped?

Because, in order to heal ourselves, there are a series of intermediate steps that are necessary, it doesn't happen all at once.

Is it reasonable to not enjoy the small achievements, because we don't get the bigger prize?

After hearing about it, I incorporated that idea into my practice.

I explain to my patients everything we must achieve to reach the goal of healing and ask them what they want to do while they undergo treatment and wait for healing with those small necessary steps.

Not everyone can be cured, but we can all be a little better while we undergo treatment and hope to benefit from it.

That is incorporating optimism as a treatment, which is the next topic.

12.14   Optimism as Therapy

Reality is complex and part of the way we experience it is related to a single choice.

Optimism and pessimism are both the consequences of a choice.

I know that what I just said is controversial, but I ask you, dear reader, for your indulgence and to continue reading. After all, reading a thesis we disagree with is often quite enriching.

We are incapable of knowing reality as a whole. Though we do know part of reality, we must imagine other parts of it. We are not knowledgeable about the whole universe.

The intimate reality of matter is not hidden and there is ample evidence that we tend to see those parts of reality that are interesting to us (attractive), and we tend to seek confirmation of what we think and believe (biases).

Optimism (seeing the glass half full and hoping that what we long for will happen) is just one point of view. Pessimism (seeing the glass half empty and waiting for what we hate to happen) is also a point of view.

The interesting thing is that both of these have an impact on health: optimism is beneficial [50–55] and pessimism is not.

If we assume that we can choose what point of view to have, where to look, what to place one's hopes on, optimism or pessimism are alternatives that we can *choose* from.

In fact, optimism can be trained [52] and even measured [56].

Some of the reasons for optimism are scientific advances in the fight against diseases [57, 58]. And the optimists are not lacking in reason in this sense, since numerous infectious diseases that in the past decimated humanity are today controlled with antibiotics. Much progress has also been made in the fight against endocrine, cardiovascular, respiratory, digestive diseases, and cancer. Today the cities are cleaner and the foods are less toxic. In many places, humanity lives in excellent sanitary conditions.

But in addition to scientific-technological optimism, there is an existential optimism: the future is, by definition, uncertain. This means I can bet on it, and if I'm going to bet, I'll do so for whoever I think is going to win.

However, this does mean we should keep one thing in mind:

How much do we bet?

In 1992, at one of the symposiums at the American Society Congress of Clinical Oncology (ASCO), Dr. Tannock presented the following result from a study that had not yet been published: with his team they had tried to study what the efficacy and toxicity of oncological treatments would be acceptable for a population.

With this objective, they designed, as in a game of cards, 50 scenarios that went from heaven to hell: in the first scenario, a person had a fatal cancer, which was cured by simply taking one tablet orally without adverse effects; in the last scenario, the person had 2 months to survive and the treatment offered had a 1% chance of relieving their symptoms, but they had to be hospitalized for a month with frequent vomiting. Between 1 and 50, the effectiveness gradually decreased, increasing the complexity and toxicity of the treatments.

The objective of the study was to see which scenario caused someone to stand up and say *"Enough."* The study didn't concern itself just with patients: doctors, nurses, and family members were also studied.

Those who were in good health stopped at different stages (doctors at 28, nurses at 32 and family members at 36) but 72% of the patients in that cohort reached stage 50.

In other words, seven out of ten patients in this study would accept a treatment with a 1% chance of relieving their symptoms, even if that meant spending 1 month of their last 2 months of life hospitalized and vomiting.

What was the authors' conclusion?

Illness changes our point of view.

Our breaking points are different when we're healthy than when we're sick.

That is why we must treat the patient and not just the tumor [59, 60].

What other conclusions can we draw from this information?

(a) That patients can accept almost any treatment we propose, so we must be very careful with what we offer.

(b) That the decisions we make when we are healthy may not be very representative of those we make when we are sick, which questions the validity of very old wills.

(c) That decisions must be made at the moment in which we must act and not beforehand.

Therefore, while optimism is the most reasonable option when deciding to undergo a treatment, we have to make sure that it is not blind, especially when we are in a more vulnerable mindset.

12.15 The Chess Pawn

This is one of the stories I use when options are very limited. It is inspired by a writing by the Spanish academic Arturo Perez Reverte, author of numerous novels [61–63] and also a weekly letter that is distributed in numerous Spanish-speaking newspapers.

In one of those weekly letters, Don Arturo analyzes the dignity of the chess pawn.

It is the lowest value piece in the game, easily sacrificed, it can only move forward one square at a time (or two, at the very start), and it can only threaten and capture pieces in the two squares diagonally in front of it.

It is, to put it mildly, extremely limited.

And yet Don Arturo points out the honor of the pawn rests in its ability to defend its square, at all costs, even at the cost of its own sacrifice.

He also points out the pawn's importance increases toward the end of the game, where it can mean the difference between victory and defeat. This is especially true if it reaches the rank in the opposite end of the board, where it can be transformed into any other piece.

Many times in life, we seem like chess pawns. We have very few moves and very few alternatives, sometimes the only thing we can do is tenaciously defend our dignity, cling to it with all our strength, sometimes it is not enough and unfortunately we lose... but other times, other glorious times, we reach that last rank and we win the game.

12.16 The Word as Medicine

We already analyzed the word as a medicine in previous chapters, but with my patients, and especially with my students and younger colleagues, I frequently use this metaphor.

During our medical training, we are taught to be careful with medical prescriptions: to know the active ingredients, excipients, pharmaceutical forms, methods of administration, doses, routes, intervals, concomitant medication, and family drugs (which may have similar effects and different tolerance).

Our art consists not only in knowing when and how to manage them, but above all, when not to manage them.

However, we are not trained in using our word in the same way.

The word also has active principles: what we should say.

It has excipients: the place in which we say it, how we introduce the topic and the silences that accompany it.

It has therapeutic effects, placebos, and nocebos.

It has forms of administration: abruptly, in small doses, incrementally.

It has routes of administration: the ways we say things, suggest them, hint at them.

It has adjuvants: strengthening or downplaying some aspects of the truth.

Taking care of our word as if it were medicine is, above all, remembering that the purpose of medical communication is essentially therapeutic.

12.17 The Meaning of Life

Nietzsche, quoted by Viktor Frankl, [64–68] maintained that *"He who has a why to live for can bear almost any how."*

It is in that sense of life where the strength to survive all misfortune lies.

The search for the meaning of life is a lifelong task, but after the diagnosis of a serious illness, that meaning becomes crucial.

Why must I endure this?

Why am I doing what I do?

What do I want to live for?

What tasks do I want to stop doing?

What tasks that I have put off all my life do I want to do now?

Most of our lives we chase carrots. That is to say, we bank moments of present happiness in exchange for future ones.

After a cancer diagnosis, living in the present means enjoying what each day can give us, but it also means having a reason to live with daily limitations and sufferings.

The meaning of our life is what gives us lucidity to enjoy the former and strength to endure the latter.

Each person has a reason to continue living: it will be their spouse, their children, their grandchildren, their job, seeing a relative marry, the birth of someone, seeing someone graduate or even finishing that one tv series or book.

There are very varied reasons and there is no one that is better than another, each one of us in their own private thoughts knows what that reason is today.

That is also where our hope and our strength lies.

12.18   Three Reasons to be Thankful for

There is a great professor at Harvard Business School, Thomas J. DeLong, [69–71] probably the most renowned expert in case-based teaching, who regularly does an exercise of finding three moments in the day for which to give thanks.

This exercise is both extremely interesting and deeply healing.

Firstly, because it forces us to look for three good things to remember about our day before resting.

It could be a word, a gesture, some form of recognition, an achievement, good news, a moment of joy.

No matter how bad your day has been, you always have to find three moments to give thanks for.

What happens is that our memory doesn't always register them if we don't go looking for them, because the bad events of the day overwhelm our consciousness.

DeLong invites us to get out of that haze and shine a light on three good moments.

Secondly, it motivates us to be grateful, to realize the gifts that have been given to us, the luck we have had, the hands that have helped us.

Being grateful is one of the wisest human attitudes.

A notebook on the nightstand, a pencil, and this exercise is a wonderful activity to end the day.

I highly recommend them to my patients.

12.19   The Advantages of Illness (or the Wise Man and the Bicycle)

This is a story taken from the narratives of the Sufis [72–74]. These narratives do not have the structure of fables, but are often teachings drawn from everyday life.

The one I heard from one of my teachers is the one about the Wise Man and the bicycle.

This story takes place in a small town in northern India in the twentieth century:

In a very poor family, made up of a father, a mother and a son, after great effort the parents manage to save a few rupees to buy their son a used bicycle.

The father cleans it, paints it, greases its chain and bearings and on the child's sixth birthday they give it to him as a gift.

Full of pride, they take the boy and his shiny bicycle to see the Wise Man who lives frugally at the end of the town.

When they see him, they show him the beautiful gift they have given their son and ask him: This is very good, right?

To which the wise man responds: it depends.

Surprised by the response, they return home confused.

Years pass, the boy handles his bicycle with great skill, moving at sometimes dizzying speeds, and when he is fifteen years old he suffers a terrible accident for which his leg has to be amputated.

Distressed parents go with their son on crutches to see the wise man and ask him.

This is very bad, right?
To which the wise man responds: it depends.
Once again surprised by the response, they return home even more confused.
Years pass again and a very bloody war breaks out between Pakistan and India.
The state institutes a draft, and takes everyone over 18 years of age to the front lines
...except the crippled.

Every time I remember this story, the inflections with which my teacher, Don Carlos Landa, who was a wonderful clinician who taught at the Faculty in Tucumán, told the story resonate in my brain and in my heart.

When he finished the story he left us this reflection: life is necessarily a tale of pain and joy, both are two sides of the same coin.

No one finds joy without having known pain and no one who has known pain stops finding joy.

Each illness has a mysterious component related to the person's existence that helps them grow. When we believe that everything is a reason for joy, we should think "*it depends.*" In the same way, when we believe that everything is a reason for pain, let's think: "*it depends.*"

12.20   The Surprises of Life (or the Prince and Death)

This is a story that José María Cabodevilla wrote in his book "December 32" about death and what happens after death.

It is a Persian legend and I transcribe it exactly as he writes it on page 6 of his text:

A gardener, still a teenager, begged his prince:

–   I found Death this morning. He threatened me! Save me! I would like to find myself far away, I would like to find myself tonight in Ispahan .

Magnanimous and affectionate , he provided him with his fastest horse. The next day the Prince encounters Death:
"Why?" he asks, "did you make a threatening gesture toward my gardener yesterday?"
-It was not so much a gesture of threat - answers Death -, but rather one of astonishment. Because I saw him in Ispahan, far away and I had to kidnap him in Ispahan that same night.

The same thing happens to us many times in life, we flee believing that we are moving away from our destination only to discover, often too late, that we were only running toward our destination.

I believe that in that sense, the most reasonable attitude is to try to look at our fears, and even at our own death, with the greatest serenity possible, because, at least in this sense, I am a fatalist: I believe that the day of our arrival into this world and the day we should leave it are probably not something we can change.

We all have our own Ispahan where we will inevitably be kidnapped at the appointed time.

But I completely understand if you don't share that idea.

12.21   The Objective of a Consultation

Finally, there is the objective of a consultation.

As we saw in one of the previous chapters, after completing a patient's medical history, I ask them what they expect from this consultation. What would they like us to answer first? What doubt would they like us to clarify?

Behind those questions is a genuine search for the patient to get what they came for in the first place.

But there is something else that motivates me to act that way, to write these tips or testimonies and ultimately to write this book.

The main objective of a consultation is for the patient to leave a little better than when they entered.

In many unfortunate cases, I may have to give the patient some bad news. That is why I make sure my patients find in me a person who wants to convey those news with care, with respect, with humanity.

In other, more fortunate cases, I can give the patient good news, calming their fears and alleviating their sorrows.

Whether the news are good or bad doesn't depend on either myself or my patient, but the way I give those news completely depends on me.

That the patient finds a person willing to listen to them, understand them, accompany them, and advise them honestly. **That** depends exclusively on me.

That my office environment is a safe environment in which the patient is treated with respect, **that** depends exclusively on me.

That the patient can speak freely knowing that what they say will be kept secret. **That** depends only on me.

That whoever leaves my consultation leaves a little better than when they came in, **that** gives meaning to my work and I hope it also gives meaning to yours.

12.22   Teaching Exercises

1. Personal

    (a) Do you have a personal communications kit?
    (b) Do you collect anecdotes from your patients?
    (c) What are your favorite readings besides those related with medicine?
    (d) Do you draw ideas from the arts or your readings for dialogue with your patients?

2. Group Activities

    (a) Get together in a writing club with your colleagues to put their experiences with patients on paper.

(b) Select a movie that reflects the emotions you feel in a specific clinical situation.

(c) Create a book club and select a text that raises an ethical issue related to medical practice.

References

1. Sontag S. Illness as metaphor and AIDS and its metaphors. Soc Sci Med. 1989;29:11.
2. Hui D, Zhukovsky DS, Bruera E. Serious illness conversations: paving the road with metaphors. Oncologist. 2018;23(6):730–3. https://doi.org/10.1634/theoncologist.2017-0448.
3. Childress JF, Siegler M. Metaphors and models of doctor-patient relationship: their implications for autonomy. Theor Med. 1984;5:17–30.
4. Sontag S. Illness as metaphor and AIDS and its metaphors. Anchor Books. 1990.
5. Uhlen M, Zhang C, Lee S, et al. A pathology atlas of the human cancer transcriptome. Science (1979). 2017;357(6352) https://doi.org/10.1126/science.aan2507.
6. Bertrand N, Wu J, Xu X, Kamaly N, Farokhzad OC. Cancer nanotechnology: the impact of passive and active targeting in the era of modern cancer biology. Adv Drug Deliv Rev. 2014:66. https://doi.org/10.1016/j.addr.2013.11.009.
7. Lambin P, Leijenaar RTH, Deist TM, et al. Radiomics: the bridge between medical imaging and personalized medicine. Nat Rev Clin Oncol. 2017;14(12) https://doi.org/10.1038/nrclinonc.2017.141.
8. Gerlinger M, Rowan AJ, Horswell S, et al. Intratumor heterogeneity and branched evolution revealed by multiregion sequencing. N Engl J Med. 2012;366(10) https://doi.org/10.1056/nejmoa1113205.
9. Kaye R. Unforgettable patients. J Pediatr. 1992;120 https://doi.org/10.1016/S0022-3476(05)81977-8.
10. Helming B. Unforgettable patient lessons from the heart. Nursing (Brux). 2001;31(9) https://doi.org/10.1097/00152193-200131090-00021.
11. Grange SL. Unforgettable patient. Going home. Nursing (Brux). 2001;31(2) https://doi.org/10.1097/00152193-200131020-00021.
12. Gunther M, Thomas SP. Nurses' narratives of unforgettable patient care events. J Nurs Scholarsh. 2006;38(4) https://doi.org/10.1111/j.1547-5069.2006.00129.x.
13. Ziegelstein RC. Personomics. *JAMA*. Intern Med. 2015;175:6. https://doi.org/10.1001/jamainternmed.2015.0861.
14. Rygiel K. Personomics—an innovative tool of precision medicine and its role in the individualized treatment of patients with breast cancer. Asia-Pac J Oncol. Published online. 2020; https://doi.org/10.32948/ajo.2020.01.10.
15. Ziegelstein RC. Personomics: the missing link in the evolution from precision medicine to personalized medicine. J Pers Med. 2017;7(4) https://doi.org/10.3390/jpm7040011.
16. Tavares T, Oliveira M, Gonçalves J, et al. Predicting prognosis in patients with advanced cancer: a prospective study. Palliat Med. 2018;32(2):413–6. https://doi.org/10.1177/0269216317705788.
17. Thomas JM, Cooney LM, Fried TR. Prognosis reconsidered in light of ancient insights-from Hippocrates to modern medicine. JAMA Intern Med. 2019;179(6) https://doi.org/10.1001/jamainternmed.2019.0302.
18. Brown R, Bylund CL, Eddington J, Gueguen JA, Kissane DW. Discussing prognosis in an oncology setting: initial evaluation of a communication skills training module. Psychooncology. 2010;19(4) https://doi.org/10.1002/pon.1580.

19. Rich BA. Prognosis terminal: truth-telling in the context of end-of-life care. Camb Q Healthc Ethics. 2014;23(2):209–19. https://doi.org/10.1017/S0963180113000741.
20. Nakazawa E, Yamamoto K, Ozeki-Hayashi R, Shaw MH, Akabayashi A. Is it worth knowing that you might die tomorrow? Revisiting the ethics of prognosis disclosure. Clin Pract. 2022;12(5):803–8. https://doi.org/10.3390/clinpract12050084.
21. Ogawa Y, Furukawa TA, Takeshima N, et al. Efficacy of antidepressants over placebo is similar in two-armed versus three-armed or more-armed randomized placebo-controlled trials. Int Clin Psychopharmacol. 2018;33(2):66–72. https://doi.org/10.1097/YIC.0000000000000201.
22. Shapiro AK, Shapiro E. The powerful placebo. From ancient priest to modern physician. The Johns Hopkins University Press; 1997.
23. Pardo-Cabello AJ, Manzano-Gamero V, Puche-Cañas E. Placebo: a brief updated review. Naunyn Schmiedeberg's Arch Pharmacol. 2022;395(11):1343–56. https://doi.org/10.1007/s00210-022-02280-w.
24. Harrington, A. (Ed.). The placebo effect: an interdisciplinary exploration. Harvard University Press. 1997.
25. Colloca L, Howick J. Placebos without deception: outcomes, mechanisms, and ethics. In: International review of neurobiology, vol. 138. Academic Press Inc.; 2018. p. 219–40. https://doi.org/10.1016/bs.irn.2018.01.005.
26. Kabat-Zinn M, Kabat-Zinn J. Everyday Blessings: The Inner Work of Mindful Parenting. New York: Hyperion. 1997.
27. Kabat-Zinn J. Coming to Our Senses: Healing Ourselves and the World through Mindfulness. New York: Hyperion. 2005.
28. Ga-Eun (Grace) Oh. LIFE AS A JOURNEY: A VIEW OF LIFE AS A JOURNEY MODERATES THE RELATIONSHIP BETWEEN SUBJECTIVE AGE AND SUBJECTIVE HEALTH. Innovation in Aging. 2019;3(Supplement_1):S454–S55. https://doi.org/10.1093/geroni/igz038.1702.
29. Madry H. Life is a journey. J Exp Orthop. 2019;6(1) https://doi.org/10.1186/s40634-019-0202-8.
30. Poppi F, Kravanja P. Sic vita est: visual representation in painting of the conceptual metaphor LIFE IS A JOURNEY. Semiotica . Published online. 2019; https://doi.org/10.1515/sem-2018-0009.
31. Rogers BA, Chicas H, Kelly JM, et al. Seeing your life story as a hero's journey increases meaning in life. J Pers Soc Psychol. Published online. 2023; https://doi.org/10.1037/pspa0000341.
32. Pogonowski J. Mathematics is the logic of the infinite": Zermelo's project of infinitary logic. Studies in Logic, Grammar and Rhetoric 2021;66(3). https://doi.org/10.2478/slgr-2021-0042.
33. Wenmackers S, Benci V, Di Nasso M. How to measure the infinite: mathematics with infinite and infinitesimal numbers. Philos Math. 2022;30(1) https://doi.org/10.1093/philmat/nkab030.
34. Díaz-Pachón DA, Hössjer O, Marks RJ. Sometimes size does not matter. Found Phys. 2023;53(1) https://doi.org/10.1007/s10701-022-00650-1.
35. Worthington EL, Sandage SJ. Forgiveness and spirituality in psychotherapy: a relational approach; 2015. https://doi.org/10.1037/14712-000.
36. Aten JD, McMinn MR, Worthington EL. Spiritually oriented interventions for counseling and psychotherapy; 2011. https://doi.org/10.1037/12313-000.
37. Aten JD, O'Grady KA, Worthington EL. The psychology of religion and spirituality for clinicians: using research in your practice. 2013. https://doi.org/10.4324/9780203864920.
38. Davis EB, Worthington EL, Schnitker SA. Handbook of positive psychology, religion, and spirituality; 2022. https://doi.org/10.1007/978-3-031-10274-5.
39. Woodyatt L, Worthington EL, Wenzel M, Griffin BJ. Handbook of the psychology of self-forgiveness; 2017. https://doi.org/10.1007/978-3-319-60573-9.
40. Toussaint LL, Worthington EL, Williams DR. Forgiveness and health: scientific evidence and theories relating forgiveness to better health; 2015. https://doi.org/10.1007/978-94-017-9993-5.
41. Worthington EL. Forgiveness and reconciliation: theory and application. 2014. https://doi.org/10.4324/9780203942734.

42. McCullough ME, Rachal KC, Worthington EL. Interpersonal forgiving in close relationships. J Pers Soc Psychol. 1997;73(2) https://doi.org/10.1037/0022-3514.73.2.321.

43. Leget C. Forgiveness and reconciliation in palliative care: the gap between the psychological and moral approaches. Religions (Basel). 2020;11(9) https://doi.org/10.3390/rel11090440.

44. Wittenberg E, Ferrell B, Goldsmith J, Buller H. Provider difficulties with spiritual and forgiveness communication at the end of life. Am J Hosp Palliat Med. 2016;33(9) https://doi.org/10.1177/1049909115591811.

45. Goman CC. A narrative framework for forgiveness at the end of life: suggestions for future research in health communication. Rev Commun. 2017;17(3) https://doi.org/10.1080/15358593.2017.1331256.

46. Ferrell B, Otis-Green S, Baird RP, Garcia A. Nurses' responses to requests for forgiveness at the end of life. J Pain Symptom Manag. 2014;47(3) https://doi.org/10.1016/j.jpainsymman.2013.05.009.

47. Thankaraj J. Time in Ecclesiastes and the Mahabharata. Ecum Rev. 2022;74(5) https://doi.org/10.1111/erev.12748.

48. Kabat-Zinn J. Full catastrophe living: using the wisdom of your body and mind to face stress, pain, and illness, 15th Anniversary Ed.; 2005.

49. Back A, Arnold R, Tulsky J. Mastering communication with seriously ill patients: balancing honesty with empathy and hope; 2009. https://doi.org/10.1017/CBO9780511576454.

50. Macgowan MJ, Engle B. Evidence for optimism: behavior therapies and motivational interviewing in adolescent substance abuse treatment. Child Adolesc Psychiatr Clin N Am. 2010;19(3) https://doi.org/10.1016/j.chc.2010.03.006.

51. Moloud R, Saeed Y, Mahmonir H, Rasool GA. Cognitive-behavioral group therapy in major depressive disorder with focus on self-esteem and optimism: an interventional study. BMC Psychiatry. 2022;22(1) https://doi.org/10.1186/s12888-022-03918-y.

52. Asani S, Panahali A, Abdi R, Badri GR. The effectiveness of mindfulness-based cognitive therapy on academic emotions and academic optimism of procrastinating students. Mod Care J. 2022;20(1) https://doi.org/10.5812/modernc-129819.

53. Martens WHJ. Optimism therapy: an adapted psychotherapeutic strategy for adult female survivors of childhood sexual abuse. Ann Am Psychother Assoc. 2007;10(2)

54. Werdani YDW. Spiritual Well-being and optimism as contributing factors that influence the subjective Well-being of cancer patients. Indones J Cancer. 2022;16(1) https://doi.org/10.33371/ijoc.v16i1.819.

55. Matzka M, Köck-Hódi S, Jahn P, Mayer H. Relationship among symptom clusters, quality of life, and treatment-specific optimism in patients with cancer. Support Care Cancer. 2018;26(8) https://doi.org/10.1007/s00520-018-4102-8.

56. Pujol SP, Guiteras AF. Proposal for an instrument for the detection of strategic optimism in breast cancer. Psicooncologia (Pozuelo de Alarcon). 2019;16(2) https://doi.org/10.5209/psic.65593.

57. Schenk EL, Patil T, Pacheco J, Bunn PA. 2020 Innovation-based optimism for lung cancer outcomes. Oncologist. 2021;26:3. https://doi.org/10.1002/onco.13590.

58. Belete TM. The current status of gene therapy for the treatment of cancer. Biologics. 2021:15. https://doi.org/10.2147/BTT.S302095.

59. Tannock IF. Treating the patient, not just the cancer. N Engl J Med. 1987;317(24) https://doi.org/10.1056/nejm198712103172409.

60. Tannock I. Will increases in chemotherapy dose intensity improve outcome of patients with common malignancies? Am J Med. 1995;99(6 SUPPL.1)

61. Pérez-Reverte A. Corsarios de Levante. 1ª ed. Madrid, España: Alfaguara. 2006.

62. Pérez-Reverte A. El club Dumas. 1ª ed. Madrid, España: Alfaguara. 1993.

63. Pérez-Reverte A. El maestro de esgrima. 1ª ed. Madrid, España: Alfaguara. 1988.

64. Frankl VE. The Unheard Cry for Meaning. Psychotherapy and Humanism. New York: Simon and Schuster. 1978.

65. Frankl VE. The Will to Meaning: Foundations and Applications of Logotherapy. New York: New American Library. 1969.

66. Frankl VE. Man's search for meaning: An introduction to logotherapy (4th ed.) (I. Lasch, Trans.). Beacon Press. 1992.
67. Frankl VE. On the theory and therapy of mental disorders : an introduction to logotherapy and existential analysis; 2004. doi:https://doi.org/10.4324/9780203005897.
68. Frankl VE. Psychotherapy and existentialism: Selected papers on logotherapy. New York: Simon and Schuster. 1967.
69. DeLong TJ. CASE STUDY: when your star player asks to go part-time. Harv Bus Rev. 2021;99:1.
70. DeLong TJ, DeLong S. The paradox of excellence. Harv Bus Rev. 2011;89:6.
71. Anderson-Gough F. When professionals have to lead: a new model for high performance. Eur Account Rev. 2011;20(1) https://doi.org/10.1080/09638180.2011.566680.
72. Seck M. Wolof Sufi Oral narratives' structure and function. Uskudar university mysticism research Institute Magazine. 2023;2023(3) https://doi.org/10.32739/ustad.2023.3.40.
73. King JR. Religious and therapeutic elements in Sufi teaching stories. J Relig Health. 1988;27(3) https://doi.org/10.1007/BF01533183.
74. Zsom D. Sufi Stories from the Cairo Genizah. *The Arabist: Budapest Studies in Arabic*. 2015; 36. https://doi.org/10.58513/arabist.2015.36.4.

Chapter 13
Teaching Communication Skills

13.1 Introduction

We have reached the final chapter. First of all, I want to thank you all for your patience in reading the previous chapters, I hope you have enjoyed them and that they were useful to you.

If we consider that communication, in addition to being a gift, is a skill that is learned, acquired, and perfected, then the time has come to finally teach it.

Let us remember that the first barrier that we must overcome is the belief that communication is innate and is not in fact a type of knowledge that can be provided [1].

This chapter is not placed here randomly. I've placed it here at the end in order to encourage all of my readers to flex their teaching muscles.

Allow me to explain: for me, teaching is the most human art of all. It is an art that humanizes both the person who imparts knowledge and those who receive it.

Why?

Because when we teach, we all learn from each other. Teachers from their students and vice versa. Every question that challenges established knowledge and every creative response that helps us understand or solve a problem enriches us deeply. It makes us all better.

Evolutionarily, teaching and learning have been the two most extraordinary tools for the progress of our species. By the same token, moral sensitivity has been integral for the care of other living beings and the environment.

There are some extraordinary texts on teaching communication concepts and skills in medicine, one of them is the one written by Ellen J. Belzer [2]. I highly recommend reading it to those interested in delving deeper into this topic.

Guided by many of their recommendations, I am going to develop in this chapter the teaching strategies that I use in my undergraduate and graduate courses relating to communication in medicine.

E. Gil Deza, *Improving Clinical Communication*, https://doi.org/10.1007/978-3-031-62446-9_13

To do this, we must understand what the barriers are to teaching this skill.

The work of Ruiz Moral and collaborators is very instructive regarding Latin American medical culture [3].

Among the outstanding points are the following:

(a) He highlights the negative attitude of teachers: they don't believe the topic to be practical or necessary.
(b) He also highlights the difficulty in incorporating the topic into students' curricula, since authorities believe that it'll take time away from other subjects, or they mention the topic is already included in other humanities subjects (Ethics, History of Medicine, Anthropology, or Psychology).
(c) The students also hold negative opinions of the topic: it is not an important subject because it is not "scientific." It is not taken into account for admission to residences. It is subjective and innate.
(d) He highlights the difficulty of professors equipped to teach the subject.
(e) Finally, Ruiz Moral talks about the restrictions placed on the use of proven methods designed to test the effectiveness of learning and skill assessment.

Each and every one of these statements can be dealt with, but only after we recognize what the barriers are to implementing this discipline in undergraduate and postgraduate health sciences careers in our current social and cultural environment.

This chapter will focus on teaching communication skills in a sequential manner, beginning with one-on-one teaching and ending in how to create a syllabus for a communication course.

13.2   Teaching at the Office (Shadow Observer)

Observing the activity of a doctor with greater experience in dealing with patients is an inexhaustible source of knowledge [4].

From this perspective, it continues to be one of the most important teaching–learning modes in all medical schools, and is very useful for the acquisition of diagnostic, therapeutic, communication, and teaching skills [5–7].

It is crucial to take advantage of the moment of student observation to clarify the communication strategies used.

Between each patient, the time is used to analyze the technical aspects (diagnosis, therapy, and prognosis) [8] as well as the ethical and communication aspects.

What did the patient want to know?

What did we say, how did we say it, how did we begin and end the dialogue?

What did the patient understand?

What do we perceive from what they felt?

What do we feel?

What made you feel comfortable?

What made you uncomfortable?

What did you learn?

What would they have done differently?

Each encounter, each patient, and each doctor is different and has different ways of approaching the same problem.

That is why it is good for the student to go through different experiences during their career: emergency rooms, obstetrics, pediatrics, adult clinic, neurology, oncology, psychiatry, chronic care, palliative care, end-of-life care [9]. These are all circumstances where communication not only covers different topics, but the way in which we approach the patient is different, making them all invaluable steps in the students' path.

In one of our graduate seminars, I ask students to describe the patient who had the most impact on your life.

Eight out of ten doctors or dentists remember patients they met at the end of medical school or right after graduation, many of them were seen during hospital shifts or their rural rotation. In many cases, that memory conditioned their choice of medical specialty. Some of those meetings happened decades ago, but the memory still burns bright.

We must take advantage of these opportunities so that the student can observe not just our clinical [10] or surgical skills [11, 12] but also our communication skills [13–15].

It will do them a lot of good and we will collaborate in their training [12].

It will also improve our practice, as it encourages us to do things better by knowing that we are being observed and can be role models for others, regardless of the fact theory and practice are hardly ever comparable [16, 17].

13.3 Using Real Patients as Teachers

This is perhaps one of the best strategies when teaching communication skills [10, 18–20]. Select those patients who can get involved in teaching and ask them to interact with the students.

Each of them is not only an expert in the ailment that affects them but also in the evaluation of the students' strengths and areas to improve [8].

There are numerous advantages to patient collaboration in medical education:

(a) Patients suffering from rare diseases allow students to come into contact with people who suffer from these conditions, which would otherwise be highly unlikely [21].
(b) It breaks the social stigma that students carry by allowing them to interact with people affected by different conditions, especially mental ones [22].
(c) It allows the patient's narrative, their personal experience, to be recorded by the student, which is crucial when the patient's story may be affected by mental disability [23].
(d) The impact of the disease on the patient's life can be evaluated, including emotional and spiritual aspects [24].

(e) It allows patients from other regions or cultures to be selected and help expand the student's cultural competence [25].

(f) In certain specialties, such as rheumatology, patients can not only report the development of their disease but also teach how to perform semiological maneuvers as effectively as medical consultants [26, 27].

Of course, this involves, first of all, training those patients, as well as their care during class [28].

The patient is providing us with an enormous service by providing their body, history, time, and person for medical training. At a minimum, we must use the parameters established in the Association of Standardized Patients [29] when it comes to their wellbeing.

These guides are based on five principles: safety, quality, professionalism, accountability, and collaboration, each of them are further developed in lists that we must consider when designing the activity we want to carry out.

The patient will be exposed to remembering his or her history, may undergo procedures or maneuvers [30], may be physically or psychologically vulnerable, therefore it is the educator's duty to ensure that everything that will be done will be both useful for learning and safe for the patient.

The moment of debriefing, when the patient evaluates a medical student, is usually a highly emotional and unforgettable moment for the student.

13.4 Teaching in Small Groups

Teaching in small groups (committees), in which no more than ten students are guided by a coordinator, is the core of teaching clinical skills [31].

In small groups, teaching is established in three pillars: interaction with the patient, interaction with the coordinator, and interaction with our peers.

The small group allows us to share experiences, points of view, doubts, and observations so that almost nothing gets overlooked.

It allows ideas to be shared and different points of view to be selected, where different members of the group can defend their points of view and enrich the rest.

That is why group design is a back and forth between homogeneity and heterogeneity: the group must be homogeneous enough to share communication codes and heterogeneous enough for different ideas and points of view to emerge.

The group dynamic is unique because alliances between students are usually not permanent but circumstantial and that is why they are the natural environment for problem-based learning.

Problems are often, unfortunately, reduced to dilemmas in classes or large groups, since it is very difficult to analyze all points of view and solutions, but in small groups, this is feasible.

The committee in which one studies thus becomes a safe environment for the expression and discussion of ideas.

On the other hand, there are synthesis works such as posters or murals that, when done in groups, tend to be enriched by the multiple skills that the group possesses: creativity, imagination, ideation, writing.

13.5   Classroom Teaching to Large Groups

Teaching in classrooms to relatively large groups continues to be the most used method in medical education to transmit knowledge [32–37].

I have selected the word knowledge on purpose, because during class, the teacher exercises leadership in teaching. A leader, as Henry Kissinger argues in his book *Leadership: six studies in world strategy* [38], takes the public from the past to the future.

In their classes, the teacher guides their students along five different paths: from ignorance to knowledge, from the superfluous to the essential, from the incoherent to the coherent, from the complex to the simple, from the past to the future.

What's more, although the traditional class continues to be superior to online classes, and its role is maintained despite the changes introduced by technology, it is a challenge to avoid the exodus of students from classes [39]. Especially the exodus of attention, increasingly hijacked by various networks.

There are some interesting experiences about the participation of students in classes in which the roles are reversed, which is called "flipping." [40–45]. In these, the teacher, instead of giving information, asks questions whose answers must be investigated by the students and then shared. This technique can be very interesting to apply in certain cases [46].

We must also consider that online classes were born of the need to implement teaching regimes at times when in-person attendance is not recommended, both in a pandemic and in war [47–49].

There are numerous tips for implementing a class [50], but two are truly essential: mastery of the topic and inspiration for students.

Mastery of the subject should be an obvious requirement, meanwhile, inspiring the students should be done at the end of the class, in order to entice them for the next lesson.

No matter how focused the topic we are looking at, it is an opportunity to learn the language of medicine [51], especially for students whose first language isn't one of the romance languages, or, at the very least, has words rooted in Latin and Greek [52].

Learning medicine is learning a new language, made up of more than 20,000 terms that are not in the common vocabulary of most people. A single medical word can indicate the pathology of the disease, origin of the injury, its location, and type. In one sentence, we can summarize an entire story that can take years to develop. A single sign gives us the key to what is happening.

But also each word has a history and each story has a name, a time, a way of practicing medicine, a doctor behind it.

Each of our students is called to write their name in the history of medicine: it can be universal, national, regional, or institutional history. If not, at the very least, they'll write their name in the history of their patients. But without understanding that history, there is no inspiration or motivation to study or improve. That is what the teacher must provide.

They must put their chosen topic in context: historical, ethical, epidemiological, and pathophysiological. They must explain how to diagnose a disease, be it clinically or with other techniques. They must analyze the evidence to justify the treatments they recommend.

Synthesize. Explain. Define. Choose. Inspire. They are all verbs and actions that apply to a great teacher and an unforgettable class.

If the class is in-person, the teacher also deploys their arts of conjuring and stagecraft: their gestures, body language, and words must work in concert to relay their teachings to the audience.

Learning is not just understanding but also getting excited about understanding.

A good class is truly unforgettable. I still remember the tone of my teacher's voice when he transmitted knowledge to us, the reverence with which he pronounced a name, the simplicity of a transcendent discovery, the apparent inconsequentiality in the eyes of his contemporaries of revolutionary knowledge (such as when William Harvey described blood circulation, a fact that had no immediate effect, but had ended the Galenic reign of fourteen centuries) [53].

Only a teacher has this possibility of perspective.

That is why class preparation is crucial, and is the topic of the next section.

13.6   Designing a Class

Of all the fundamental aspects of designing a class, the most important is mastery of the topic: this means that you must know the topic that you are going to teach in depth and, if it is a skill, you must have experience in what you are going to transmit.

A teacher has the opportunity to transform a good moment into an unforgettable moment. Don't waste it.

Theoretical mastery of a topic assumes many things. First, you must be able to *"define"* it precisely. By this, I don't mean you have to know the dictionary definition (though you certainly should), but rather you must know the history of the topic: how it started, which ideas and viewpoints competed throughout history, and finally, why one (if any) prevailed over the others. You must also know the biography of the men and women behind those ideas. The class can go from the general (the panorama) to the particular (the microscopic) or vice versa. The important thing is that you should reach your endpoints, whether general or particular, in a small number of steps (ideally, five).

Practical mastery of the subject involves the confrontation of the abstract, theoretical model with concrete reality: this adjustment is called experience [54]. When did theory work, when did it need some adjusting, what mistakes you made, and ultimately, what you learned by applying that knowledge.

That is what the student is going to take away from you.

When planning the class, I use the three-stage model:

(a) I start with the conclusions you wish to reach, because the students' attention falters after the first minutes. *This is what I want you to take home today.*
(b) I continue with demonstrations: the entire theoretical, historical, ethical, and biographical framework. It is essentially information. I do it in the form of questions and point out where they can find the answers.
(c) I finish by repeating the conclusions, if possible in the form of images and sometimes with music, so that it's easier to remember.

Since topic that brings us together in this chapter is a class on communication, I'll use this time to explain the exercises I use most frequently in my own classes:

13.6.1 Role Play

A role-playing exercise is essentially a continuation of children's games, such as playing house, playing doctor, cops and robbers, etc.

In short, role-playing allows us to physically and mentally assume the representation of a communicational instance [21, 55–58].

In communication, it is a great exercise because there are four roles that you can study:

(a) The Sender, aka the one who has to broadcast the news.
(b) The receiver, aka the one who has to receive the news.
(c) Observers, aka the rest of the class.
(d) The one who selected the topic.

In practice, it is a very simple exercise: two or more students are selected (depending on how much noise is desired between sender and receiver) and then whoever has the role of sender is given a card with the topic that must be communicated: *"the diagnosis is malignant/benign," "unfortunately the patient died," "the patient is cured,"* and so on. The receiver gets a card with the emotion with which they must respond: *"relief," "disappointment," "regret," "guilt," "gratitude," "distress,"* etc.

Allow them to interact for 10 min and then begin interacting with the class:

What did they feel?
What did they think?
How would they have done it differently?
Who has had a similar experience?
What seemed right to you?
What seemed wrong to you?

And if it is feasible, those who think it could have been done differently should come and show how they think it should've been done.

Finally, you should ask the whole class what they thought of the topic and the chosen emotion. Is there another name for that emotion? What would it be? How would they represent it?

13.6.2   Charades

Charades [59, 60] is a game designed to evaluate non-verbal communication skills, both in the transmission and interpretation of a message.

It is a very common game at children's birthdays and family gatherings, where you have to try to guess something (usually an object, a movie, or something similar) by interpreting non-verbal signals from a partner .

It is essentially a game about transmitting information through body language, and how to interpret it. Which means it can easily be adapted for use in class.

There are at least three variants:

1. The classic one in which one gives an emotion to the sender, and they must explain what it is to the class without speaking, everything must be communicated gesturally. The class, meanwhile, must try to interpret the actor's state of mind. The first person to correctly detect the mood must explain what was the key that led them to that conclusion.
2. A second variant consists of the exercise of watching a videoclip. This can be from the news, a movie, a YouTube video, or some other piece of audiovisual media [61–63]. The trick, however, is that the class must watch it without sound. Ideally, the video should be around 5 min long, during which the class should record the emotions that the speaker is transmitting. Afterwards, they can watch the video with sound and compare and contrast everyone's perception and how well it held up when the full video was experienced. If you want to make it more of a game, pause the video at times of your choosing and have students write down the main emotion they see in the image, then award points based on accuracy when the full video is played.
3. The third exercise is that of the *deaf class* [64, 65]. Students are instructed to come to class with earplugs or sound-attenuating headphones. The teacher, with the class *"deafened"* thus, gives a ten-minute speech on a topic. The class challenge is similar to the previous one: the students must write down the topic they believe was being discussed, the emotions that the teacher brought into play and the ideas that accompanied that emotion.

In all cases, we seek to stimulate understanding of non-verbal signals, which will ideally also bring to the forefront the amount of information we transmit without realizing it through our own non-verbal cues.

13.6.3 Media Interview

The idea of this exercise is to teach students how to compress their messages without losing detail [66–68]. Media, whether it be printed, radio, television, and so on, usually have limited time (or space) with which to transmit an idea, which means you're incentivized to transmit the message with as few words as possible.

In this exercise, each student is given a published paper to read, while being told they'll need to act as the researchers' spokesperson. They will have to summarize the paper, first in 10 m, then 5 m, and finally, in a minute and a half. The other students should pay attention to:

What did they elect to say in each case?
How did they say it?
How do they start and end that message?

It should be patently obvious that the minute and a half summary will be the most demanding, as it must be focused on the most important discovery, finding, conclusion, or challenge of the entire work.

Aside from teaching compression, this exercise is also good in teaching correction.

Everything can be said, but not everything can be said in the same manner.

The problem is not how much time you have, but how you use it.

Everyone has the opportunity for their "five minutes of fame," but few know how to take advantage of it.

13.6.4 Debates

Debates are one of the most valuable communication exercises [69, 70]. Firstly, because they allow the dynamic exchange of ideas, and secondly, because the objective of the debate is not to fight and defeat the other, but to argue in such a way as to convince the audience.

Once students understand the reason for this dynamic, they acquire the ability to look for interesting arguments and ways to say them in a convincing way for the audience.

For the first debate, teams of four members with a captain are chosen according to their affinity with their own ideas, making it easier for them to study the arguments for and against.

For the second debate, a topic is selected and teams are formed like for the first debate, but each team needs to defend ideas that they personally oppose, with the aim of studying the elements in favor of the opposite position in a more in-depth way.

For the third debate, teams should comprise people both for *and* against the topic selected, though each team overall must of course present a position either in favor or in opposition, as dictated by the teacher.

The rules of the debate are established: opening, development, cross-questions, and closing. The rules of behavior are established: what is allowed and what is not allowed. After the debate, the audience is asked to vote for which position was most convincing. As a bonus, you can ask two members of the audience to come forth and explain the arguments for and against, to see how well the audience actually understood the topic.

This kind of exercise is particularly well suited to studying bioethical concerns.

13.6.5   Scientific Writing: Abstract, Case Report, Paper

Scientific writing is a necessary and useful skill [71–76].

Knowing how to write in an impersonal manner, how to use the correct tenses, and how to use the correct acronyms in order to save space are all invaluable aspects of our profession.

The initial structure (the first draft) should have these writing rules:

(a) Three paragraphs for the introduction (one for the explaining of the problem, one for what we know so far, and one to explain what we were looking for and the reason why we were interested).
(b) Two paragraphs for material and methods (One for selection criteria and one for statistical analysis).
(c) Four paragraphs, two tables and two figures for results (One for population characteristics, one for implementation of the study, one for main results, and one for secondary findings; the tables and figures should complement these topics).
(d) Four paragraphs for discussion (one for those who agree with what was discovered, one for those who disagree with what was discovered, one to highlight what was discovered, and one for future research needed).
(e) A paragraph for conclusions.
(f) A five word title.
(g) Authors.

The work can be done individually or in a group. Both ways are appropriate as long as the roles and efforts of each of the members are equitably distributed in group work.

Students choose the topic they want to research and once it has been approved, they have 1 week to make their first draft and present it. After that they have a month to finish it, presenting their progress each week to get feedback. At the end of the month, each group must present their research to the class. For this, they should write an abstract (consisting of: Title, Authors and a paragraph for four topics: Objectives, Material and methods, Results, and Conclusions) as well as make a ten-minute oral presentation (With a maximum of seven slides: Title (1), Work Description (5), Acknowledgments (1).

This exercise helps in stimulating an interest in bibliographic research, clinical histories, or clinical cases and to write following the rules stipulated for scientific publications, while at the same time helping students with "clarity of language," that is, to transmit ideas with the greatest simplicity possible. Above all, it helps them appreciate scientific literature from a new perspective.

13.6.6 Writing to a Colleague

Writing to a colleague is about a clinical case [77–81] and consists of writing two handwritten notes: in one, you agree with your colleague's choice of treatment. In the other, you don't. Each note should have the following paragraphs:

1. Personalized greeting.
2. Description of the problem.
3. Explanation of our recommendation.
4. Farewell and leaving open a communication channel in case of doubt or disagreement.

This practice, which today seems a bit outdated, helps in establishing respect for the absent colleague and lays the foundations for a potentially conflictive situation that is the oft-feared "second opinion."

Many patients today seek a second opinion, and it is very reasonable to assume that we'll not always agree with our colleague's assessment (whether we're the "second opinion" ourselves or the "first" one, as it were).

We should never assume that our colleague is wrong in their assessment, especially if we're seeing the patient after them.

We must consider that it is possible that we are seeing the patient at a different evolutionary stage of the disease, or we're seeing them after they've carried out a new study that our colleague had no access to.

When we explain our findings we must highlight these circumstances.

The tone must be friendly, otherwise our colleague can feel judged or criticized.

If our indication differs from what our colleague made, it is not necessary for us to emphasize that we disagree, our duty is to rationally justify what we think is correct.

Finally, we must say goodbye with respect and leave an interpersonal communication channel open so that, if they so wish, they can contact us.

The fact that it is handwritten gives it an air of greater professional respect, as long as our handwriting is legible.

A variant of this exercise is to establish beforehand whether the student's relationship with the colleague is friendly or unfriendly, which sometimes influences the choice of words and makes the class more interesting.

13.6.7   Emotional Writing

This exercise is triggered by an emotion. Two that I frequently use in class are gratitude [82–85] and forgiveness [86, 87] (though many others can be used), which are
two very powerful emotions.

For the thank you letter, we must begin by keeping in mind the person we want
to thank, then write the reasons why we want to thank them and finally the way we
want to do it.

Many times this letter is addressed to someone that is alive, so the exercise ends
by having the student deliver that letter.

Voluntarily, those who wish to share their letter can do so in the classroom, but
the objective of the exercise is to focus on the study of the emotion of gratitude.

What is a gift?

Why do we feel undeserving of receiving it?

What impact did it have on our lives?

Have we thanked the person we're writing the letter to before?

Why do we want to thank them?

How do we want to do it?

What do we expect to happen?

How do we feel after writing that note?

Something similar happens with the letter of forgiveness.

Again, this is an intimate letter that can only be shared if the interested party
wishes to do so.

We address this letter to someone who, knowingly or not, has caused us harm.

Therefore, if the person is not aware of what they have done to us, this will be an
unpleasant surprise for them.

This means that if the person we're writing to is alive, it is not essential to hand
her over; it must be an exercise in prudence that leads us to do so.

This letter describes history, as we remember it, to capture on paper the facts and
circumstances in which such an event occurred.

It should also describe what the damage we suffered consisted of, and how it
marked our life or our behavior.

Finally, it should include why we have we now decided to forgive this fact, what
has changed in our lives that gives us the strength to leave this situation in the past.

Once again the exercise consists of connecting with the emotion of forgiveness.

What does forgiveness mean?

Why do we give it?

What do we hope will happen to us?

What do we hope will happen to the other if they receive this letter?

What words do we use to describe the events and what were the damages?

13.6.8   Reverse, Mirror, or Unskilled Handwriting

These are exercises to practice at home to see how our mind works [88–90].

Reverse writing is training with our dominant hand so that we can write upside down, meaning someone sitting in front of us can read it without issue.

This is an interesting exercise because usually, our patients sit in front of us. Meaning if we practice enough, we can write for *them* and not for us.

It is something that many patients appreciate, because as you speak you write so that they understand the alternatives, the numbers, the acronyms of the studies we order, or the treatments we recommend.

The extra challenge this represents tends to generate admiration and confidence in the patient, which leads to our analysis of their case and our therapeutic recommendation being more understandable. Especially because these are notes patients usually take with them.

On more than one occasion, the patient has returned, several years later, with the note I wrote, which has been with them ever since.

Mirror writing is the exercise of writing, just as Leonardo did in his notebooks, so that it can only be read in a mirror.

In addition to being a difficult exercise, it is a diversion that helps improve handwriting and spelling, but above all, it helps synthesize ideas, since one ends up writing only what one considers essential.

This exercise has helped me bring more than one abstract below the maximum number of words allowed.

Writing with our non-dominant hand is an exercise in creativity; the slowness and difficulty involved in knowing what one wants to say but not being able to write it correctly is notable.

It helps us face a difficulty similar to that suffered by many of our neurological patients or our young children.

All these exercises seek to get us out of our automatic mindset and rediscover the pleasure of writing for communication, which is so important in medicine.

13.6.9   Discussing Clinical Cases

Most of the time, the discussion of clinical cases is focused on the pathology and the greater or lesser difficulty of establishing the diagnosis, therapy, or prognosis.

In short, the discussion is about whether a case is unusual or not.

In communication, on the other hand, the clinical case is fundamentally used to see how we approach a person who has a particular history, ideas, values, and desires that are specific to that person.

Therefore, the discussion does not focus on the complexity of the case in question, but rather on the adaptability of medical discourse to communicate with the patient.

We can use real patients or cases in which the teacher guides the class.

It is an exercise that allows us to see how the student asks questions and how they refine the question to obtain the answer to what they are looking for.

Why is what you ask important?

Why do you have difficulty asking it directly?

Why do you ask it this way?

Is there another way to ask it?

How would the student like to be asked?

13.6.10   Testimonials from Colleagues

Many journals, including the most important oncology journal, the Journal of Clinical Oncology (JCO) , have among their chapters testimonials where doctors write about their experience with patients [91].

In the case of the JCO, it is called "Art of Oncology," and previously it had an even more explicit subtitle "When the tumor is not the target," to differentiate it from the articles intended to inform us about certain treatments or molecular targets.

I frequently use the testimonies in this section in my classes to show my students how doctors around the world feel more or less the same, have more or less the same difficulties and are going through more or less the same feelings.

How patients who die affect us all. How pediatric patients tend to give us lessons of wisdom for our entire lives and, above all, how experiences that have happened decades before the author sat down to write the testimony we read, have stayed with them all this time.

The same will undoubtedly happen to them throughout their career.

They are moments of great common enrichment in the class. It is as if we are all receiving the same lesson that a colleague has generously decided to put into writing.

13.6.11   Meditation

The meditation class is an exercise that I give toward the mid-point of the course.

In our country, this means it happens during winter, before mid-terms in July.

Most students are anxious and worried about those mid-terms, so it is a good time to see how to deal with worries.

I use Dr. Jon Kabat-Zinn's seated meditation tapes for the exercise [92], all of which are available online.

Normally, in a class of fifty students, there are about ten who practice meditation, about ten who think it is a huge nonsense and make fun of it, and about thirty who have not tried it.

We put the chairs in a circle, and I invite students to make themselves comfortable, put away all electronic items and follow Kabat-Zinn's voice.

There are usually moments of discomfort and, on more than one occasion, I have had to impose my authority as a teacher and "force" them to do it and even change places with some joker who makes it difficult for his colleagues to attempt the exercise.

After 5 min, the mood of the group usually changes and we begin to see the benefits of the ability to calm down.

At the end of this activity, I explain the difference between the left and right hemispheres of the brain when it comes to attention, memory, and perception of reality.

Meditation forces us to concentrate our attention on breathing and that, in some way, manages to lower anxiety levels, allowing us to see more clearly the problem(s) that afflict us.

Just as dawn makes the threatening shadows cast on the ceiling of a child's room disappear, so does the tranquility of our mind in a safe space makes the monsters of the imagination disappear.

Then we talk about what we fear about exams: not having tried too hard, losing face, jeopardizing a scholarship.

What affects our mood?

Where did our mind travel?

What recurring idea affected our concentration?

How much did it cost us to keep cell phones off?

I later explain that an increasing number of doctors are also everyday meditators, and that helps us stay sane in the midst of some chaotic days.

13.6.12   Theater

Theater as we know it, was born in Greece and it is therefore not surprising that the word "person" derives from the mask they used and that Greece is also the cradle of democracy [93].

This relationship between an area closely related to people's expression and democratic deliberation is no mere accident.

One of the texts I use is that of Armand Nicholi, professor of psychiatry at Harvard, who wrote the work "The Question of God" [94] in which he imagines a meeting between Sigmund Freud and CS Lewis.

In that play, these two giants analyze the problem of God, the meaning of life, and the question of death and they do it in a masterful way.

The dialogues of the actors present us in an original way the problem of the existence of God, using the myths, fictions, and realities presented by two giants of thought, both distinguished writers. Nicholi extracts his ideas from the profuse correspondence that both authors had with different people and presents them to us, the audience.

To read or better yet, to act out this work, is to go through the finest arguments on this problem.

The theatrical experience is one of the richest to learn empathy [95, 96].

13.6.13 Movies

The use of films for teaching communication in medicine is widespread and there are many interesting and profound topics that have been put up on the silver screen [97].

The death of a smoker is represented by Jason Robards in a superlative way in the film "Magnolia" and his dialogue with his nurse, represented by Philip Seymour Hoffman, is excellent.

Another excellent film is "The Diving Bell and the Butterfly" which describes the experience of a locked-in syndrome suffered by Jean-Dominique Bauby.

Assisted fertilization and the limit to treatments is explored in a wonderful way in the film "My sister's Keeper" with Cameron Diaz, Alec Baldwin, the masterful Abigail Breslin, and Sofía Vassilieva. It is not only fun but also very deep and it allows us to see the different perspectives from which a problem must be faced.

But, from my perspective, one of the most useful films for doctor–patient communication is "The Doctor," [98] a 1991 film where there is a masterful interaction between William Hunt and Wendy Crewson (it can be seen on YouTube under the title "First exam") .

In that scene, everything that is of a technical nature is done perfectly: the office is spotless, hands are washed, the endoscopy maneuver is carried out flawlessly and yet, at the same time, everything that pertains to communication is a disaster: there is zero empathy, no care for the information provided, and no care is taken about what the patient feels.

Additionally, it helps to reflect on the sexism present in medical practice in the last century.

It is a scene that I usually use in my classes, because it allows us to see, in an objective way and with the help of two great actors, the gestures and words that we use in our consultations and how to correct some defects.

13.6.14 Analyzing a Photograph

Photography is an extraordinary art that immortalizes a moment. The refinement of semiology means recovering the ability to observe the moment [99, 100].

Throughout my teaching experience, I have a series of photographs of different moments taken by great photographers. Robert Capa [101, 102] is one of my favorites, especially for his series of photographs documenting the Spanish Civil War and the Second World War. He is particularly fascinating when we realize he took all his pictures with a 35 mm camera and a single 50 mm lens, although his whole life is extraordinary.

There are numerous photographs to analyze: rampaging crowds, destroyed soldiers, profiles of people in deep loneliness, depression or pain, dying people, faces overflowing with pride at the triumph, faces dejected for not having achieved their goals. Thousands upon thousands of gestures, looks, postures, clothing... in colorful, bright, sordid, pristine, grimy, enviable, nauseating environments.

Post a photograph and listen to the comments that arise, the way of analyzing it, the feelings it generates, the attractiveness or repulsion, the details, the composition.

This entire exercise is an act of communication where one sees how the student dives into his own reactions.

A variant that is also widely used is the observation of a painting and Prof. Helen Shield organizes a visit to the museum for her students in Boston in order to carry out this very exercise.

13.6.15   Poetry

Poetry is the most beautiful of all arts.

It is capable of translating emotion, feeling, and thought into metrics and syllables, being the perfect metaphor that exposes, almost without altering them, those conditions to the brain and heart of the reader.

A good poem is both unforgettable and untranslatable, even in its own language.

Of all the good poems, some are extraordinary for communication.

I frequently use what, for me, is the summit of all of them: The Golem by Jorge Luis Borges [103–107], I don't know which is the best translation of the first two stanzas, but to read it in Spanish is to be crossed in each line by an indescribable idea and feeling of amazement and humility. What a marvel of inspiration, erudition, and work that achieves such perfection!

I help my students understand the genius of their author who takes us from Platonic dialogues to molecular biology; from cabbalistic myths to the modern laboratory.

Which teaches us how the inevitable consequence of Hubris is humiliation.

Plato is dead, but his word lives on. Borges has died, but his word lives on. The myth of the Golem is an increasingly closer reality.

Have we learned our lesson?

13.6.16   Music

Music is also an excellent art.

There are a large number of musical compositions ideal for sharing in class: Mozart's requiem, written shortly after his father's death; the "Stabat Mater," a hymn from the thirteenth century that recounts the suffering of the Virgin Mary in the face of the suffering of her crucified son; modern compositions that talk about drug use, health losses, or recoveries.

Analyze the illnesses of composers and the effect on their music: depression in Chopin, syphilis in Mozart, tuberculosis in many of them, AIDS in Freddy Mercury.

The history of castrati and the use of desiderative medicine in the health of children in religious choirs of the eighteenth century.

The paradox between music and deafness as is the case of Beethoven.

There is enormous material available to teachers who want to teach communication and develop listening skills in music.

Opera is a genre that students are not usually fond of.

Some arias, however, are undeniably sublime.

The one I use the most is the "Nessun Dorma."

I start by telling them the story of Turandot and Kalaf and I make them listen to the Nessun Dorma performed by Pavarotti, which in most cases generates a group that thinks it is beautiful and another that considers it good, but not so good.

Then I tell you the story of Puccini and how he wrote the music for the opera, but was unable to finish it because he was undergoing radiotherapy in Brussels and died during treatment in 1924 from head and neck cancer [108–111].

In fact, maestro Toscanini, who premiered the opera, ended it before finishing the third act, saying "this is as far as the maestro wrote," the opera would be completed by Alfano, a friend of Puccini, at the request of his family.

Then I tell my students the story of José Carreras, a great tenor, who was on the verge of ending his career as a singer due to leukemia, for which he had to undergo a bone marrow transplant in 1987. I tell them of how he told us at a congress of the American Society of Clinical Oncology how he found solace by listening to Nessun Dorma in the lonely nights leading up to his transplant. After that story, I make them listen to it a second time and I translate what he says.

Now all the students are paying attention and they are all excited about the end.

That fragment is an example of the progress of medicine: an opera written by a patient who unfortunately died from his cancer, being sung by a patient who survived his cancer.

This usually transforms the class into an unforgettable moment for the students and the teacher.

As a side effect, some students become interested in opera, which is a very nice side effect.

All of these exercises are designed to be applied in class and one can use them freely.

When you design a communication course, it is a very good idea to keep them in mind.

13.7   Designing a Communications Course for Medicine

Depending on the duration of the course, one can plan four, eight, twelve or more classes.

The duration of the classes should not be less than 45 minutes and should not be more than 2 h. Less than 45 min means students won't be able to participate in a meaningful manner, and more than 2 h usually leads to disinterest and wandering minds.

The core idea that the course needs to present and reinforce is that communication is a learnable and perfectible skill.

That, as happens in many other disciplines, there are people for whom it is easier or harder, but everyone can benefit from acquiring the knowledge to communicate better.

If I only have four classes, I will focus on chapter seven of this book: What is the communication map that the doctor must have in mind to satisfy the patient's needs?

If I can extend a little more I will incorporate chapters four, five, and six.

If I have 12 classes, I expand on the other chapters of this book.

We must think that, as teachers, we only have one opportunity for our students to understand that a skill that we consider "Soft" is actually the *hardest* and most useful skill in their professional life.

13.8   The Syllabus

When I have to design a health communication course, I develop all topics we've discussed in this book, adapting them for the intended audience: emergency medicine, intensive care, chronic care, palliative care, nursing, administrative, and so on.

All of them have as a fundamental element of their professional life the need to communicate with patients, family members, and/or members of the work team and they must all develop these capabilities to the maximum.

Understanding the origin and value of the word, the beneficial effect that a word said at the right time can produce or the harmful effect of a word spoken rashly are integral to this development.

Learning how the truth was handled throughout history and the history behind words is for a member of the health team what knowing about food is for a Chef: it is what we must work with every day.

Distinguishing information from communication, learning to convey information clearly and communicate humanely, adapting to the needs of our patients, reducing burnout, developing our personal communication kit, that is the main objective of a course and of this book.

My hope is that it is useful to you, my dear reader, and above all, that it is useful to your patients and their families.

I hope you have very good days ahead.

References

1. Perron NJ, Sommer J, Louis-Simonet M, Nendaz M. Teaching communication skills: beyond wishful thinking. Swiss Med Wkly. 2015:145. https://doi.org/10.4414/smw.2015.14064.

2. Dosser I. Skills training in communication and related topics part 1: dealing with conflict and change. Ellen J Belzer Radcliffe £29.99 326 pp 9781846192777 1846192773. Cancer Nurs Pract. 2010;9(2) https://doi.org/10.7748/cnp.9.2.9.s13.

3. Ruiz Moral R, García De Leonardo C, Cerro Pérez A, Caballero Martínez F, Monge MD. Barriers to teaching communication skills in Spanish medical schools: a qualitative study with academic leaders. BMC Med Educ. 2020;20(1) https://doi.org/10.1186/s12909-020-1944-9.

4. Gordon J. ABC of learning and teaching in medicine: one to one teaching and feedback. Br Med J. 2003;326(7388) https://doi.org/10.1136/bmj.326.7388.543.

5. Bergus GR, Woodhead JC, Kreiter CD. Using systematically observed clinical encounters (Soces) to assess medical students' skills in clinical settings. Adv Med Educ Pract. 2010:1. https://doi.org/10.2147/AMEP.S12962.

6. Hofmeister EH. Nonparticipant student observation of faculty classroomteaching. J Vet Med Educ. 2021;48(1) https://doi.org/10.3138/JVME.2019-0025.

7. Alford CL, Currie DM. Introducing first-year medical students to clinical practice by having them "shadow" third-year clerks. Teach Learn Med. 2004;16(3) https://doi.org/10.1207/s15328015tlm1603_7.

8. Hernandez C, Mermelstein R, Robinson JK, Yudkowsky R. Assessing students' ability to detect melanomas using standardized patients and moulage. J Am Acad Dermatol. 2013;68(3) https://doi.org/10.1016/j.jaad.2011.10.032.

9. Tan XH, Foo MA, Lim LHS, et al. Teaching and assessing communication skills in palliative medicine: a systematic scoping review. Palliat Med. 2021;35(1 SUPPL)

10. Golden BP, Tackett S, Kobayashi K, et al. Sitting at the bedside: patient and internal medicine trainee perceptions. J Gen Intern Med. 2022;37(12) https://doi.org/10.1007/s11606-021-07231-4.

11. Clark BW, Niessen T, Apfel A, et al. Relationship of physical examination technique to associated clinical skills: results from a direct observation assessment. Am J Med. 2022;135(6) https://doi.org/10.1016/j.amjmed.2021.11.021.

12. Conroy M, Chilaka J, Colucci G. The education of medical students in human factors—a National Survey. Int J Med Stud. Published online. 2022; https://doi.org/10.5195/ijms.2022.1189.

13. Peterson EB, Calhoun AW, Rider EA. The reliability of a modified Kalamazoo consensus statement checklist for assessing the communication skills of multidisciplinary clinicians in the simulated environment. Patient Educ Couns. 2014;96(3):411–8. https://doi.org/10.1016/j.pec.2014.07.013.

14. Simpson JG, Furnace J, Crosby J, et al. The Scottish doctor—learning outcomes for the medical undergraduate in Scotland: a foundation for competent and reflective practitioners. Med Teach. 2002;24(2):136–43. https://doi.org/10.1080/01421590220120713.

15. Duffy FD, Gordon GH, Whelan G, Cole-Kelly K, Frankel R, Participants A. Assessing competence in communication and interpersonal skills: the Kalamazoo II Report. Vol 79; 2004.

16. Kovacs-Litman A, Wong K, Shojania KG, Callery S, Vearncombe M, Leis JA. Do physicians clean their hands? Insights from a covert observational study. J Hosp Med. 2016;11(12) https://doi.org/10.1002/jhm.2632.

17. Driever EM, Stiggelbout AM, Brand PLP. Do consultants do what they say they do? Observational study of the extent to which clinicians involve their patients in the decision-making process. BMJ Open. 2022;12(1) https://doi.org/10.1136/bmjopen-2021-056471.

18. Belzer EJ. Improving patient communication in no time. Fam Pract Manag. 1999;6(5):23–8. PMID: 10537793.

19. Geoffroy PA, Delyon J, Strullu M, et al. Standardized patients or conventional lecture for teaching communication skills to undergraduate medical students: a randomized controlled study. Psychiatry Investig. 2020;17(4):299–310. https://doi.org/10.30773/pi.2019.0258.

20. Carvalho IP, Pais VG, Silva FR, et al. Teaching communication skills in clinical settings: comparing two applications of a comprehensive program with standardized and real patients. BMC Med Educ. 2014;14(1) https://doi.org/10.1186/1472-6920-14-92.

21. Sanges S, Sanges S, Sanges S, et al. Raising rare disease awareness using red flags, role play simulation and patient educators: results of a novel educational workshop on Raynaud phenomenon and systemic sclerosis. Orphanet J Rare Dis. 2020;15(1) https://doi.org/10.1186/s13023-020-01439-z.

22. Atienza-Carbonell B, Hernández-Évole H, Balanzá-Martínez V. A "patient as educator" intervention: reducing stigmatizing attitudes toward mental illness among medical students. Front Public Health. 2022:10. https://doi.org/10.3389/fpubh.2022.1020929.

23. Coret A, Boyd K, Hobbs K, Zazulak J, McConnell M. Patient narratives as a teaching tool: a pilot study of first-year medical students and patient educators affected by intellectual/developmental disabilities. Teach Learn Med. 2018;30(3) https://doi.org/10.1080/10401334.2017.1398653.

24. Ehman JW, Ott BB, Short TH, Ciampa RC, Hansen-Flaschen J. Do patients want physicians to inquire about their spiritual or religious beliefs if they become gravely ill? Arch Intern Med. 1999;159(15) https://doi.org/10.1001/archinte.159.15.1803.

25. Watt K, Abbott P, Reath J. Developing cultural competence in general practitioners: an integrative review of the literature. BMC Fam Pract. 2016;17(1) https://doi.org/10.1186/s12875-016-0560-6.

26. Gruppen LD, Branch VK, Laing TJ. The use of trained patient educators with rheumatoid arthritis to teach medical students. Arthritis Rheum. 1996;9(4) https://doi.org/10.1002/1529-0131(199608)9:4<302::AID-ANR1790090415>3.0.CO;2-R.

27. Raj N, Badcock LJ, Brown GA, Deighton CM, O'Reilly SC. Undergraduate musculoskeletal examination teaching by trained patient educators—a comparison with doctor-led teaching. Rheumatology. 2006;45(11) https://doi.org/10.1093/rheumatology/kel126.

28. Lauckner H, Doucet S, Wells S. Patients as educators: the challenges and benefits of sharing experiences with students. Med Educ. 2012;46(10) https://doi.org/10.1111/j.1365-2923.2012.04356.x.

29. Lewis KL, Bohnert CA, Gammon WL, et al. The Association of Standardized Patient Educators (ASPE) Standards of Best Practice (SOBP). Adv Simul. 2017;2(1) https://doi.org/10.1186/s41077-017-0043-4.

30. Hopkins H, Weaks C, Webster T, Elcin M. The association of standardized patient educators (ASPE) gynecological teaching associate (GTA) and male urogenital teaching associate (MUTA) standards of best practice. Adv Simul. 2021;6(1) https://doi.org/10.1186/s41077-021-00162-4.

31. Jaques D. ABC of learning and teaching in medicine: teaching small groups. BMJ. 2003;326(7387) https://doi.org/10.1136/bmj.326.7387.492.

32. Joshi P, Bodkha P. A comparative evaluation of students' insight of face to face classroom lectures and virtual online lectures. Natl J Physiol Pharm Pharmacol. 2021;11(1) https://doi.org/10.5455/njppp.2021.10.08225202026082020.

33. Petersen K, Dong T, Hemmer PA, Kelly WF. Online virtual patient cases vs. weekly classroom lectures in an internal medicine clerkship: effects on military learner outcomes. Mil Med. 2023;188(5-6) https://doi.org/10.1093/milmed/usac136.

34. Cantillon P. ABC of learning and teaching in medicine teaching large groups helping students to learn in lectures. BMJ Br Med J. 2003:326.

35. Stackhouse AA, Rafi D, Walls R, et al. Knowledge attainment and engagement among medical students: a comparison of three forms of online learning. Adv Med Educ Pract. 2023:14. https://doi.org/10.2147/AMEP.S391816.

36. Hughes JDM, Azzi E, Rose GW, Ramnanan CJ, Khamisa K. A survey of senior medical students' attitudes and awareness toward teaching and participation in a formal clinical teaching elective: a Canadian perspective. Med Educ Online. 2017;22(1) https://doi.org/10.108 0/10872981.2016.1270022.

37. Cantillon P. ABC of learning and teaching in medicine: teaching large groups. Br Med J. 2003;326(7386) https://doi.org/10.1136/bmj.326.7386.437.

38. Boček M. Henry Kissinger: leadership: six studies in world strategy. Czech J Int Relations/ Mezinarodni vztahy. 2023;58(1) https://doi.org/10.32422/mv-cjir.719.

39. Ikonne U, Campbell AM, Whelihan KE, Bay RC, Lewis JH. Exodus from the classroom: student perceptions, lecture capture technology, and the inception of on-demand preclinical medical education. J Am Osteopath Assoc. 2018;118(12) https://doi.org/10.7556/jaoa.2018.174.

40. King AM, Mayer C, Barrie M, Greenberger S, Way DP. Replacing lectures with small groups: the impact of flipping the residency conference day. West J Emerg Med. 2018;19(1) https://doi.org/10.5811/westjem.2017.10.35235.

41. Young TP, Bailey CJ, Guptill M, Thorp AW, Thomas TL. The flipped classroom: a modality for mixed asynchronous and synchronous learning in a residency program. West J Emerg Med. 2014;15(7) https://doi.org/10.5811/westjem.2014.10.23515.

42. Khanittanuphong P, Iamthanaporn K, Bvonpanttarananon J. The impact of the transition from flipped classroom to online lectures on learning outcomes and student satisfaction in a rehabilitation medicine clerkship during the COVID-19 pandemic. BMC Med Educ. 2022;22(1) https://doi.org/10.1186/s12909-022-03959-7.

43. Hu X, Zhang H, Song Y, et al. Implementation of flipped classroom combined with problem-based learning: an approach to promote learning about hyperthyroidism in the endocrinology internship. BMC Med Educ. 2019;19(1) https://doi.org/10.1186/s12909-019-1714-8.

44. Sourg HAA, Satti S, Ahmed N, Ahmed ABM. Impact of flipped classroom model in increasing the achievement for medical students. BMC Med Educ. 2023;23(1) https://doi.org/10.1186/s12909-023-04276-3.

45. Riddell J, Jhun P, Fung CC, et al. Does the flipped classroom improve learning in graduate medical education? J Grad Med Educ. 2017;9(4) https://doi.org/10.4300/JGME-D-16-00817.1.

46. Pejin I, Oroz S, Milojković Đ, Milić N, Milić N, Rajović N. Flipped classroom: the novel learning environment for medical students. Medicinski podmladak. 2022;73(4) https://doi.org/10.5937/mp73-39285.

47. Tang B, Coret A, Qureshi A, Barron H, Ayala AP, Law M. Online lectures in undergraduate medical education: scoping review. JMIR Med Educ. 2018;20(4) https://doi.org/10.2196/mededu.9091.

48. Kumar A, Sarkar M, Davis E, et al. Impact of the COVID-19 pandemic on teaching and learning in health professional education: a mixed methods study protocol. BMC Med Educ. 2021;21(1) https://doi.org/10.1186/s12909-021-02871-w.

49. Khaniukov OO, Smolianova OV, Shchukina OS. Distance learning during the war in Ukraine: experience of internal medicine department (organisation and challenges). Art Med. 2022;23(3) https://doi.org/10.21802/artm.2022.3.23.134.

50. Chandra A, Schmitt G, Ganjoo R. Twelve tips for structuring classes in higher education: lessons learned from a biology premedical class. MedEdPublish. 2019:8. https://doi.org/10.15694/mep.2019.000129.1.

51. Lee SS, Foong CC, Choon SK, Vadivelu J. Language in medicine: a necessity or redundancy for medical undergraduates? Int Med J. 2020;27:5.

52. Pshenychna M, Heorhievska V, Khaustova M. Problems of teaching latin to foreign medical students and ways to solve them. Zhytomyr Ivan Franko State University Journal Pedagogical Sciences. 2023;1(112) https://doi.org/10.35433/pedagogy.1(112).2023.76-87.

53. Nuland SB. Doctors: the illustrated history of medical pioneers. Black Dog and Leventhal Publisher, Inc.; 2008.

54. Farrow R. ABC of learning and teaching in medicine: creating teaching materials. BMJ. 2003;326(7395) https://doi.org/10.1136/bmj.326.7395.921.

55. Jackson VA, Back AL. Teaching communication skills using role-play: an experience-based guide for educators. J Palliat Med. 2011;14(6):775–80. https://doi.org/10.1089/jpm.2010.0493.

56. Elhilu AH, El-Setouhy M, Mobarki AS, Abualgasem MM, Ahmed MA. Peer role-play simulation: a valuable alternative to bedside teaching during the COVID-19 pandemic. Adv Med Educ Pract. 2023:14. https://doi.org/10.2147/AMEP.S399531.

57. Sepúlveda HÁ. Promoting significant learnings in the university teaching of history through a role play. Estudios Pedagogicos. 2020;46(2) https://doi.org/10.4067/S0718-07052020000200097.

58. Krishnan DG, Keloth AV, Ahmad S, Mohandas PG. Role play versus small group discussion in teaching prescription communication skills: a comparative study on students of phase two of the bachelor of medicine and bachelor of surgery (MBBS) course. J Adv Med Educ Prof. 2022;11(1) https://doi.org/10.30476/jamp.2022.96136.1679.

59. Amirthalingam SD, Ramasamy S, Aznal SSHS. Gamification through collaborative learning in medical education. Asia Pac Sch. 2023;8(3) https://doi.org/10.29060/TAPS.2023-8-3/SC2921.

60. Ahmad M, Gharatya A, Law S, et al. Modified surgical heads-up charades-can gamification of surgical topics promote learning and make revision enjoyable and useful? Br J Surg. 2020;107(SUPPL 3)

61. Budiastuti RE, Wijayatiningsih TD. Analysing communication strategies of Youtube video by students of English Department in Unimus. Surakarta English and Literature Journal. 2019;2(1) https://doi.org/10.52429/selju.v2i1.228.

62. Belova N, Zowada C. Innovating higher education via game-based learning on misconceptions. Educ Sci (Basel). 2020;10(9) https://doi.org/10.3390/educsci10090221.

63. Nfor S. Improving communicative competence through mime: bringing students' 'out-of-school' literacy practices into Japanese University EFL Oral Communication Classes. Scenario: A Journal of Performative Teaching, Learning, Research. 2018;XII:2. https://doi.org/10.33178/scenario.12.2.2.

64. Roberts G, Lewandowski J, Galantucci B. How communication changes when we cannot mime the world: experimental evidence for the effect of iconicity on combinatoriality. Cognition. 2015:141. https://doi.org/10.1016/j.cognition.2015.04.001.

65. Santos AS, Portes AJF. Perceptions of deaf subjects about communication in primary health care. Rev Lat Am Enfermagem. 2019:27. https://doi.org/10.1590/1518-8345.2612.3127.

66. Mauriello TP. Preparing for news media interviews and entertainment documentaries. In: *Public speaking for criminal justice professionals*; 2020. doi:https://doi.org/10.4324/9781003047957-11.

67. Iman N, Ramli M, Saridewi N. Kahoot as an assessment tools: students' perception of game-based learning platform. Jurnal Penelitian dan Pembelajaran IPA. 2021;7(2) https://doi.org/10.30870/jppi.v7i2.8304.

68. Gilman A. Preparing for a media interview. J Commun Healthc. 2010;3(2) https://doi.org/10.1179/175380710x12688262020678.

69. Samaha R, Kattan C, Rassy E, Kattan J. Learning by debate: innovative tool in the hematology-oncology fellowship program. J Cancer Educ. 2022;37(6) https://doi.org/10.1007/s13187-021-02002-5.

70. Feito GL. Hacia una mejor comprensión del papel de la naturaleza en los debates bioéticos. Veritas. 2010:23. https://doi.org/10.4067/s0718-92732010000200006.

71. Iyengar S, Massey DS. Scientific communication in a post-truth society. Proc Natl Acad Sci USA. 2019;116(16) https://doi.org/10.1073/pnas.1805868115.

72. Oktasari D, Jumadi W, Hariadi MH, Syari EL. 3d page-flipped worksheet on impulse-momentum to develop students' scientific communication skills. J Pendidik IPA Indonesia. 2019;8(2) https://doi.org/10.15294/jpii.v8i2.15737.

73. Malik A, Ubaidillah M. Multiple skill laboratory activities: how to improve students' scientific communication and collaboration skills. J Pendidik IPA Indonesia. 2021;10(4) https://doi.org/10.15294/jpii.v10i4.31442.

74. Taufiq M, Rokhman F. Scientific communication skills profile of prospective science teachers based on sociocultural aspects. J Pendidik IPA Indonesia. 2020;9(2) https://doi.org/10.15294/jpii.v9i2.24366.

75. Mattox KL, Allen MK. Scientific communications. J Am Coll Emerg Physicians. 1978;7(9) https://doi.org/10.1016/S0361-1124(78)80358-X.

76. DeJesus JM, Callanan MA, Solis G, Gelman SA. Generic language in scientific communication. Proc Natl Acad Sci USA. 2019;116(37) https://doi.org/10.1073/pnas.1817706116.

77. Sargeant J, Macleod T, Sinclair D, Power M. How do physicians assess their family physician colleagues' performance? Creating a rubric to inform assessment and feedback. J Contin Educ Health Prof. 2011;31(2) https://doi.org/10.1002/chp.20111.

78. Robinson D, Dearman S. Still room for improvement: standardisation of clinical correspondence and experience in a rural crisis and home treatment service. BJPsych Bull. 2019;43(3) https://doi.org/10.1192/bjb.2019.29.

79. Cahilog Z, Lei HYH, Al-Musawi S. 'Creating assessments as an active learning strategy: what are students' perceptions? A mixed methods study'–a supplementary letter. Med Educ Online. 2019;24(1) https://doi.org/10.1080/10872981.2019.1677392.

80. Nordlund C. Letters to colleagues: a community of practice for navigating and reshaping identity. Visual Inquiry. 2019;8(1) https://doi.org/10.1386/vi.8.1.49_1.

81. Box-Steffensmeier JM, Christenson DP, Craig AW. Cue-taking in congress: interest group signals from dear colleague letters. Am J Pol Sci. 2019;63(1) https://doi.org/10.1111/ajps.12399.

82. Christanto SA, Brenda D, Assisiansi C, Pangestu MJ, Sarita I, Sulistiani V. Gratitude letter: an effort to increase subjective well-being in college. ANIMA Indonesian Psychol J. 2017;32(3) https://doi.org/10.24123/aipj.v32i3.630.

83. Stefan D, Lefdahl-Davis E, Alayan A, et al. The impact of gratitude letters and visits on relationships, happiness, well-being, and meaning of graduate students. J Positive Sch Psychol. 2021;5(2) https://doi.org/10.47602/jpsp.v5i2.256.

84. Seligman MEP, Steen TA, Park N, Peterson C. Gratitude Letter. Character Lab Playbook . Published online. 2018; https://doi.org/10.53776/playbooks-activities-gratitude-letter.

85. Stone BM, Lindt JD, Rabinovich NE, Gilbert DG. Effects of the gratitude letter and positive attention bias modification on attentional deployment and emotional states. J Happiness Stud. 2022;23(1) https://doi.org/10.1007/s10902-021-00377-2.

86. Schumann K, Walton GM. Rehumanizing the self after victimization: the roles of forgiveness versus revenge. J Pers Soc Psychol. 2022;122(3) https://doi.org/10.1037/pspi0000367.

87. Rashid T. Positive psychotherapy. In: Encyclopedia of quality of life and well-being research. 2020. doi:https://doi.org/10.1007/978-3-319-69909-7_3378-2.

88. McIntosh RD, Hillary K, Brennan A, Lechowicz M. Developmental mirror-writing is paralleled by orientation recognition errors. Laterality. 2018;23(6) https://doi.org/10.1080/1357650X.2018.1445748.

89. Vecchini A, Buratta L, Fogassi L. Grapho-motor imitation training in children with handwriting difficulties: a single-center pilot study. Cogent Educ. 2023;10(1) https://doi.org/10.1080/2331186X.2023.2192152.

90. Cunningham H, Taylor DS, Desai UA, et al. Reading the self: medical students' experience of reflecting on their writing over time. Acad Med. 2021;96(8) https://doi.org/10.1097/ACM.0000000000003814.

91. Steensma DP. Stories we tell one another: narrative reflection and the art of oncology. Am Soc Clin Oncol Educ Book; 2013. p. 33. https://doi.org/10.1200/edbook_am.2013.33.e331.

92. Kabat-Zinn M, Kabat-Zinn J. Everyday Blessings: The Inner Work of Mindful Parenting. New York: Hyperion. 1997.

93. Csapo E, Goette HR, Green JR, et al. *Theatre and autocracy in the ancient world*; 2022. doi:https://doi.org/10.1515/9783110980356.

94. Arceci RJ. The question of god: C.S. Lewis and Sigmund Freud debate god, love, sex, and the meaning of life. J Pediatr Hematol Oncol. 2003;25(4) https://doi.org/10.1097/00043426-200304000-00020.

95. Dow AW, Leong D, Anderson A, et al. Using theater to teach clinical empathy: a pilot study. J Gen Intern Med. 2007;22(8) https://doi.org/10.1007/s11606-007-0224-2.

96. Sevrain-Goideau M, Gohier B, Bellanger W, Annweiler C, Campone M, Coutant R. Forum theater staging of difficult encounters with patients to increase empathy in students: evaluation of efficacy at the University of Angers Medical School. BMC Med Educ. 2020;20(1) https://doi.org/10.1186/s12909-020-1965-4.

97. Smith A. Doctors on film. BMJ . Published online. 2022; https://doi.org/10.1136/bmj.o2720.

98. Bottasso O. When doctors become patients. About the film, The Doctor (1991). Revista de Medicina y Cine. 2022;18(3) https://doi.org/10.14201/rmc.29543.

99. Milam EC, Leger MC. Use of medical photography among dermatologists: a nationwide online survey study. J Eur Acad Dermatol Venereol. 2018;32(10) https://doi.org/10.1111/jdv.14839.

100. Subramaniam S, Gopichandran V. A picture speaks a thousand words: using participant photography in environmental pedagogy for medical students. Educ Health Change Learn Pract. 2018;31(3) https://doi.org/10.4103/efh.EfH_124_17.

101. Clavería LR. Social value of war photography: Robert Capa in the Spanish civil war. Doc Inf Sci. 2015:38. https://doi.org/10.5209/rev_dcin.2015.v38.50817.

102. Hidalgo CV. The photographs of Robert Capa and Gerda Taro during the siege of the Alcazar of Toledo (1936). Review of the magnum photos catalog. Gen J Info Documentation. 2020;30(1) https://doi.org/10.5209/RGID.70067.

103. Ángeles B. Paradoja y deconstrucción en "El golem" de Jorge Luis Borges. Revista chilena de literatura. 2022:531–51. https://doi.org/10.4067/S0718-22952022000100531.

104. Henricksen W. Why Jorge Luis Borges still matters, even though he hoped to be forgotten. Middle Atlantic Rev Lat Am Stud. 2022;6(1) https://doi.org/10.23870/mars.386.

105. Kozicki K, Cardoso LG. Verbal realism in a magic world: Carlos Santiago Nino vs. Jorge Luis Borges. Anamorphosis—International Magazine of Direito e Literature. 2020;6(1) https://doi.org/10.21119/anamps.61.79-99.

106. Chinchilla SK. Between the Adam and the golem, regarding a poem by Jorge Luis Borges. J Philol Linguist Univ Costa Rica. 2015;17(1-2) https://doi.org/10.15517/rfl.v17i1-2.20974.

107. Soud SE. Borges the golem-maker: intimations of "presence" in "the circular ruins". MLN. 1995;110(4) https://doi.org/10.1353/mln.1995.0078.

108. Lima NS. The (bio)ethical narrative: a lyrical-analytical approach. Ethics Cinema J. 2011;1(1)

109. Espinosa Reynoso JJ. Nessun slept. Int Med Mex. 2007;23:2.

110. Georgieva G, Enchev M, Stoykov M, Milkov M, Baycheva S. Giacomo Puccini—a great composer and a genius. Scripta Scientifica Medica. 2022;54 https://doi.org/10.14748/ssm.v54i0.9001.

111. Semkin D, Bushueva L. Giacomo Puccini's operatic legacy and its study in the practice of vocalists. Wisdom. 2020;15(2) https://doi.org/10.24234/WISDOM.V15I2.355.

Index

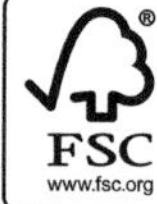

FSC
www.fsc.org
MIX
Papier aus verantwortungsvollen Quellen
Paper from responsible sources
FSC® C105338